Michael M. Polimus DDS
1717 Penn Ave., Apt. #902
Pittsburgh, PA 15221
(412) 243-7030

ENDODONTICS

ENDODONTICS
SECOND EDITION

CHRISTOPHER J R STOCK
MSc, BDS, DGDP (UK)
Senior Research Fellow
Department of Conservative Dentistry
Eastman Dental Hospital and Institute
London, UK

KISHOR GULABIVALA
BDS, MSc, FDS RCS (EDIN.)
Consultant and Lecturer
Department of Conservative Dentistry
Eastman Dental Hospital and Institute
London, UK

RICHARD T WALKER
RD, BDS, PhD, MSc, FDS RCPS (GLASG.)
Senior Lecturer
Leeds Dental Institute
Honorary Consultant
United Leeds Teaching Hospitals Trust, UK

JANE R GOODMAN
BDS, FDS RCS (EDIN.)
Consultant
Department of Children's Dentistry
Eastman Dental Hospital and Institute
London, UK

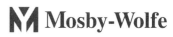

London Baltimore Barcelona Bogotá Boston Buenos Aires Carlsbad, CA Chicago Madrid Mexico City Milan Naples, FL New York
Philadelphia St. Louis Seoul Singapore Sydney Taipei Tokyo Toronto Wiesbaden

Copyright © 1995 Times Mirror International Publishers Limited

Published in 1995 by Mosby-Wolfe, an imprint of Times Mirror International Publishers Limited

Reprinted in 1997.

Printed by Grafos, S.A. Arte sobre papel, Barcelona, Spain.

ISBN 0 7234 1890 X

All rights reserved. No part of this publication may be reproduced, stored in a retrieval system, copied or transmitted, in any form or by any means, electronic, mechanical, photocopying, recording or otherwise without written permission from the Publisher or in accordance with the provisions of the Copyright Act 1988, or under the terms of any licence permitting limited copying issued by the Copyright Licensing Agency, 33–34 Alfred Place, London, WC1E 7DP.

Any person who does any unauthorised act in relation to this publication may be liable to criminal prosecution and civil claims for damages.

Permission to photocopy or reproduce solely for internal or personal use is permitted for libraries or other users registered with the Copyright Clearance Center, provided that the base fee of $4.00 per chapter plus $.10 per page is paid directly to the Copyright Clearance Center, 21 Congress Street, Salem, MA 01970. This consent does not extend to other kinds of copying, such as copying for general distribution, for advertising or promotional purposes, for creating new collected works, or for resale.

For full details of all Times Mirror International Publishers Limited titles, please write to Times Mirror International Publishers Limited, Lynton House, 7–12 Tavistock Square, London WC1H 9LB, England.

A CIP catalogue record for this book is available from the British Library.

Library of Congress Cataloging-in-Publication Data applied for.

Contents

Preface		iv
Acknowledgements		v
1	Biological basis for endodontics *K. Gulabivala*	1
2	Patient assessment *C.J.R. Stock*	39
3	Radiography *R.T. Walker*	51
4	Treatment planning *R.T. Walker*	69
5	Pre-endodontic management *R.T. Walker and C.J.R. Stock*	77
6	Root canal morphology *R.T. Walker*	89
7	Preparation of the root canal *K. Gulabivala and C.J.R. Stock*	95
8	Intracanal medication and temporary seal *K. Gulabivala*	145
9	Obturation of the root canal system *K. Gulabivala*	151
10	Perio-endo lesions *C.J.R. Stock*	177
11	Surgical endodontics *R.T. Walker*	185
12	Emergency endodontics *R.T. Walker*	195
13	Tooth resorption *C.J.R. Stock*	201
14	Endodontic problems *K. Gulabivala and C.J.R. Stock*	209
15	Restoration of the root-filled tooth *K. Gulabivala*	241
16	Primary dentition *J.R. Goodman*	273
17	Medicolegal aspects *C.J.R. Stock*	279
	References and further reading	281
	Index	285

Preface

Rational endodontic therapy must be founded upon a sound understanding of the biological concepts of disease, its natural history and the physical, chemical and therapeutic basis of dealing with infection. Much fundamental biological research still remains to be undertaken in endodontics and although the principles of endodontic therapy have not changed, the research findings and collective clinical experience of the authors has prompted a re-evaluation of the treatment concepts. This, together with the large array of new equipment and materials, has resulted in a need to rewrite rather than update this edition. Two new authors have brought a broader view to the book without losing the emphasis on the practical approach.

The book is directed at both the undergraduate student and the general dental practitioner, leading them in logical steps through the subject of endodontics. The first chapter outlines the biological basis for endodontics, so far as we understand it today. The remaining chapters are based on a more practical approach describing the current techniques and materials used in the treatment of patients. The text is liberally illustrated with numerous photographs and colour diagrams to convey the message more effectively.

The standard of endodontics taught in dental schools has improved considerably over the past few years with many more teachers taking an interest in the subject. It is appreciated that endodontics together with periodontics forms the essential foundation for any restorative management. Students must therefore be competent to carry out root canal treatment of both anterior and posterior teeth.

The demand from patients for root canal treatment has increased together with the expectation of success, even later into life, when disease or problems of wear and tear intervene. The general dental practitioner is therefore continually being faced with increasingly difficult cases to treat which require practical expertise.

Book learning alone cannot convey practical skills, however practical the information. Theoretical knowledge has to be assimilated into a working knowledge by vigilant practice. Some individuals have an innate ability to make this transition, whereas for others the process is facilitated by further hands-on instruction. The acquisition of practical skills is a matter of constant disciplined effort in achieving a preconceived end result. The scientific rationale for both this process and the preconceived end result should be continuously reviewed in the light of new knowledge. There is nothing new in this general concept which is embodied in the following age old passage from Aristotle,

'Excellence is an art won by training and habituation. We do not act rightly because we have virtue or excellence, rather we have those because we acted rightly. We are what we repeatedly do. Excellence then is not an act but a habit'.

The authors hope that this book will form only the basis for the readers development in this interesting field.

Acknowledgements

The authors gratefully acknowledge the valuable direct and indirect contributions made by the following at the Eastman Dental Institute and Hospital in the completion of this textbook:

The staff and MSc students (in both Endodontics and Conservative Dentistry) of the department of Conservative Dentistry who in the course of many discussions over the years have helped to critically evaluate our working practices in Endodontics and have contributed in producing much of our teaching material.

Mr J.F. Roberts for providing illustrations 16.6, 16.8, 16.9, 16.11, 16.14, 16.15, 16.16, 16.17 and 16.20, Mr F.J. Hill for illustration 16.23 and Professor G.B. Winter for allowing the use of departmental material.

The departments of Children's Dentistry and Oral Pathology (in particular Drs P. Speight and J. Bennett) who gave permission to use their photographic slide material. The department of Electron Microscopy and specifically Mrs P. Barber and Mrs N. Mordan whose expertise enabled the production of SEM micrographs reproduced in the book. The audio-visual department and specifically Mr J. Morgan for their expertise in producing numerous photographs of equipment, materials and teeth.

In addition, the authors would like to thank the following: Angela Christie for the expertly produced artwork. Dr Ramachandran Nair, Dr E. Saunders, Professor M Tagger, Dr P. Dummer and Dr T. Pitt Ford for permission to use some of their slide material.

Numerous other contributors have helped in the collection of the clinical and other illustrative material, and their assistance is greatly appreciated and acknowledged by name in the text.

1 Biological basis for endodontics

Endodontology and endodontics

Endodontology may be defined as the branch of dental science concerned with the study of form, function, health of, injuries to and diseases of the dental pulp and periradicular region and their treatment. The aetiology and diagnosis of dental pain and disease are considered to be integral to endodontic practice. *Endodontic treatment* encompasses any procedure designed to maintain the health of all, or part of, the pulp. When the pulp is diseased or injured treatment is aimed at maintaining or restoring the health of the periradicular tissues, usually by root canal treatment but occasionally in combination with endodontic surgery.[1]

The need for endodontic treatment

A general increase in awareness of the benefits of dental care has seen a rise in the demand for procedures that help to retain teeth longer. Although the rate of caries has declined in some parts of the world, it has not been eliminated and this, along with an increase in the presentation of problems due to attrition, abrasion, erosion and trauma, has resulted in an increased demand for fixed restorative treatment which aims to restore aesthetics and function. Restorative procedures may damage the pulp, and consequently problems related to the pulp and periradicular tissues have also increased.

The few epidemiological surveys of treatment needs that have been conducted suggest that periradicular lesions are often undiagnosed or untreated. The large proportion of patients referred to departments of restorative dentistry for advice and treatment of endodontic problems[2] represent untreated cases and also those in whom treatment has been unsuccessful. The Dental Practice Board records show that over a million teeth are treated endodontically on the National Health Service in England and Wales every year.

Conventional root canal treatment has an overall success rate of 65–95%, which may incline to the lower end of the range where follow-up periods exceed 10 years. Outcome is influenced by the quality of treatment[3] and the design and quality of the subsequent restoration [4]: poorly adapted root fillings, and those short by more than 2 mm from the root apex, have higher failure rates. Endodontic failure may necessitate tooth extraction; poor endodontic treatment therefore increases the risk of tooth loss.

A rational approach to the treatment of disease requires an understanding of the pathological process, which in turn demands a knowledge of the normal anatomy and physiology of the tissues involved.

ANATOMY AND PHYSIOLOGY

The dental pulp

The dental pulp is a connective tissue like any other in the body and consists of cells, ground substance and neural and vascular supplies. Its unique characteristic is that it is encased in a rigid hard tissue (**1.1**). The pulp, in conjunction with the dentine which surrounds it, is referred to as the *pulp–dentine complex* (**1.2, 1.3**).

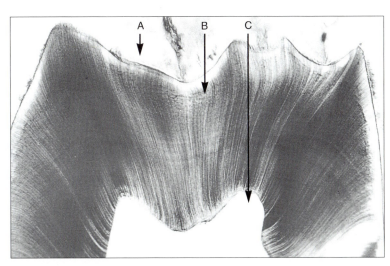

1.1 Ground section of crown of tooth: A = enamel; B = dentine; C = pulp

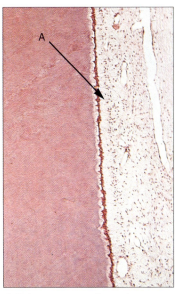

1.2 Low-power view of pulp–dentine complex: A = cell–free zone

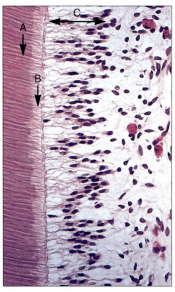

1.3 High-power view of pulp–dentine complex: A = mineralised dentine; B = predentine; C = odontoblasts

Dentine is a specialized connective tissue of mesenchymal origin. It is laid down by the highly differentiated and specialized odontoblasts and forms the bulk of the mineralized portion of the tooth. Dentine consists of thousands of tubules radiating outwards from the dental pulp to the enamel in the crown and the cementum in the root (**1.4**): up to 65 000 tubules/mm^2 at the pulpal end and 15 000/mm^2 at the dentine–enamel junction. The diameter of the tubules is about 3 µm near the pulp and less than 1 µm peripherally. The dentinal tubules account for 45% of the surface area near the pulp and 1% of the total surface area near the dentine–enamel junction. The dentinal tubules, which are interconnected by lateral tubules (**1.5, 1.6**), make up 20–30% of the volume of dentine. In the crown the tubules follow a gentle S-shaped curve (**1.4**) and therefore trauma to one part of the crown affects the pulp at a more apical level (**1.7, 1.8**): a deeper cavity would traumatize more tubules and cause greater damage.

Tubules contain the long narrow *odontoblastic processes* (**1.9**). Whether these processes traverse the dentine midway to the enamel–dentine junction or the full distance is not clear. The remainder of the tubule is filled with fluid and fluid exchange may occur from the pulp outwards or from the enamel towards the pulp.

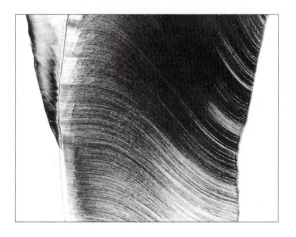

1.4 Ground section of tooth at the cemento-enamel junction

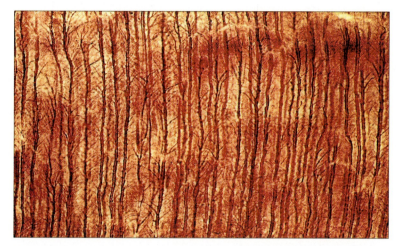

1.5 Low-power view of lateral communication between dentinal tubules

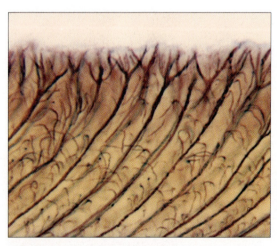

1.6 High-power view of lateral communication between dentinal tubules

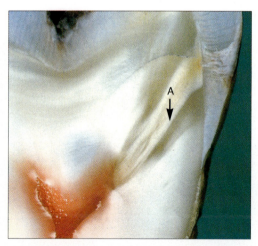

1.7 Sclerosis of dentine caused by caries: A = sclerosed dentine

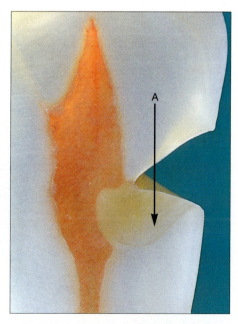

1.8 Sclerosis of dentine and pulp calcification caused by cervical abrasion: A = sclerosed dentine

Peritubular dentine (**1.10**) lines the tubules and is laid down by the odontoblast process. It is 40% more mineralized than intertubular dentine (the mineralized tissue between the tubules). Peritubular dentine is thought to form as a normal consequence of aging and may be accelerated by stimuli such as caries (**1.7**), attrition (**1.50**) and abrasion (**1.8**). Occlusion of dentinal tubules by this process and by mineral crystals is called *sclerosis* and gives aged root apices their characteristic translucency (**1.11**).

Primary dentine (**1.12**) forms during tooth development at a rate of 4 µm per day. *Secondary dentine* (**1.12**) forms once the teeth are fully developed and is laid down evenly over the entire pulpal surface at about 0.8 µm per day; it is also known as physiological or regular secondary dentine. Secondary dentine may be distinguished from primary dentine by the slight and sudden change in direction of tubules. Irregular secondary dentine is laid down unevenly in response to noxious external stimuli such as dental caries, attrition and abrasion (**1.13–1.15**) at a rate of 3 µm per day.

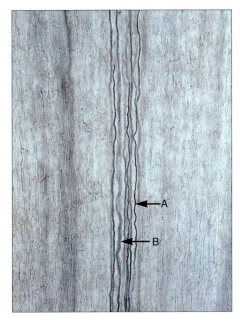

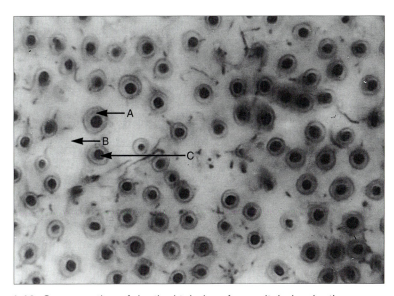

1.9 High-power view of odontoblast process in dentinal tubule: A = tubule; B = odontoblast process

1.10 Cross-section of dentinal tubules: A = peritubular dentine; B = intertubular dentine; C = odontoblast process

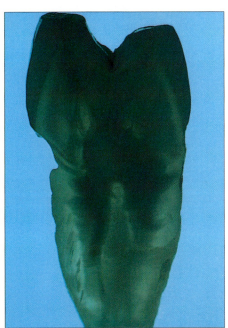

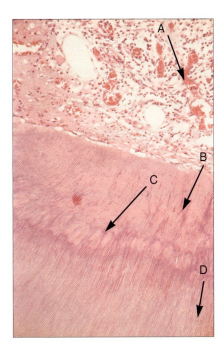

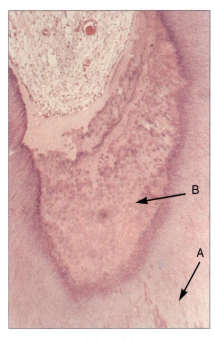

1.11 Translucency of root caused by sclerosis of dentine

1.12 Change in direction of secondary dentinal tubules: A = pulp; B = secondary dentine; C = change in direction of tubules; D = primary dentine

1.13 Primary (A) and irregular secondary dentine (B)

Odontoblast cell bodies are separated from mineralized dentine by an unmineralized layer, 15 μm wide, known as *predentine* (**1.16**). Odontoblasts form a single layer of cells, but in histological section appear as a multilayered structure (**1.16**) because their nuclei are at different levels. Odontoblasts are incapable of further division once fully mature and if damaged may be replaced from undifferentiated mesenchymal cells.

Immediately adjacent to the odontoblast layer is a zone of connective tissue, the *Cell-free zone*, which is relatively free of cells (**1.2**). It disappears during periods of cellular activity in a young pulp or in older pulps where new dentine is being formed.

The remainder of the pulp consists of *ground substance* into which are embedded fibroblasts and inflammatory cells, collagen fibres and a complex network of blood vessels and nerve fibres (**1.17**).

Functions of the pulp

The primary functions of the pulp are formative and defensive, but may be broader. It is unlikely that the pulp is a vestigial organ. The difference in the rate of deposition of primary and secondary dentine suggests that pulp tissue has a lifetime role. Defence reactions, including the initial inflammatory response, blockage of dentinal tubules by large molecular substances, sclerosis of dentinal tubules by formation of peritubular dentine and laying down of secondary dentine, are essential to the survival of the pulp.

The pulp has also been thought of as a sensory organ that warns against disease (i.e. caries or the loss of tooth tissue) by eliciting pain, but this is a relatively poor warning system considering the number of teeth whose pulps become irreversibly inflamed apparently without warning.

Two further points are of speculative interest: (1) hypothetically, if secondary dentine deposition progressed at the same rate as primary dentine the pulp would rapidly become obliterated, rendering a tooth with very different mechanical properties and by inference the raison d'être of the pulp and dentine may be to give the tooth resilience; (2) any tooth deformation resulting from loads may be detected by proprioceptors in the pulp. Although the existence of a proprioceptive mechanism has not been proved, it is an attractive explanation for the susceptibility of pulpless teeth to fracture.

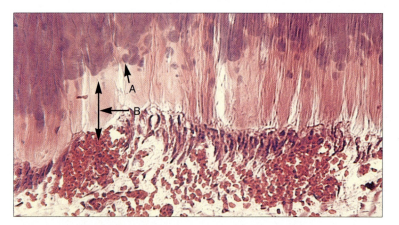

1.14 Active deposition of irregular secondary dentine: A = globular dentine at mineralising front; B = widened predentine

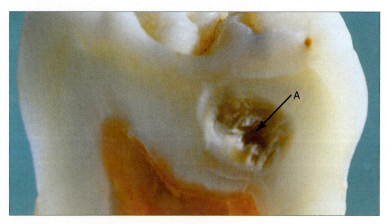

1.15 Irregular deposition of secondary dentine due to caries: A = caries

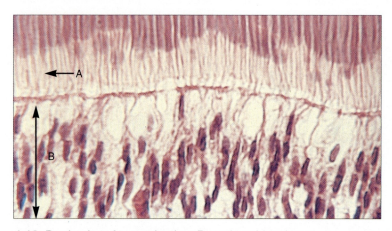

1.16 Predentine: A = predentine; B = odontoblast layer

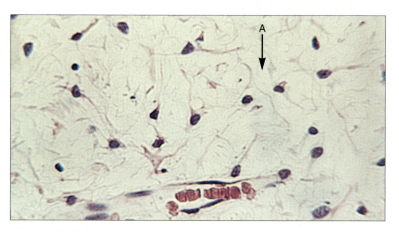

1.17 Pulp tissue elements: A = ground substance

Vascular supply to the pulp

The unique vascular system of the pulp helps to overcome the problems of encapsulation in a rigid cage (1.18–1.20). Arterioles from the dental arteries enter through the apical foramen and pass centrally through the pulp, giving off lateral branches which divide further into capillaries. Minor vessels may enter through lateral canals (1.21), but are unlikely to provide sufficient collateral circulation. Smaller vessels reach the odontoblast layer, where they divide extensively to form a plexus below (1.22) and within (1.23) the odontoblast layer. Venous return is collected by a network of capillaries which unite to form venules coursing down the central portion of the pulp (1.24). The unique feature in this arrangement is the arteriovenous shunt which prevents build-up of unsustainable pressure in the rigid environment. The presence of lymphatic vessels has not been definitely confirmed. In general, with age the blood supply diminishes and its architecture becomes simpler. This diminished blood supply may render a pulp more susceptible to irreversible damage.

1.18 Network of blood vessels in the pulp (courtesy of Prof. I. Kramer)

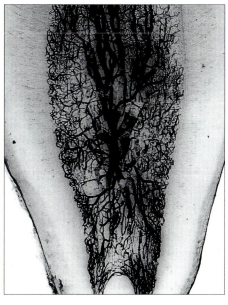

1.19 High-power view of network of blood vessels in the pulp (courtesy of Prof. I. Kramer)

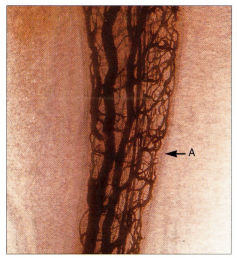

1.20 Relationship of arterioles and capillaries in the pulp to dentine: A = dentine (courtesy of Prof. I. Kramer)

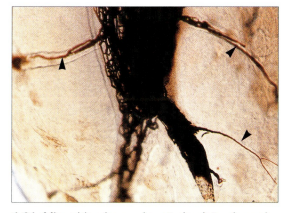

1.21 Minor blood vessels entering lateral canals (courtesy of Prof. I. Kramer)

1.22 Capillary plexus adjacent to the dentine (courtesy of Prof. I. Kramer)

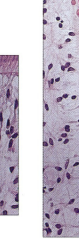

1.23 Capillary from the subodontoblastic plexus: A = capillary

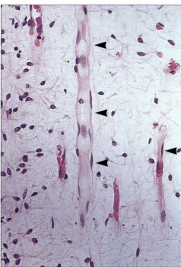

1.24 Venules (arrowed) coursing through centre of pulp

Functional aspects

Inflammation of the pulp in a localized coronal zone does not cause immediate strangulation of apical vessels and death of the pulp. A localized area of inflammation is confined by a combination of ground substance and unique blood supply, which redistributes blood via arteriovenous shunts.

Nerve supply to the pulp

The dental pulp is richly innervated with both sensory and autonomic nerves fibres. These enter the pulp with the blood vessels through the apical foramen. As the nerve bundles pass coronally they divide into smaller branches until ultimately single axons terminate as free nerve endings in the pulp–dentine border area. Here the nerve fibres form the dense *plexus of Raschow* (**1.25**). Individual axons may branch into many terminal filaments, which in turn may enter the dentinal tubules (**1.26**): one axon may innervate up to 100 dentinal tubules which usually penetrate the tubules by only 100–200 μm. Some tubules may contain several nerve fibres.

Functional aspects

Autonomic supply

The autonomic nerve supply consists of sympathetic fibres which control the microcirculation.

Sensory supply

The sensory innervation consists of two (possibly three) types of fibre. The faster conducting myelinated *A-δ-fibres* are thought to be responsible for sharp, localized dentinal pain experienced during drilling, probing, air drying, application of hyperosmotic fluids, and heating or cooling the dentine. The common feature of these stimuli is that they all cause rapid movement of fluid in the dentinal tubules, which causes mechanical distortion of tissue in the pulp–dentine border and stimulates the A-δ-fibres (*the hydrodynamic theory*) (**1.27**). Sensitivity of dentine may be increased by opening dentinal tubules by acid etching. Conversely, blocking the tubules, for example by composite resin, potassium oxalate crystals or naturally by sclerosis, prevents fluid flow and desensitizes dentine.

Stimulation of the slower conducting, unmyelinated *C-fibres* is thought to give rise to the duller, throbbing, less localized pain. The C-fibres are activated by thermal, mechanical or chemical stimuli reaching the deeper parts of the pulp. Dentinal stimulation does not activate the C-fibres unless it causes damage to the pulp tissue (such as raising the pulp temperature to about 44°C or subjecting it to extreme cold).

The A-δ–fibres have a lower threshold than the C-fibres and are stimulated first during electric pulp testing. As the stimulus intensity increases more A-δ-fibres are activated and some C-fibres may be recruited, giving rise to a strong unpleasant sensation. Young teeth with immature roots have very few A-δ-fibres, which may explain the relative unreliability of electric pulp testing in these teeth.

A third type of nerve, the *A-β-fibres*, are myelinated and have the most rapid conduction velocity. These fibres are thought to respond to non-noxious mechanical stimulation of the intact crown and may be important in regulating mastication and loading of teeth, but they also respond to stimulation of dentine.

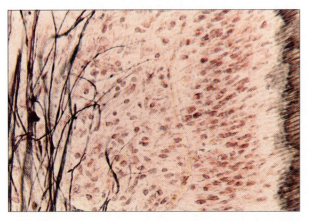

1.25 Plexus of Raschow

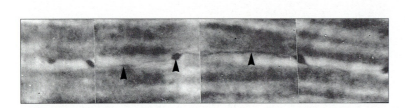

1.26 Nerve axon in dentinal tubule (arrowed)

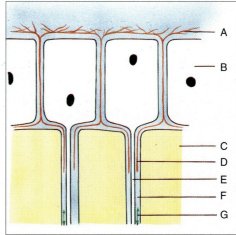

1.27 Hydrodynamic theory: A = nerve plexus; B = odontoblast; C = dentine; D = A-δ nerve fibre; E = odontoblast process; F = dentinal tubule; G = fluid movement stimulates A-δ nerve fibre

The different nerve fibres and variations in types and threshold of stimulation, combined with the patient's perception and tolerance of pain, gives rise to a wide range of descriptions of pain. This, together with poor correlation between symptoms and histopathology, makes diagnosis of conditions of the pulp difficult.

The periradicular tissues

These consist of cementum, periodontal ligament and alveolar bone.

Cementum

Cementum covers the radicular dentine (**1.28**). It abuts the enamel in 30% of teeth, overlaps it in 60% and is separated from it by a gap in about 10%, which may explain cervical sensitivity in young teeth without abrasion. The cementum is principally an inorganic tissue and is more impervious than dentine.

Cellular cementum contains cementocytes (**1.29**) which communicate with each other via canaliculi and with dentine. It is usually found in the apical and furcation regions of the tooth. Sharpey's fibres may be embedded in cellular cementum (**1.30**).

Acellular cementum (**1.31**) forms the innermost layer of the cementum and is devoid of cells. It covers almost the whole root surface in a thin hyaline layer which has incremental lines running parallel to the root surface. It contains closely packed mineralized periodontal fibres.

Intermediate cementum is found at the cementodentinal junction, and has characteristics of both cementum and dentine. Near the enamel it may have characteristics of aprismatic enamel.

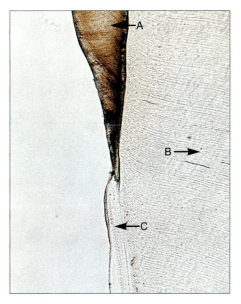

1.28 Ground section showing the relationship between cementum, radicular dentine and enamel: A = enamel; B = dentine; C = cementum

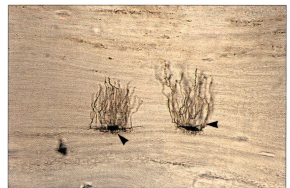

1.29 Cementocytes in cellular cementum (arrowed)

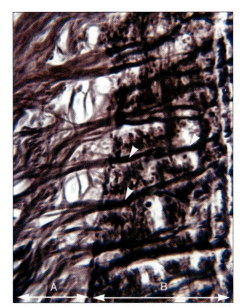

1.30 Sharpey's fibres in cementum (arrowed): A = unmineralized tissue; B = mineralized tissue

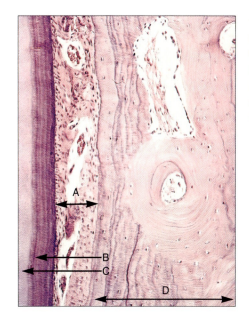

1.31 Cementum, dentine, periodontal ligament and alveolar bone: A = periodontal ligament; B = acellular cementum; C = dentine; D = alveolar bone

Functions

Cementum provides attachment for the periodontal ligament fibres which suspend the tooth from the alveolar bone. It is laid down through life in compensation for loss of occlusal tooth substance and plays a most important physiological role in the repair of resorbed cementum and dentine. The breakdown in this normal mechanism may result in external root resorption which may manifest clinically if extensive enough. Cementum formation around the apical foramen is thought to be an important end result of successful healing following root canal therapy (**1.32**).

Periodontal ligament

The periodontal ligament is a dense fibrous connective tissue which supports the tooth and attaches it to its socket (**1.33**). Its principal component is collagen, which is embedded in a gel-like matrix. The fibres are arranged in specific groups with individual functions. These include *gingival, transseptal, alveolar crest* (**1.34**), *horizontal, oblique* (**1.35, 1.36**) and *apical* fibres. Another important component is the *oxytalan* fibre. Functional adaptation may take place in the broad zone known as the *intermediate plexus* (**1.37**). The main cells of the ligament are fibroblasts, with occa-

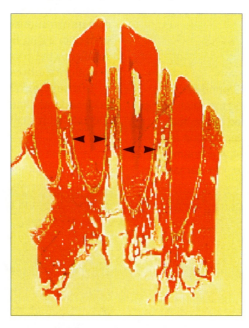

1.32 Healing of periapex with cementum formation (arrowed): A = periodontal ligament; B = root canal; C = alveolar bone (courtesy of Dr T. Pitt Ford)

1.33 Periodontal ligament supporting teeth in alveolar bone (arrowed)

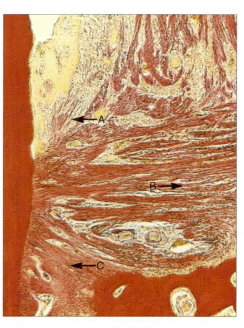

1.34 Gingival, transseptal and alveolar crest fibres: longitudinal view: A = gingival fibres; B = transeptal fibres; C = alveolar crest fibres

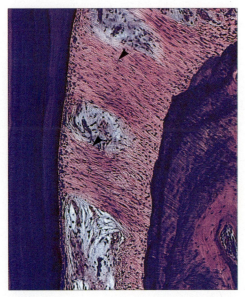

1.35 Oblique fibres: longitudinal view

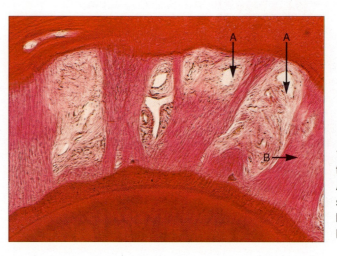

1.36 Oblique fibres: transverse view: A = polyhedric spaces containing blood vessels; B = ligament fibres

sional defence cells. The *root sheath of Hertwig*, which helps root formation, does not totally involute once root formation is complete but degenerates into what resembles a perforated bag of epithelial cells (**1.38**), sometimes described as the *rests of Malassez* (**1.39**). The perforations are quite large, and the intercommunicating strands of epithelial tissue may not all be visible in a given histological section. These cells can proliferate when stimulated by inflammation to form a cyst.

Blood supply

The periodontal ligament's blood supply originates from the inferior dental artery. Arterioles enter the ligament near the apex of the root and from the lateral aspects of the alveolar socket and branch into capillaries within the ligament in a polyhedric pattern along the long axis of the root (**1.36**). Collagen fibres run through the spaces. The blood vessels are closer to the bone than to the cementum. Communications may be seen between the vasculature of the pulp and the periodontal ligament, especially near the apex and furcation (**1.40**). Venules drain to the apex or through apertures in the bony wall of the socket and into the marrow spaces.

Nerve supply

Nerve bundles enter the periodontal ligament through numerous foramina in the alveolar bone. They branch and end in small rounded bodies near the cementum. The nerves carry pain, touch and pressure sensations and form an important part of the feedback mechanism of the masticatory apparatus.

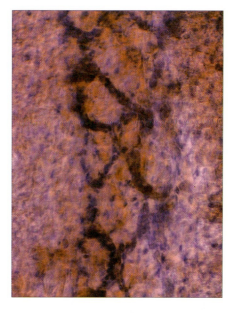

1.38 'Perforated bag' appearance of epithelial Malassez cells

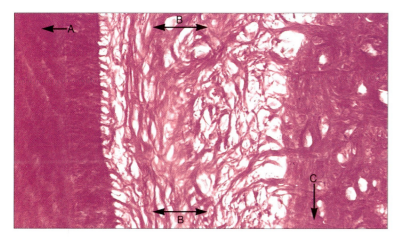

1.37 Intermediate plexus: A = dentine; B = intermediate plexus; C = alveolar bone

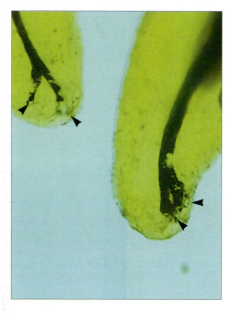

1.40 Vascular communications at the root apex

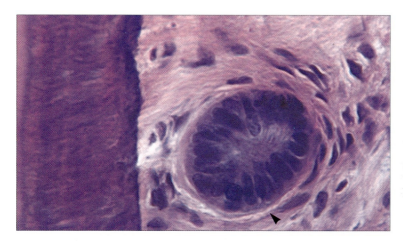

1.39 Rest of Malassez

Functions

The ligament has a proprioceptive function and acts as a viscoelastic cushion because of its fibres and hydraulic fluid systems (blood vessels and their communications with vessel reservoirs in the bone marrow and interstitial fluid of the ligament). The ligament has great adaptive capacity; it responds to functional overload by widening to relieve the load on the tooth (**1.41–1.44**).

The radiographs in **1.41** and **1.42** show the same tooth before and after placement of a crown with a premature occlusal contact: in **1.42**, the periodontal ligament space is noticeably wider. **1.43** shows a histological view of a disused tooth with a lack of proper orientation of fibres in a narrow ligament. **1.44** shows the periodontal ligament of a tooth under heavy occlusal load, with evidence of adjacent bone resorption causing the ligament to widen: this widening should be distinguished from that which occurs in response to pathological irritation. The periodontal ligament also plays an important part in the eruption of teeth and healing, for example following surgery or trauma. Vascular communications between the pulp and periodontium form pathways for transmission of inflammation and micro-organisms between the tissues.

Alveolar bone

Alveolar bone supports the teeth (**1.45**) by forming the other attachment for fibres of the periodontal ligament. It consists of two plates of *cortical bone* separated by *spongy bone* (**1.46**). In some areas the alveolar bone is thin with no spongy bone (**1.45**). The alveolar bone and cortical plates are thickest in the mandible. The spaces between trabeculae of spongy bone are filled with marrow, which consists of haematopoietic tissue in early life and later of fatty tissue (**1.46**). The shape and structure of the trabeculae reflect the stress-bearing requirements of a particular site. The surfaces of the inorganic parts of bone are lined by *osteoblasts* responsible for bone formation: those which become incorporated within the mineral tissue are called *osteocytes* and maintain contact with each other via canaliculi; *osteoclasts* are responsible for bone resorption and may be seen in the *Howship's lacunae* (**1.47**). Cortical bone adjacent to the ligament gives the radiographic appearance of a dense white line next to the dark line of the ligament (**1.41, 1.42**). Bone is a dynamic tissue, continually forming and resorbing in response to functional requirements. In addition to such local response to needs, bone metabolism is under hormonal control. It is easily resorbed by inflammatory mediators, at either the periapex or the marginal attachment. In health the crest of the

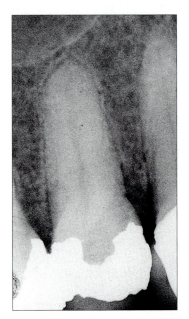

1.41 Normal periodontal ligament

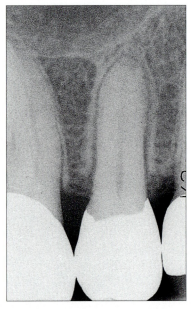

1.42 The tooth in **1.41** following crown placement. Premature occlusal contact caused overloading and widening of periodontal ligament

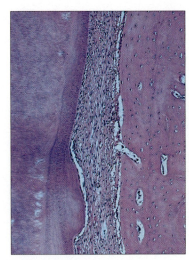

1.43 Disused periodontal ligament. Note the lack of proper orientation of fibres in a narrow ligament

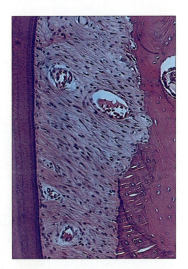

1.44 Overloaded periodontal ligament with oblique fibre orientation and resorption of bone

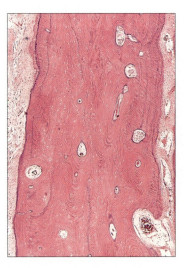

1.45 Alveolar bone

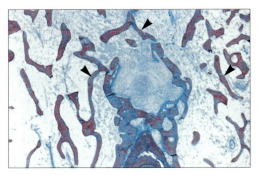

1.46 Trabeculae in spongy bone

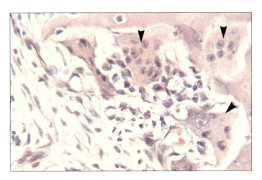

1.47 Osteoclasts (arrowed) in Howship's lacunae

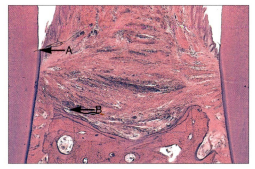

1.48 Relationship between alveolar bone and cementoenamel junction in health: A = cementeonamel junction; B = alveolar bone

alveolus lies about 2 mm apical to the cementoenamel junction (**1.48**) but in periodontal disease it may lie much more towards the apex of the root.

PATHOLOGY AND THERAPY

The dental pulp

Pathogenesis of pulpal pathology

Dental pulps may become inflamed in response to a variety of factors and can ultimately become necrotic. Factors that may cause pulp inflammation include the following:

Tooth tissue loss

Caries (**1.49**) is the most common cause of pulpal damage but abrasion, attrition (**1.50**), erosion and restorative procedures may also elicit inflammation by exposing dentinal tubules to bacteria and their products.

Restorative procedures

Procedures that cut into dentine cause damage by transecting odontoblast processes, generating heat and causing dehydration (**1.51**). The amount of damage is related to the type of handpiece used, the speed of rotation, the type of bur (diamond or tungsten, large or small), interfacial force, vibration and use of an effective coolant (lack of coolant can cause high surface temperatures, sometimes causing incandescence: **1.52**). Other procedures such as cavity cleaning, acid etching, electrosurgery, impression taking, direct construction of temporary restorations and cementation may also damage the pulp.

Restorative materials

The toxicity of materials, their acidity, the amount of heat they generate on setting and their ability to cause dehydration may all cause pulp damage and inflammation (**1.53**). The effect of these

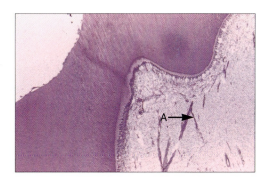

1.49 Effect of caries on the pulp: A = inflamed pulp tissue

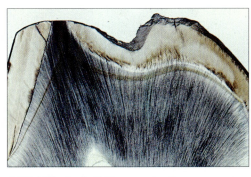

1.50 Effect of attrition on dentine

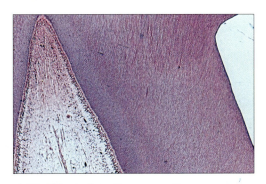

1.51 Effect of cavity preparation on pulp

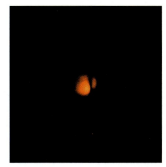

1.52 Incandescence caused by dry cutting of dentine

factors on the pulp has been gauged from studies on animal teeth and young human premolars scheduled for extraction.

The immediate response of the pulp to these factors is aspiration/displacement of the odontoblast or its nucleus into the tubule (**1.54**) and localized inflammation of the pulp confined to the zone subjacent to the involved tubules (**1.55**). Later responses include deposition of secondary dentine (**1.56**) and tubule sclerosis (**1.57**). The severity of response increases if superimposition of a sequence of factors occurs. The healthy young pulp is able to recover from minor insults in 3–8 weeks.

The main cause of lasting pulp inflammation is not the trauma caused by restorative procedures but the presence of bacteria in cavities as a result of incomplete removal of caries (**1.58, 1.59**), contamination from saliva (**1.60**) or incorporation in the smear layer dur-

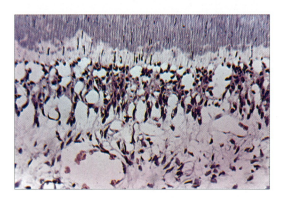

1.53 Effect of cavity preparation and toxic restorative material on pulp

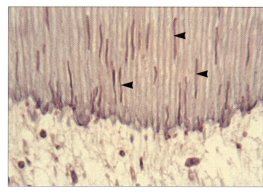

1.54 Aspiration of odontoblasts into dentinal tubules (arrowed)

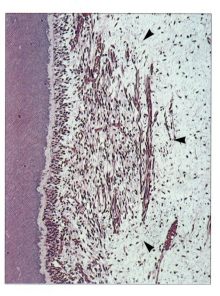

1.55 Localized inflammation of pulp (arrowed)

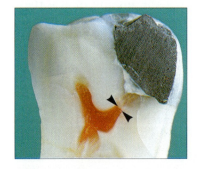

1.56 Secondary dentine deposition caused by caries and its treatment

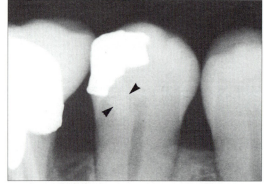

1.57 Sclerosed dentinal tubules (arrowed)

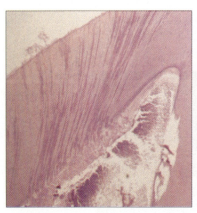

1.58 Bacteria in dentinal tubules (low-power view)

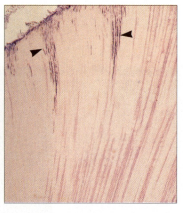

1.59 Bacteria in dentinal tubules (high-power view)

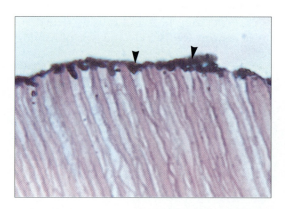

1.60 Bacteria lining the surface of cut dentine

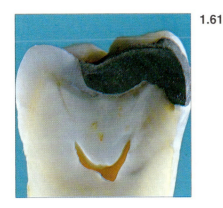

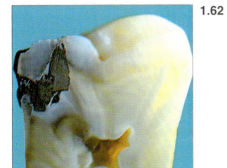

1.61, 1.62 Microleakage under restorations

ing cavity preparation. A more important source of bacteria is microleakage (**1.61, 1.62**): bacteria and their products are capable of diffusing through dentinal tubules to induce an inflammatory response. If the pulp is healthy it is able to block the path of diffusion, initially by producing high molecular weight proteins and later by calcification and secondary dentine formation. The effect of restorative procedures may, however, be significant if moderate to severe inflammation is already present in the pulp. It is therefore extremely important to take steps during clinical procedures to reduce their effect.

Thorough cavity cleaning may help to reduce bacterial damage and should involve removing the smear layer (**1.63**) using weak acids (**1.64**) or a chelating agent such as ethylenediaminetetra-acetic acid (EDTA) (**1.65**), but this leaves dentinal tubules open and the pulp susceptible to bacterial attack. Absolute control of contamination by this approach is not possible using current techniques and materials, which reduce but do not eliminate microleakage. Although the smear layer reduces adaptation of the restorative material it may be best to retain it to protect the pulp from the effects of microleakage. A reasonable compromise is to partially remove the surface of the smear layer only, leaving the dentinal plugs intact (**1.66**): 3% hydrogen peroxide is sufficient for this purpose in most instances. Another way of reducing bacterial contamination is to use an antibacterial restorative or lining material; however, none of the permanent restorative materials exhibits lasting antibacterial effects. Calcium hydroxide and zinc oxide/eugenol materials are noted for their antibacterial properties but they lack durability if exposed to the oral environ-

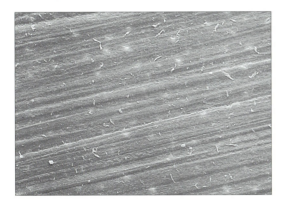

1.63 Smear layer produced by cavity preparation (scanning electron microsocope (SEM) view)

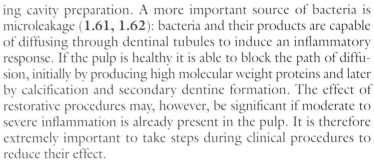

1.64 Removal of smear layer by phosphoric acid to reveal dentinal tubule openings (SEM view)

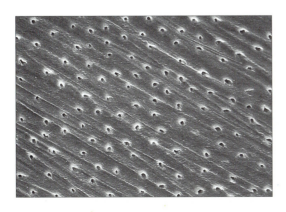

1.65 Removal of smear layer by EDTA (SEM view)

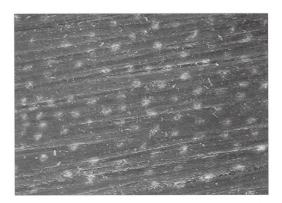

1.66 Partial removal of smear layer using 3% hydrogen peroxide (SEM view)

ment. It is therefore recommended that one of these materials is used as simply a base for a cavity and covered by a compatible but more durable, permanent material, though even under these circumstances calcium hydroxide may be lost by microleakage. It is important to minimize microleakage by achieving the best marginal adaptation possible (**1.67–1.72**).

Severe inflammatory and degenerative changes in the pulp

Spread of inflammation

The way inflammation spreads from a localized site (**1.73**) to the rest of the pulp (**1.74**) is not fully understood. It may be related to the ability of the pulp to close off dentinal tubules, and to wall off the inflammatory lesion if this fails. The localized response progresses to more severe inflammation if the provoking factors are not controlled. Progression of inflammation may produce a wide range of histological pictures, including areas of chronic inflammation coexisting with microabscesses and partial necrosis, which do not correlate with clinical signs and symptoms, a fact which makes clinical diagnosis of the state of the pulp extremely difficult. Added to this picture of uncertainty is the finding that in some cases periapical changes associated with localized inflammation of the pulp are visible on radiographs, even in the pres-

1.67 Carious lesion

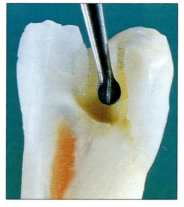

1.68 Removal of carious dentine

1.69 Completed preparation

1.70 Sub-lining with calcium hydroxide

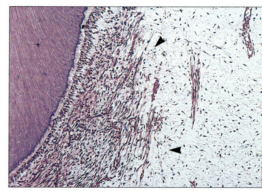

1.73 Localized pulp inflammation

1.71 Lining with zinc oxide/eugenol

1.72 Placement of amalgam

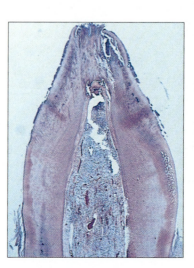

1.74 Severe inflammation affecting most of the pulp

ence of vital healthy pulp tissue in the roots or in the pulp chamber (**1.75, 1.76**). A reasonably clear distinction is possible only between vital (although inflamed) and completely necrotic pulps using the tests currently available, which are crude and aim to stimulate only specific nerve fibres in the pulp.

Under the specific condition of injury caused by traumatic impact, sudden severance of the blood supply can result in total necrosis of the pulp without any periradicular change. Such change would then become evident only if the necrotic pulp becomes infected (**1.77, 1.78**).

Mineral deposits

A common finding in the pulp is the presence of mineral deposits or stones, most commonly in teeth with diseased pulps but also in unerupted teeth. The cause of calcification is unknown. Calcification is of two types: smooth and rounded deposits are formed by concentric laminations and are found in the coronal pulp (**1.79, 1.80**); the irregular calcifications without laminations are more likely to be found in the radicular pulp (**1.81, 1.82**) and may be rod- or leaf-shaped. Laminated stones grow by the addition of collagen fibrils to their surface, the irregular variety by calcification of pre-existing collagen fibre bundles. The calcifications may be a dystrophic change, but are not always found in association with degenerative

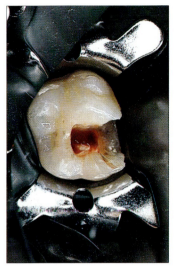

1.75 Pulp chamber containing vital pulp tissue

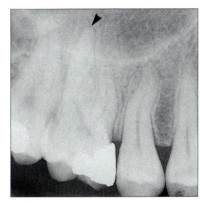

1.76 Radiograph of tooth seen in **1.75**, showing periapical area around palatal root before opening into the pulp (arrowed)

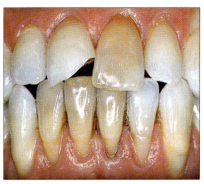

1.77 Discoloration of teeth caused by pulp calcification and dentine sclerosis following trauma; although nonresponsive to pulp tests there was no periapical change

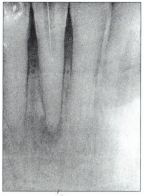

1.78 This tooth presented with a periapical area many years after giving negative readings to pulp testing

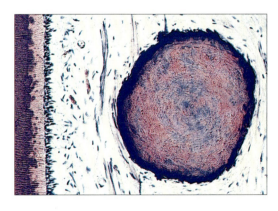

1.79 Calcified stone in the pulp chamber

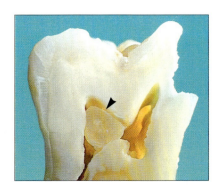

1.80 Longitudinal section of tooth, showing a large round stone in the pulp chamber

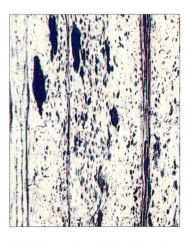

1.81 Irregular calcifications in the radicular pulp

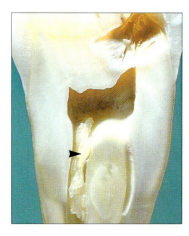

1.82 Longitudinal section of tooth: note irregular calcification in the root canal

changes. The main clinical significance of pulp calcification lies in the difficulty it can cause during root canal therapy. Sometimes calcification may almost obliterate the pulp space (**1.83–85**), which can make location and negotiation of canals difficult. Furthermore, dislodged stones may be pushed apically causing a blockage. Irregular calcification in the canal also has the potential to harbour bacteria and make their elimination more difficult.

Treatment of the compromised pulp

Pulp compromised by exposure or near exposure due to deep caries or trauma may be treated by pulp therapy or removed by root canal treatment. The approach chosen depends on the operator's perceived chances of success, the long-term prognosis and overall treatment planning considerations: a single damaged tooth in an otherwise intact arch, to be restored with amalgam, lends itself easily to corrective measures and therefore allows a conservative approach; a tooth scheduled for a cast restoration, however, is less easily corrected and a pragmatic approach may be root canal treatment.

Opinion differs on whether to preserve or eliminate the pulp if restorative considerations are less important. Root canal treatment has a high success rate (80–95%) and may be preferable because the pulp is susceptible to long-term failure; further, irregular calcification and internal resorption in a canal treated by pulp therapy may render root canal treatment more difficult at a later stage. Many practitioners would consider pulp therapy only to treat an incompletely formed root in order to encourage its complete formation. However, pulp therapy has a success rate of 85–90% and evidence of pulp calcification and significant internal resorption is lacking. In addition, a tooth with a vital pulp may be less susceptible to fracture.

Rationale for pulp therapy

When dealing with a deep carious lesion, a number of clinical assessments must be made. First, the histological state of the pulp must be assessed from the history of pain, examination findings, pulp tests and radiographs. A poor correlation between the histopathology of the pulp and clinical signs and symptoms means that the operator has to make an educated guess, but despite this it has often been stated that teeth exhibiting no pain or periradicular pathology stand a good chance of survival following pulpal therapy. The second assessment is to estimate the proximity of the carious lesion to the pulp and the third to guess the extent to which the superficial pulp may be necrotic and contaminated by bacteria (**1.86**).

The aim of treatment is to remove all infected tissue and to produce a bacteria-tight restoration.

Types of therapy

Indirect pulp capping

This technique (**1.87–1.91**) is used if excavation of all the carious dentine from the pulpal surface would lead to a traumatic exposure of the pulp through sound dentine (**1.87**). Some of the soft carious dentine over the pulp is left (**1.88**) and dressed with an antibacterial material in order to kill residual bacteria and to remineralize the dentine. The tooth is restored with a permanent material (**1.91**) that excludes microleakage to prevent reactivation of the lesion. It is widely accepted that a calcium hydroxide material should be used to cover the carious dentine (**1.89**) and a base of zinc oxide/eugenol placed over this (**1.90**). Calcium

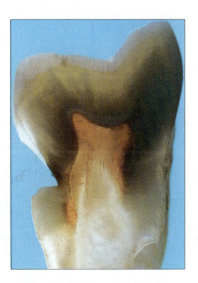

1.83 Almost complete obliteration of pulp space by calcification: low-power view

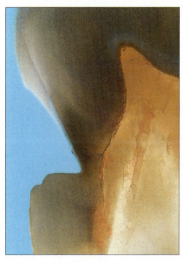

1.84 High-power view of tooth in **1.83**

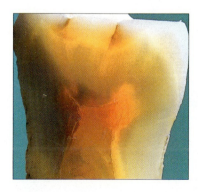

1.85

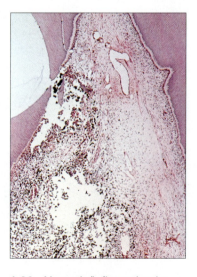

1.86 Necrotic/inflamed pulp below pulp exposure

1.87–1.91 Indirect pulp capping

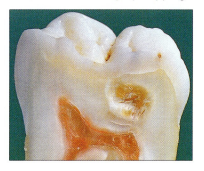
1.87

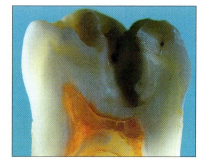
1.88

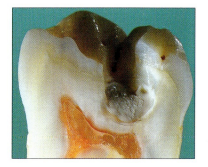
1.89

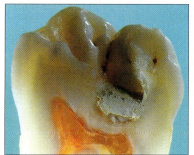
1.90

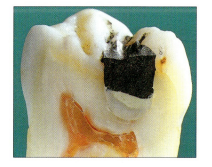
1.91

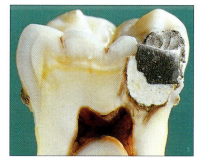
1.92 Necrosis of pulp due to microleakage

1.93–1.104 Direct pulp capping

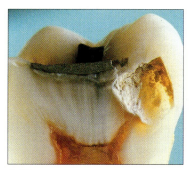
1.93

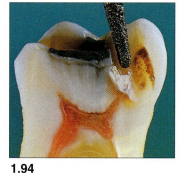
1.94

hydroxide is more acceptable directly over the pulp than zinc oxide/eugenol in the presence of micro-exposures and may make the residual dentine harder. If there are no subsequent clinical symptoms and the tooth shows signs of continuing vitality, two approaches may be adopted: the tooth may be restored permanently or the dressing may be removed after an arbitrary period (usually 3 months) and residual carious dentine excavated in the hope that secondary dentine formed during this period might prevent exposure. However, at the rate of secondary dentine formation (3 μm per day), only 0.27 mm of dentine would be formed in 3 months, which is unlikely to prevent a traumatic exposure.

The practical problem with this technique is that the depth of carious lesion remaining is not easily gauged. An unacceptable thickness of carious dentine may be left behind and be reactivated by microleakage leading to pulp necrosis (**1.92**). Dentine softening and staining do not necessarily precede bacterial invasion and bacterial invasion of hard dentine is possible. Indirect pulp capping is therefore an unpredictable procedure. Its success relies on correctly diagnosing the pulpal condition, removing most of the carious dentine and preventing further microleakage.

Direct pulp capping

Successful treatment of pulpal exposure by direct pulp capping (**1.93–1.104**) depends on the pulp being healthy, contamination by bacteria low and no subsequent microleakage. The most important factor in successful treatment is a healthy pulp. The pulp is likely to be healthier in younger teeth but, although success rates may be higher in younger teeth, age is not always a good prognostic indicator. If excavation of deep caries (**1.93, 1.94, 1.100**) leads to traumatic pulp exposure (**1.95, 1.101**), bacterial contamination of pulp tissue is assumed to be relatively minor. Treatment of pulps exposed to salivary contamination for several hours following traumatic injury may be successful, and minor contamination by saliva during operative procedures is unlikely to affect the outcome.

There is no apparent relationship between size of exposure and success rate, although it was once firmly believed that larger exposures gave a poorer prognosis. Treatment of carious exposures might be expected to be less successful than treatment of traumatic exposures but studies indicate that, in the absence of previous pulpal symptoms, the success rates are similar.

Technique

The surface of the exposed pulp is gently washed with sterile water or saline to remove contaminants, debris and dentine chips. Haemostasis is achieved using slightly moist cotton pellets: dry pellets are not recommended as their removal will cause further bleeding. Profuse bleeding for longer than about 5 min is a sign of severe pulp inflammation and more radical treatment should be considered (**1.102**). Once haemostasis is secure (**1.101**) the surface of the wound should be dressed with a setting or non-set-

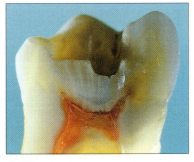
1.95

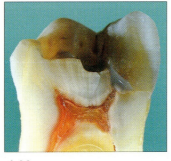
1.96

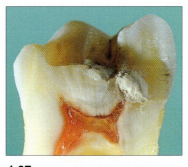
1.97

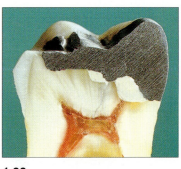
1.98

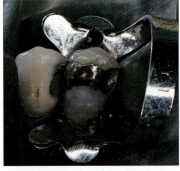
1.99 Distal filling in |3 with recurrent caries

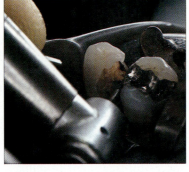
1.100

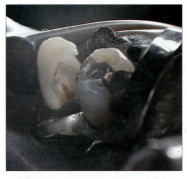
1.101

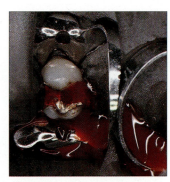
1.102 Profuse bleeding from a hyperaemic pulp

ting calcium hydroxide material (**1.96, 1.103**), placed over vital tissue, not a blood clot. The dressing is then covered with a zinc oxide/eugenol base to eliminate bacterial microleakage (**1.97**), but if a composite restorative material is to be used for the final restoration (**1.104**) a glass ionomer cement may be more suitable. The permanent, well-adapted restoration is then placed (**1.98, 1.104**).

Pulpotomy

This term is applied to removal of coronal pulp tissue that is too severely inflamed or contaminated by microorganisms to give a satisfactory result (**1.105**). The extent of tissue removed will vary depending on the amount of inflammation. For example, pulp exposed by tooth fracture may react in one of two ways: (1) the epithelium-covered pulp (pulp polyp) may proliferate and inflammation is limited to a depth of 2 mm; (2) superficial necrosis may occur, with inflammation penetrating several millimetres from the site of exposure.

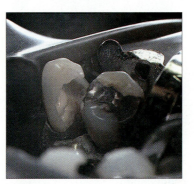
1.103

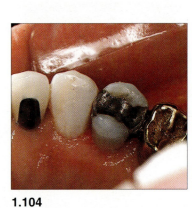
1.104

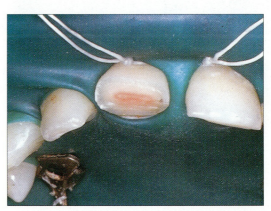
1.105 Pulp exposure due to traumatic fracture

Technique

The principles of pulpotomy are similar to those of direct pulp capping but the exposure is larger and calcium hydroxide is applied deeper in the root. The aim of the procedure is to remove superficial necrotic pulp tissue down to healthy tissue and success depends on complete removal of necrotic and inflamed tissue (**1.86**). This is thought to be most effectively achieved using an abrasive diamond bur at high speed and with adequate water cooling (**1.106**). All debris must be removed to achieve a clean healthy wound (**1.107**). Following haemostasis (**1.108**), calcium hydroxide is applied without pressure (**1.109, 1.110**) and is covered with a layer of zinc oxide/eugenol mixed to a thin consistency (**1.111**). Some practitioners advocate cutting a step in the cavity to support a plastic or Teflon disc on which the zinc oxide/eugenol dressing is placed.

Assessment of success of pulp therapy

All cases should be carefully followed up. An initial assessment 6–12 weeks after therapy is recommended, followed by 6-monthly and annual reviews. At each examination a history of symptoms should be obtained and the following assessments made: tenderness of adjacent soft tissues to palpation; tenderness of the tooth to percussion; radiographic signs of pulpal and periapical changes; response to vitality tests (vitality tests may reveal little information in pulpotomized teeth). Additional tests for teeth treated by pulp capping and pulpotomy include checking the presence and integrity of the calcific barrier radiographically and direct probing following removal of the dressing.

If early radiographic assessment shows no evidence of bridge formation (**1.112**), the treatment is considered to have failed and conventional root canal therapy should be considered. Incompletely formed roots should demonstrate radiographic evidence of pro-

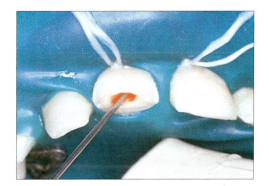

1.107 Irrigating the pulpal wound

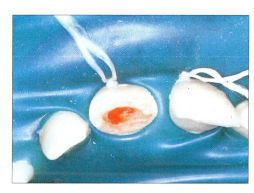

1.108 Haemostatis

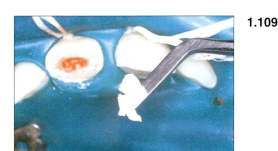

1.106 Removal of superficial necrotic pulp

1.109, 1.110 Application of calcium hydroxide

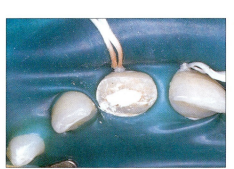

1.109

1.110

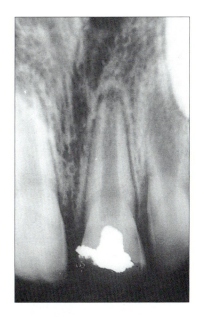

1.111 Zinc oxide/eugenol dressing

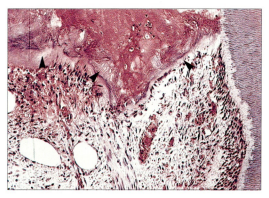

1.112 Calcific bridge formation

gressing root formation (**1.113, 1.114**). Some practitioners recommend root canal treatment as soon as root formation is complete, to prevent continued calcification of the root canal which may render the procedure more difficult later (**1.115, 1.116**). However, this technique is not universally accepted and many consider that if the residual pulp remains healthy it should be removed only if restorative requirements for retention dictate.

PERIRADICULAR PATHOLOGY AND THERAPY

Pathogenesis

The exact pathogenesis of the periradicular lesion is not clear, despite much research into the sequence of events. The periradicular lesion related to the compromised dental pulp may develop by one of two means:

1. Progressive, increasingly severe pulp inflammation can lead to an initial periradicular lesion associated with the interaction of bacteria and their products with the defence mechanisms of the pulp tissue. Bacterial toxins and inflammatory mediators carried periapically in blood vessels from the pulp may cause a periradicular lesion (**1.75, 1.76**). Pulp therapy may help to eliminate this early lesion but is an unpredictable treatment. Once pulp tissue loses its vitality, it contains no defence cells to counter the growth and spread of microorganisms and a new line of defence becomes established at the periapex of the tooth, where a ready source of defence cells is available to confine the infection within the root canal system.

2. If the dental pulp suddenly loses its vitality as a result of impact trauma, initial signs of acute trauma and disruption of apical blood vessels occur, followed by healing – or chronic inflammation if the pulp space becomes infected with bacteria.

Factors implicated in the pathogenesis of the periradicular lesion are discussed below.

Altered host tissue

The belief that necrotic pulp tissue causes periradicular pathology has been shown to be unfounded in laboratory and clinical studies. For example, intact, caries-free unrestored teeth that have been made non-vital by traumatic impact, but which have uninfected root canals, are not associated with periapical lesions. The suggestion that stagnant tissue fluid diffuses out of the root canal to cause periapical inflammation has also been disproved.

Microorganisms and their products

Microorganisms and their products have been implicated as the major factor in the development of the periradicular lesion. A variety of different microorganisms have been found in root canal systems by sampling and culturing methods (**Table 1.1**). Earlier studies did not have the advantage of advanced culturing techniques and therefore found mainly aerobic and facultative organisms and some anaerobes. The typical flora included streptococci, gram-negative cocci, lactobacilli and a range of anaerobic bacteria. As culturing techniques improved, particularly for the strict anaerobic bacteria, it was possible to isolate and identify many more strains and species. The picture of root canal infection has therefore undergone a tremendous change. Almost all of these microorganisms originate from the oral cavity, and rarely from other parts of the body. The anaerobic environment of the root canal system allows certain types of organisms to survive; hence the composition of the microbial flora in the root canal is very different from those of the oral and periodontal environments.

1.113 **1.114**

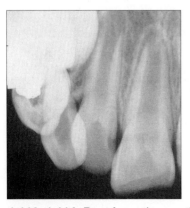 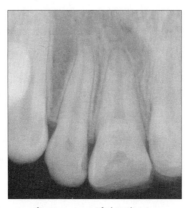

1.113, 1.114 Root formation continues after successful pulpotomy

1.115 **1.116**

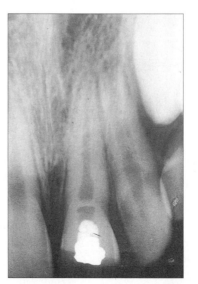 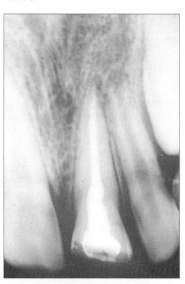

1.115, 1.116 Elective devitalization following completion of root formation is not universally performed

Table 1.1 Bacteria isolated from root canals

Aerobes	Facultative anaerobes	Obligate anaerobes
Gram Positive Cocci	**Gram Positive Cocci**	**Gram Positive Cocci**
Streptococcus salivarius	Streptococcus milleri	Streptococcus constellatus
Streptococcus viridans	Streptococcus mitis	Streptococcus intermedius
	Streptococcus mitior	Streptococcus morbillorum
	Streptococcus mutans	Peptostreptococcus anaerobius
	Streptococcus sanguis	Peptostreptococcus micros
	Streptococcus faecalis	Peptostreptococcus prevotii
	Streptococcus oralis	Peptostreptococcus magnus
	Streptococcus intermedius	Peptostreptococcus asaccharolyticus
	Enterococcus faecalis	
	Enterococcus faecium	
	Gram Positive Rods	**Gram Positive Rods**
	Actinomyces naeslundii	Actinomyces israeli
	Actinomyces viscosus	Actinomyces meyeri
	Corynebacterium xerosis	Actinomyces odontolyticus
	Lactobacillus salivarius	Arachnia propionica
	Lactobacillus fermentum	Eubacterium alactolyticum
		Eubacterium brachy
		Eubacterium lentum
		Eubacterium nodatum
		Eubacterium timidum
		Lactobacillus catenaforme
		Lactobacillus minutus
		Propionibacterium acnes
	Gram Negative Cocci	**Gram Negative Cocci**
	Neisseria	Veillonella parvula
	Gram Negative Rods	**Gram Negative Rods**
	Eikenella corrodens	Porphyromonas gingivalis
	Capnocytophaga ochracia	Porphyromonas endodontalis
	Campylobacter sputorum	Prevotella oralis
		Prevotella oris
		Prevotella buccae
		Prevotella intermedius
		Prevotella melaninogenicus
		Prevotella loeschei
		Fusobacterium nucleatum
		Fusobacterium necrophorum
		Selenomonas sputigena
		Wolinella recta
		Wolinella curva
		Treponema
		Mitsuokella dentalis

Microorganisms access the root canal system most commonly through the crown or root by carious exposure, open dentinal tubules, lateral canals and cracks; less commonly by anachoresis (an infection of chronically inflamed tissue by blood-borne bacteria). A chronically inflamed pulp may become infected in this way but it is unlikely that an empty canal would.

Experimental monoinfection of root canals shows minimal periradicular response and short-lived infection; only certain bacteria (*Pseudomonas, Enterococci*) are capable of surviving as single-strain infections. More commonly, root canal infections are mixed, containing eight or more strains with three or four strains predominating. The types and combinations of bacteria found vary greatly. Members of the genus *Bacteroides* have been reclassified as *Porphyromonas* or *Prevotella* and have been investigated most widely because they are prominent in such infections.

Mixed flora seem more able to survive than monoinfections because one strain can produce nutrients required for another (however, overgrowth of one species may cause the demise of another). As the source of nutrients and concentrations of the various metabolic products change, the microbial flora also alters, and this relationship between microorganisms and prevailing conditions determines which strains will survive. The virulence of the flora may therefore vary with time.

The size of the periradicular lesion appears to be directly related to the number of strains, and to the total numbers (10^2–10^7) of bacteria present. Some studies have also reported a correlation between symptoms and presence of certain organisms, such as *P. melaninogenicus*, *P. gingivalis*, *P. endodontalis* and *P. buccae*. These and other organisms (*P. asaccharolyticus*, *P. corporis*, *P. denticola*, *P. intermedius* and *P. loeschei*) have also been associated with severe, and sometimes rapidly spreading, abscesses. An antibiotic active against anaerobic Gram-negative organisms should overcome these infections, but will not exclude infection by Gram-positive or Gram-negative aerobic organisms.

Microorganisms may be suspended in the lumen of the root canal if it is filled with fluid (**1.117a, b**). They may be seen on root canal walls (**1.117b, d, f**) as colonies of single bacterial forms (**1.117e**) or co-aggregates of several forms (**1.117b**).

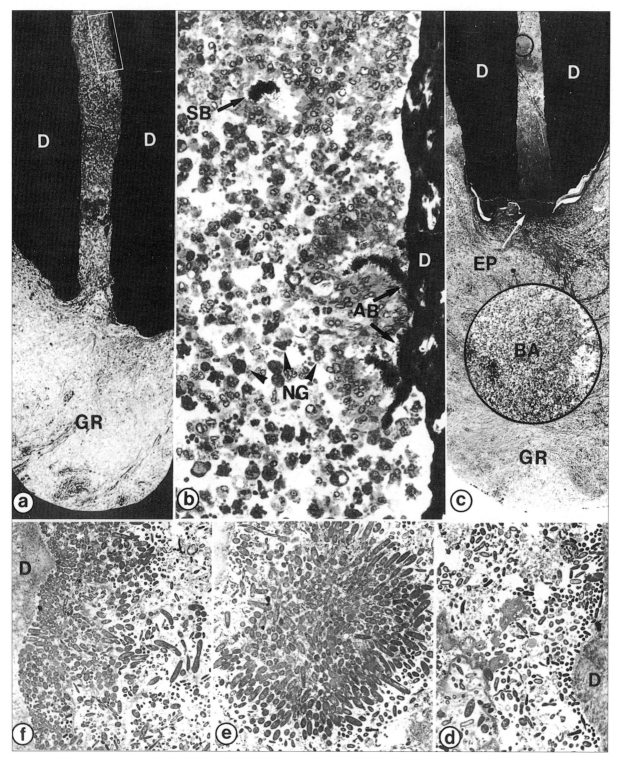

1.117 The endodontic flora in the apical third of a periapically affected human root. The flora appears to be blocked by a wall of neutrophils (NG in **b**) or an epithelial plug (EP in **c**). Note the dense aggregates of bacteria sticking to the dentine wall (AB in **b**) and similar ones (SB in **b**) along with loose collections of bacteria (insert in **c**) remaining suspended in the root canal among neutrophils. A cluster of an apparently monobacterial colony is magnified in **e**. Electron micrographs show bacterial condensation on the surface of the dentine wall, forming thin (**d**) or thick (**f**) layered bacterial plaques. The rectangular demarcated portion in a and the circular one in **c** are magnified in **b** and in the inset in **c**, respectively. GR = granuloma, D = dentine. Original magnification: **a** × 50; **b** × 400; **c** × 40 (inset × 400); **d** × 2440; **e** × 3015; **f** × 3215 (courtesy of Dr Ramachandran Nair)

Filamentous forms may sometimes be seen adhering at right angles to the dentinal walls, with coccal forms forming strings oriented in the same direction, demonstrating a symbiotic relationship. In some instances, colonies produce a plaque-like amorphous matrix with single or multilayered condensations of bacteria (**1.117d, 1.117f**). The predominant morphologic forms differ in the apical and coronal aspects of the canal: coccoids and rods are more numerous in the coronal parts, filaments and spirochaetes predominate in the apical part of the canal. The impression is of the root canal walls covered with microcolonies of single or mixed bacteria, which may be completely separate or which may coalesce, with their own unique microhabitat to support them. Microorganisms may also variably invade dentinal tubules (**1.118**), being able to penetrate predentine more easily than calcified dentine. Penetration of dentine (which may extend to its full width) by bacteria is determined by several factors, which may include duration of infection, type of organism and absence of cementum allowing ingress of nutrients from the periodontal ligament.

The apical extent of microbial growth is also subject to considerable variation. In some teeth the bulk of microorganisms may be found in the coronal part of the canal; in others microbial colonies extend up to the apical foramen where they may be seen next to an apical plug of polymorphonuclear leucocytes (PMNLs) (**1.117a**) or epithelial cells (**1.117c**). Epithelial proliferation in the periapical tissues may therefore have a protective role, as it does elsewhere in the body.

In acute exacerbation of chronic lesions bacteria (including cocci, rods, filamentous bacteria and spirochaetes) may proliferate beyond the apical foramen and into the periradicular lesion (**1.120**), overwhelming the local defences (**1.119**). Rarely, chronic periradicular lesions may contain clusters of viable bacteria, most often *Actinomyces israelii*, *A. propionica*, *A. naeslundii* and *Arachnia propionica* (**1.121**). Others, such as *Staphylococcus epidermidis*, *Fusobacterium nucleatum*, *Propionibacterium acnes*, *Peptostreptococcus micros*, *Bacteroides gracilis* and facultative streptococci, have also been implicated but are probably contaminants. Claims of finding microorganisms embedded in an extracellular plaque-like matrix covering the external surface of the root have been made, but have not been corroborated.

Most chronic periradicular lesions do not contain bacteria and are thought to be caused by certain factors (molecular substances produced by microorganisms, such as endotoxins, exotoxins, metabolic products and other virulence factors) diffusing out of the root canal. The smallest molecule likely to initiate and maintain a periradicular response is unknown but would be a useful indicator of the level of seal required to stop diffusion of noxious molecules from the root canal to the periradicular tissues. The most widely investigated of these is endotoxin, produced by Gram-negative organisms and found in root canal systems, in dentinal tubules up to 300 μm deep and in periradicular tissues (the role of exotoxins has not been studied widely). Other virulence factors implicated include coagulase, collagenase, leucocidin, haemolysin, necrotoxin and gelatinase.

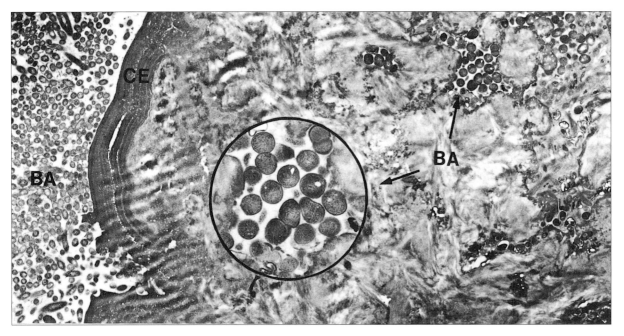

1.118 Presence of bacterial clusters in the root dentine, slightly coronal to the periapical area shown in **1.119**. Note part of the apical plaque is visible peripheral to the cementum (CD) and clusters of bacteria (BA) existing in apparently disintegrating dentinal tubules. Original magnification × 5300; inset × 12 800 (courtesy of Dr Ramachandran Nair)

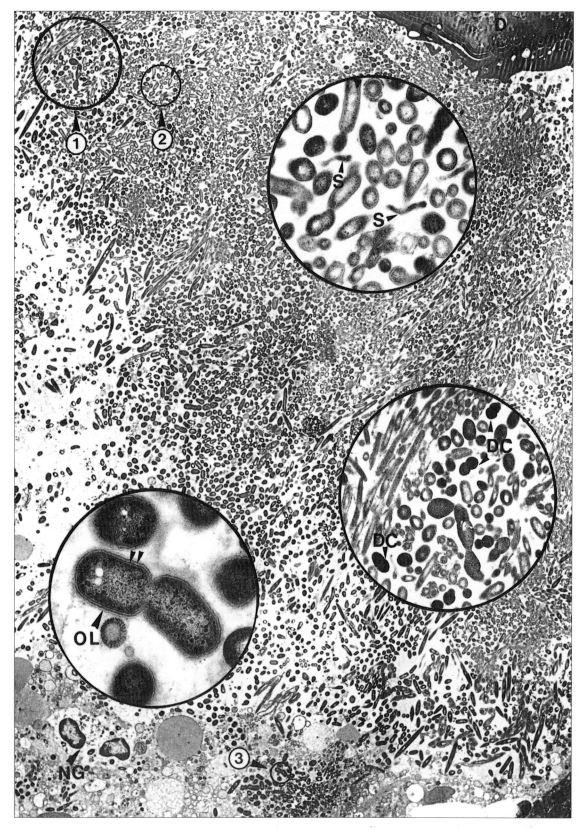

1.119 A massive periapical plaque associated with an acute lesion. Note the mixed nature of the flora. Numerous dividing cocci (DC, middle inset), rods (lower inset), filamentous bacteria and spirocaetes (S, upper inset) can be seen. Rods often reveal a Gram-negative cell wall (double arrowhead), some of them showing a third outer layer (OL). The circular areas 1, 2 and 3 are magnified in the middle, upper and lower insets, respectively. D = dentine; C = cementum; NG = neutrophils. Original magnification × 2680; upper inset × 19 200; middle inset × 11 200; lower inset × 36 400 (courtesy of Dr Ramachandran Nair)

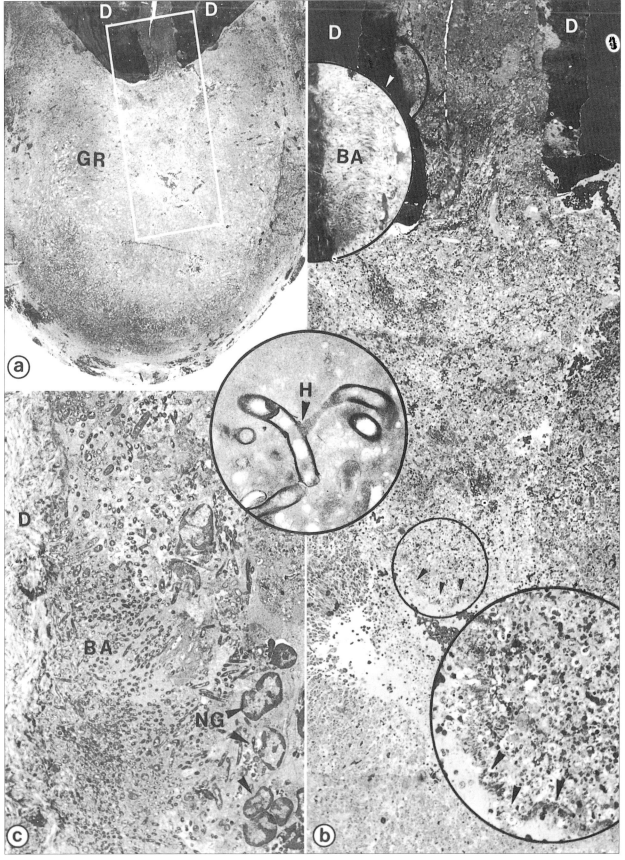

1.120 An apical plaque invading a resting granuloma. (The rectangular area in **a** is magnified in **b**.) The well encapsulated granuloma (GR) shows the bacterial front (arrowheads in **b** and lower inset) deep within the body of the lesion. Note the funnel-like area of tissue necrosis immediately in front of the apical foramen (**a** and **b**) and the plaque-like bacterial condensation (BA in **b** and upper inset) along the root dentine: **c** is an electron micrograph of this plaque. The middle inset shows a high magnification of a branching or hyphal-like structure found among the plaque flora. D = dentine; NG = neutrophilic granulocytes. Original magnification: **a** × 23; **b** × 100; **c** × 2680; upper inset × 400; middle inset × 4300; lower inset × 250 (courtesy of Dr Ramachandran Nair)

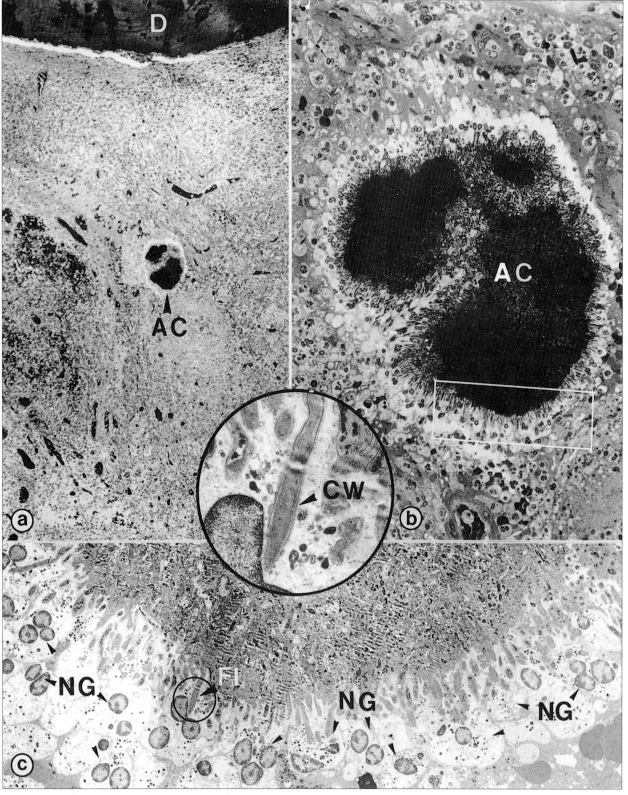

1.121 Actinomyces in the body of a human periapical granuloma. The colony (AC in **a**) is magnified in **b**. The rectangular area demarcated in **b** is magnified in **c**. Note the starburst appearance of the colony with needle-like peripheral filaments surrounded by few layers of neutrophilic granulocytes (NG), some of which contain phagocytosed bacteria. A dividing peripheral filament (FI) is magnified in the inset. Note the typical Gram-positive wall (CW). D = dentine. Original magnification: **a** × 60; **b** × 430; **c** × 1680; inset × 6700 (courtesy of Dr Ramachandran Nair)

Host defence factors

The full range of specific and non-specific defence reactions has been implicated in the development and maintenance of a periradicular lesion (**1.122**). The most important mechanism or combination of pathways in localizing microorganisms to the root canal is not clear; the reactions occurring may vary with the microorganisms present. However, it is clear that the periradicular lesion is the result of a defence reaction which prevents infection of the surrounding bone.

Non-specific responses

Non-specific responses are mediated by the direct action of some microorganisms and their products on the immune system which then initiates an inflammatory response, attracting PMNLs to the apical foramen where they phagocytose invading organisms, helping to confine them to the root canal.

Specific responses

Defence cells are drawn to the periradicular site, including the T and B lymphocytes that are usually peripheral to PMNLs and help mount the specific immune response. Endotoxin also stimulates B lymphocytes to proliferate and produce antibodies; it may also activate the complement pathway to attract more PMNLs and macrophages. IgE antibody reactions (type 1 hypersensitivity) and mast cells have been seen in the periradicular region. IgM and IgG react with cell wall antigens to activate the complement system and to cause its phagocytosis (type 2 hypersensitivity); they may also react with antigens from root canals to form immune complexes, which in turn can stimulate release of vasoactive amines and the chemotaxis of PMNLs (type 3 hypersensitivity). T lymphocytes are more predominant in the periradicular lesion than B lymphocytes and are probably involved in cell-mediated immunity (type 4 hypersensitivity). The numbers of T-helper and T-suppressor cells are equal in the chronic lesion but in a growing lesion the T-helper cells outnumber the T-suppressor cells.

Cells in the periradicular lesion

The chronic periradicular lesion may be conveniently visualised according to the *zones of Fish* (**1.123**). The *zone of infection*, which consists of PMNLs lined up almost as a membrane to prevent bacterial invasion, is seen in the apical or lateral foramen. Many of these cells die and release lysosomal enzymes, which cause further necrosis. Adjacent to this layer is the *zone of contamination*, which is affected by the diffusing antigens and irritants from the root canal. Lymphocytes and plasma cells predominate in this zone, but in the presence of root canal antigens do not survive long. Relatively large amorphous areas, known as Russell bodies, are also present; they are thought to be associated with plasma cells. Peripheral to the zone of contamination is the *zone of irritation* in which macrophages and osteoclasts predominate. This zone is distant from severe contamination and macrophages are able to scavenge and remove cellular debris. Beyond this is the *zone of stimulation*, an area of intense cellular activity, dominated by young fibroblasts and osteoblasts which produce a fibrous capsule to surround the lesion and, in an established lesion in equilibrium, produce a lining of sclerosed bone. Changes in size of a periradicular granuloma can be visualized in terms of size changes in the zones.

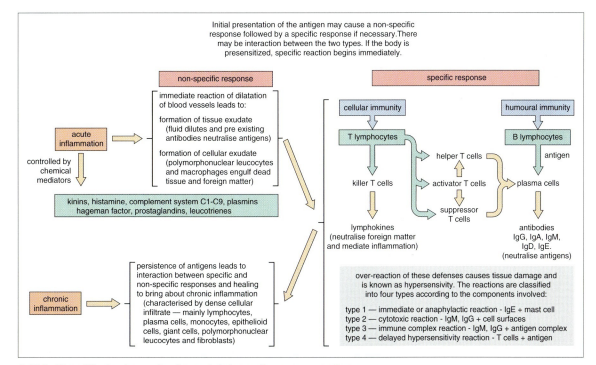

1.122 Simplified schematic chart of defence/immune reactions

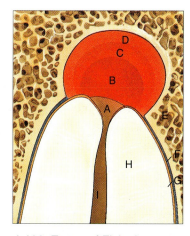

1.123 Zones of Fish: A = zone of infection; B = zone of contamination; C = zone of irritation; D = zone of stimulation; E = alveolar bone; F = periodontal ligament; G = cementum; H = dentine; I = root canal

The periapical area is richly supplied by proliferating blood vessels and nerve fibres. Complex interactions between sprouting sensory fibres, neuropeptides, immune cells and healing mechanisms are possible.

The size of the periradicular lesion may change according to the balance between microorganisms and their toxins on the one side and the host defences on the other. The irritants may dominate at any time if the root canal flora becomes more virulent or if the host defences are depleted by an unrelated systemic condition. This dynamic balance causes variations in the histological and clinical picture but there is no direct correlation between the histological and clinical pictures.

Types of lesion

A range of periradicular conditions has been identified in order to understand the different clinical presentations and to aid differential diagnosis. These conditions may be classified as follows.

Acute periradicular inflammation

This uncommon condition arises if acute pulpal inflammation spreads to the periodontal ligament more rapidly than the periradicular bone is resorbed. The result is an accumulation of PMNLs and oedema due to the vascular response in the periradicular periodontal ligament, causing severe pain. The tooth may feel raised in the socket and be acutely sensitive to touch. At an early stage no obvious periradicular tenderness to palpation is present (but may develop with time – **1.124**), and no periradicular change is demonstrable on radiographic images (**1.125**). Lessening of pain is accompanied by appearance of a periradicular area. Inflammation of the periodontal ligament may also be caused by trauma, either chronic as in bruxism or acute as in an impact injury.

Chronic periradicular inflammation

The histology of this lesion (the 'granuloma') has already been described in detail (see 'Cells in the periradicular region'). It is clinically asymptomatic and presents as a periradicular radiolucency (**1.126**). Treatment is associated with the risk of an acute flare-up, thought to be because it causes a sudden change from a predominantly anaerobic micobial flora to an aerobic one.

Chronic suppurative periradicular inflammation

In some cases the conflict between microorganisms and PMNLs causes the death of both. The accumulation of dead cells and consequent release of lysosomal enzymes produces pus, which is usually conveyed to the nearest body surface by a sinus tract which becomes lined by epithelium. The opening of a draining sinus tract is sometimes raised, forming a 'gumboil' (**1.127**). The patient may complain of a bad taste in the mouth but

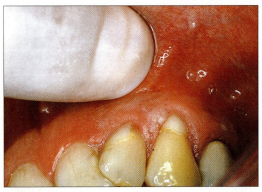

1.124 Tenderness to palpation over maxillary left lateral incisor and canine

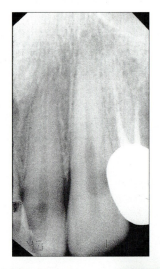

1.125 Definite evidence of radiographic periapical change is lacking

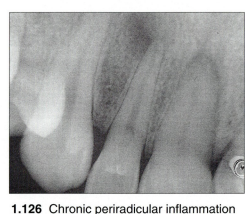

1.126 Chronic periradicular inflammation

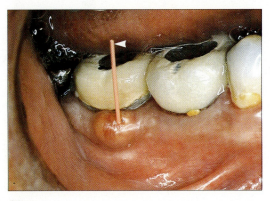

1.127 Chronic suppurative periradicular inflammation (gutta percha point in sinus)

1.128 Radiographic view of tooth in **1.127**

rarely of pain; there may be mild discomfort on palpation of the area. Periapical radiolucency (**1.128**) is obvious. It is possible to place a gutta-percha point in the sinus to locate its source.

Acute periradicular abscess/cellulitis

This is caused by an influx of bacteria into the periradicular area that overwhelm the defences (**1.118, 1.120**) and may arise from any of the categories described so far. In response, large numbers of PMNLs migrate to the lesion, and the rapid death of large numbers of cells and release of lysosomal enzymes causes an accumulation of pus. The abscess thus formed is a highly acidic environment which causes death of surrounding tissues. Various degrees of swelling and pain are seen (**1.129–1.139**). The position of the swelling depends on the tissue planes (themselves determined by muscle and fascia attachments) through which the pus spreads and accumulates. The tooth may feel elevated in its socket. Bacteria may spread through the tissue planes, causing cellulitis associated with pyrexia, and causing the patient to feel unwell. If it is associated with a maxillary tooth, the swelling may cause the ipsilateral eye to close (**1.139**); cellulitis manifests as a diffuse firm swelling and can lead to life-threatening conditions. If a maxillary tooth is involved cavernous sinus thrombosis may develop; if a mandibular tooth is involved Ludwig's angina may develop. Patients with Ludwig's angina (**1.134, 1.135**), become seriously ill, with marked pyrexia; swallowing, speaking and breathing become difficult. If the glottis becomes involved the patient may die within 12–24 hours. The condition should be identified early and the patient referred urgently for medical attention. Management involves extracting the tooth, draining the abscess and antibiotic therapy.

Periradicular osteomyelitis

This is a very serious progression of a periradicular infection. Local infection diffuses through the medullary spaces, causing bone necrosis. The spread may be limited or extensive. PMNLs fill the medullary spaces and destroy osteoblasts lining the trabeculae, starting the process of bone resorption. The patient's

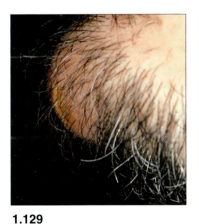
1.129

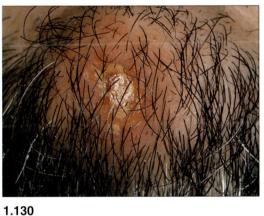
1.130

1.129–1.131 Swelling of chin associated with mandibular anterior teeth

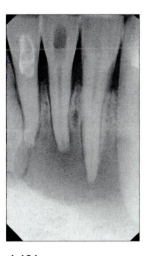
1.131

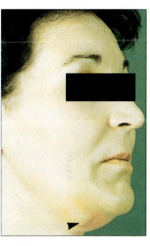
1.132 Localized sub-mandibular swelling (arrowed)

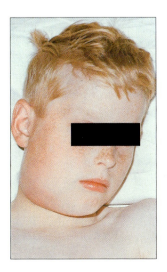
1.133 Spreading submandibular swelling

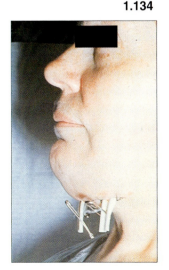
1.134

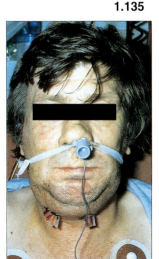
1.135

1.134, 1.135 Treatment of Ludwig's angina

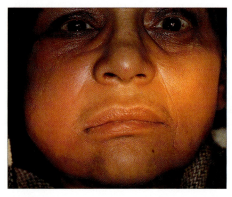
1.136

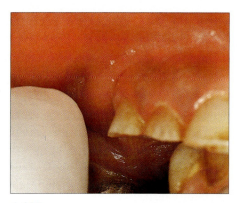
1.137

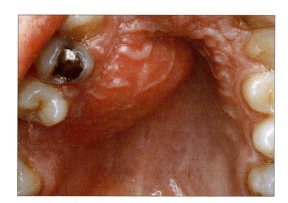
1.138 Palatal swelling associated with maxillary lateral incisor

1.136, 1.137 Right facial and infraorbital swelling associated with maxillary canine

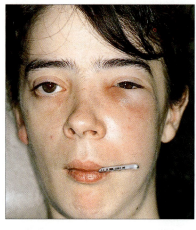
1.139 Closure of eye associated with infection thought to arise from maxillary canine

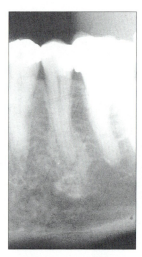
1.140 Periradicular condensing osteitis associated with 5̄

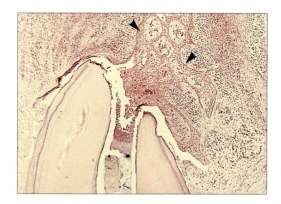
1.141 Proliferation of epithelial tissue adjacent to the apical foramen

temperature is elevated, lymph nodes are swollen and pain is severe. The teeth may be loosened but there may be no obvious swelling in the early stage.

Untreated acute osteomyelitis may progress to a chronic stage, which is less symptomatic but just as serious and merits prompt treatment.

Periradicular osteosclerosis (condensing osteitis)

Information is scarce about this uncommon lesion: it is thought to be a response to low-grade mild irritation. Density of the bone may increase and mild chronic inflammation may occur in the marrow spaces. The radio-opaque periradicular lesion (**1.140**) is asymptomatic. If it is associated with an infected pulp, it may be resolved by root canal therapy.

Granulomas, epithelial proliferation and cysts

Epithelial rests of Malassez may be stimulated by inflammation to proliferate. The pattern of proliferation is variable: they may form strands, arcades and rings at the junction of the unin-

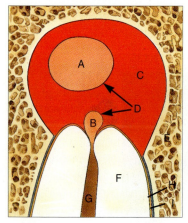
1.142 Bay and true cysts: A = true cyst; B = bay cyst; C = granuloma; D = epithelium; E = alveolar bone; F = dentine; G = root canal; H = cementum; I = periodontal ligament

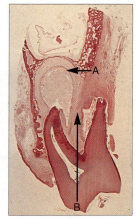
1.143 Histological section showing a bay cyst: A = bay cyst; B = granuloma

flamed connective tissue with the granulation tissue. Proliferation may also occur within the body of the granuloma, where they help to plug the apical foramen and limit egress of bacteria and toxins (**1.141**). In some instances these epithelial plugs bulge into the periradicular lesion, forming a sac connected to the root and continuous with the root canal, termed a 'Bay cyst' (**1.142, 1.143**). In these cases, microorganisms from the root canal have direct access to the 'cyst' cavity and may invade it (**1.144**).

A true cyst has been defined as a pathological, epithelium-lined cavity usually containing fluid or semisolid material. A true cyst does not communicate with the root canal or any other opening (**1.145**). The exact mechanism of cyst formation in association with the apex of a root is not clear; the epithelium may surround an abscess or granuloma, cutting off the tissues within from their nutrient source and causing their degeneration; alternatively, dividing epithelial cells may grow until the central cells are starved of nutrients and degenerate. The method of cyst enlargement is

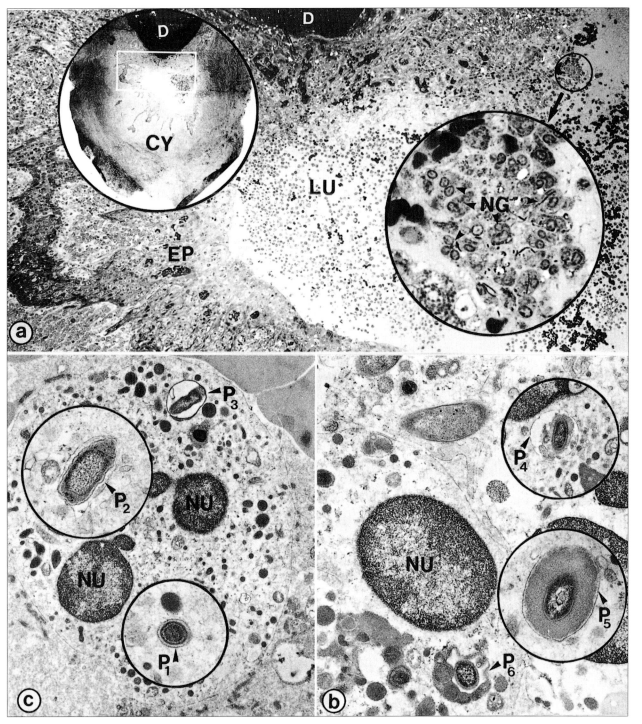

1.144 Bacteria in a radicular cyst. Note the distinct epithelial lining (EP) of the cyst lumen (LU) and a cluster of neutrophils (NG) showing phagocytosed bacteria. The upper inset in **a** shows an overview of the well encapsulated cyst (CY). The electron micrographs in **b** and **c** show the several types of membrane-delimited phagosomes (P_1 to P_6) containing bacteria. Note the close adherence of bacteria and the phagosome membrane in P_1 and P_2, although a clear space is visible between them in P_3. An electron-dense coating of varying thickness may be distinguished on the bacterial surface in P_4 and P_5. Note the bacterium in P_6 is devoid of such a coating but the phagosome contains several membrane-delimited granule-like structures. D = dentine; NU = nucleus. Original magnification: **a** × 100 (left inset × 10, right inset × 850); **b** × 12 800 (upper inset × 8900, lower inset × 17 500); **c** (lower inset) × 8900, (upper inset) × 17 500 (courtesy of Dr Ramachandran Nair)

also speculative: theories involve selective absorption of fluids and an active biochemical interaction between cyst wall and adjacent tissues. Whatever the explanation, it is clear that cysts tend to grow. The cyst is an independent pathological entity within another pathological entity, the granuloma (**1.145**), and the relative proportions of granulomatous and cystic tissue will vary.

Prevalence

The relative prevalence of cysts and granulomas in periradicular lesions associated with necrotic pulps, and the merits of surgical versus non-surgical treatment, are much debated because it is difficult clinically to differentiate a true cyst from a granuloma before beginning therapy. Large circumscribed radiographic lesions with a sclerotic border were once considered likely to be cysts, but this has not been proved.

It is not possible to diagnose a cyst by radiographic techniques alone, unless it is extremely large (**1.146**). Two studies have shown the prevalence of radicular cysts in biopsied periradicular tissues[5] to be about 50% and these workers inferred that, because the success rate of conventional root canal therapy is 85–90%, most cysts will heal by non-surgical therapy alone. However, other studies have demonstrated much lower prevalences (some as low as 7%[7]), partly because the samples studied varied, but mostly because of the criteria used to make the diagnosis: in excised biopsy specimens absence of intact epithelial lining may be attributed to surgical breakage, but bay cysts may give a similar appearance and could be misdiagnosed. The prevalence of true cysts is not known.

Treatment

There is no consensus on treatment. A bay cyst will heal once microbial contamination of the root canal system is eliminated, but successful treatment of a true cyst depends on eliminating the factors that promote its pathogenesis and sustain its growth. A granulomatous lesion would respond to removal of irritants from the canal, but a cyst (being an independent lesion) may not. Successful treatment of a cyst has been thought to require its

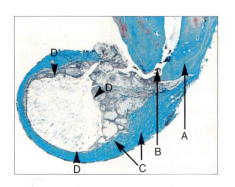

1.145 Histological section of true cyst: A = root apex; B = root canal; C = granuloma; D = cyst

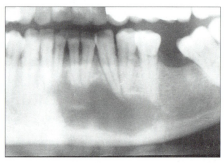

1.146 Large peri-radicular cyst associated with mandibular incisors

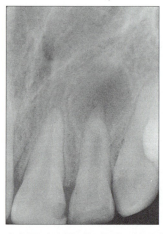

1.147, 1.148 Periapical healing by cleaning alone

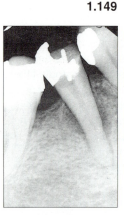
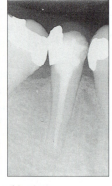

1.149, 1.150 Healing of lesions associated with lateral canals

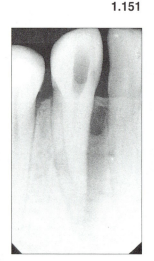
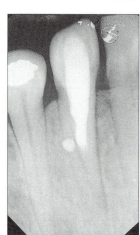

1.151, 1.152 Periradicular healing despite inability to negotiate full length of canals

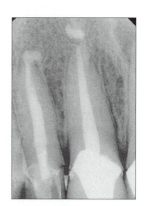

1.153 Normal healing following extrusion of filling material

enucleation, its deflation by puncture or induction of acute inflammation in the vicinity. Enucleation has been reliably tested without significant recurrence but the effectiveness of the decompression method is debatable: healing is slow, unpredictable and allows no opportunity for adequate biopsy. The third method is unpredictable and is not recommended. However, the preferred therapeutic regimen in the first instance for all periapical lesions associated with compromised pulps, in view of the inability to differentiate clinically between a granuloma and a cyst and its high success rate, is conventional non-surgical treatment. If, at follow up, adequate root canal treatment has not resolved the problem, then a surgical approach should be considered.

Treatment of periradicular lesions

Resolution is dependent on separating the invading organisms from the defence reactions. The healing process may be conceptualized using the zones of Fish. Removing the microorganisms and their products eliminates the zones of infection and contamination, allowing macrophages from the zone of irritation to move in and remove the dead cells and debris. This process also makes way for ingress of osteoblasts and fibroblasts from the outermost and active zone of stimulation, new ingrowing blood vessels and nerve fibres, which proliferate into the zone of irritation. In this way healing gradually progresses from the boundary of the lesion inwards until a normal periodontal ligament is established. Ideally, healing should result in formation of cementum over the apical foramen, isolating the root canal system from the periradicular tissues (**1.31**), but this is not always possible. Incomplete removal of the infection will reduce, but not eliminate, the inflammatory area. Healing may be modified and delayed by the method of treatment used, of which there are three in general use. These are described below.

Chemomechanical debridement

This is the most widely used, and biologically the most acceptable, method. It attempts to remove the cause from the root canal system by combining mechanical debridement (use of files) with use of acceptable antibacterial chemicals such as sodium hypochlorite – the case shown in **1.147** and **1.148** has been resolved by simple cleaning of the canal. Sterility in the canal system is not important, and is almost impossible with current techniques; fortunately, disturbing the microflora by instrumentation helps to kill enough of it to alter the pathogenicity of the flora and allow periradicular healing. Cleaning the lateral canals associated with radicular radiolucencies is impossible and, fortunately, usually is unnecessary; adequate cleaning of the main canal should encourage healing (**1.149**, **1.150**). Figures **1.151** and **1.152** show an extreme example of a mandibular canine with two canals that could not be conventionally instrumented to its full length, yet complete periradicular healing was achieved. Two explanations may be advanced for this. The first is that the coronal cleaning rendered the apical flora non-pathogenic. In this scenario, some microbial contamination would remain apical to the root filling and would have the potential to regrow, especially if the coronal seal broke down. The second explanation is that the pulp tissue apical to the root filling may be vital, the lateral radiolucency being explained by coronal necrosis and lateral canals, whereas the apical radiolucency could have been due to inflammatory mediators (as in **1.75**, **1.76**). The removal of the coronal infection resolved the inflammation (however, the apical tissue may potentially become necrotic in the future). In either scenario, the long-term endodontic prognosis for the tooth is uncertain.

Factors affecting healing

Factors that may modify healing include instrumentation through the apical foramen and extrusion of material (such as organic tissue, microorganisms, dentine chips, any chemical irrigant or medicament used) from the root canal. Over-instrumentation through the apical foramen may cause a transient acute inflammation, as may extrusion of uninfected dentine chips: if these are infected, the transient acute inflammation (accompanied by acute symptoms) may develop into chronic inflammation. The effect of extrusion of chemicals is usually short lived, but the impingement of an irritant other than the cause of the chronic periradicular response may cause an acute flare-up, involving pain and swelling. This is thought to be a manifestation of the immunological phenomenon known as the *altered adaptation syndrome*.

The final stage in treatment consists of obturating the root canal system with a material which should be as inert as possible. Extrusion of obturating material may cause transient acute symptoms followed by normal healing (**1.153**), delayed healing (**1.154**, **1.155**) or a foreign body response (see Chapter 13), depending on its toxicity and resistance to disintegration. These

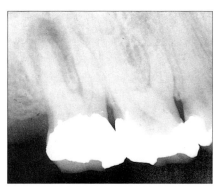

1.154

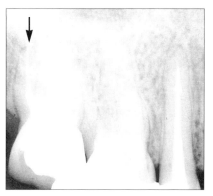

1.155

1.154, 1.155 Delayed healing caused by extruded filling material from the distobuccal canal of a maxillary second molar (arrowed)

may manifest clinically as discomfort and persistence of the periradicular lesion.

Periradicular surgery and retrograde seal

In some cases the infection is inaccessible in dentinal tubules (**1.156–1.159**), apical accessory canals (**1.160, 1.161**)) or is established extraradicularly (**1.121**) and chemomechanical treatment of the root canal alone is inadequate to resolve the lesion. These cases may require an additional surgical approach to the periapex. Healing is likely to be much more complicated in such cases: initial healing following removal of some of the primary infection from the canal, which may be seen as a reduction in the size of the periapical lesion, would be frustrated by persistent residual infection; the surgical procedure would then inflict additional trauma to the site and change the histological picture completely.

The procedure should remove the cause of infection, leaving the complicated wound to heal by organization of a blood clot. The first step in this process is formation of an epithelial seal which matures with nutrient support from developing underlying connective tissue. Reattachment of the mucoperiosteal flap may be compromised by the presence of periodontal disease.

Further connective tissue healing consists of removal and organization of the clot into periosteum, alveolar bone, cementum and periodontal ligament. The apical root resection creates a surface of exposed dentine with a root canal outline which may be large and filled with a material of variable toxicity. The exposed dentinal surface becomes covered with cementum but the root canal is usually covered with fibrous tissue. Sometimes, healing occurs by fibrous repair (**1.162**), or if the exposed dentinal tubules are contaminated by bacteria, then healing may be compromised. Sometimes normal bony healing occurs around the periapex but the cortical plates of bone do not reform (**1.163**) (this may show as a radiolucency; see **1.164**).

Some operators use a retrograde surgical approach without first carrying out conventional root canal treatment. The success of this approach relies on removing some of the infection with the resected root and curetted tissue and (most importantly) on the seal provided by the retrograde filling. Although this technique is occasionally successful (**1.165, 1.166**), failure to remove the causative agents from the canal eventually leads to relapse (**1.167–1.170**). None of the restorative materials currently available provides an absolute seal, and the probability of failure remains high. **1.171, 1.172** show the root end of a tooth with retrograde root filling but no filling in the canal. Bacterial plaque has developed in the inter-

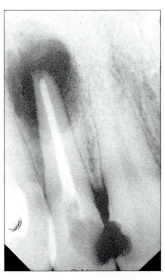

1.156 Adequate root filling demonstrated on radiograph

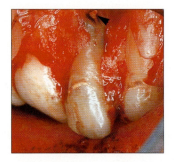

1.157 Periapical surgery and root resection of the tooth shown in **1.156** shows stained root dentine (arrowed)

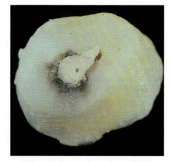

1.158 Resected root end showing stained/infected dentine

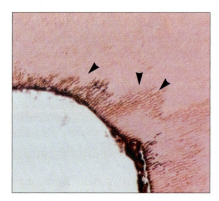

1.159 Histological view of the root end shown in **1.158**, showing infected dentinal tubules

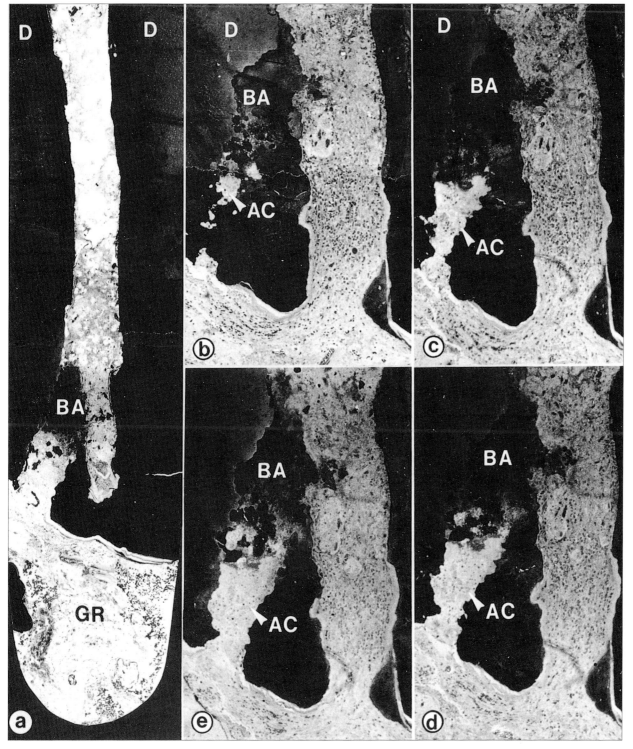

1.160 Axial sections through the surgically removed apical portion of the root with a therapy-resistant periapical lesion (GR). Note the cluster of bacteria visible in the root canal (BA). Parts **b–e** show serial semithin sections taken at varying distances from the section plane of **a** to reveal the emerging (**b**) and gradually widening (**c–e**) profiles of an accessory root canal (AC). Note that the accessory canal is clogged with bacteria (BA). Original magnification: **a** × 52; **b–e** × 62 (courtesy of Dr Ramachandran Nair)

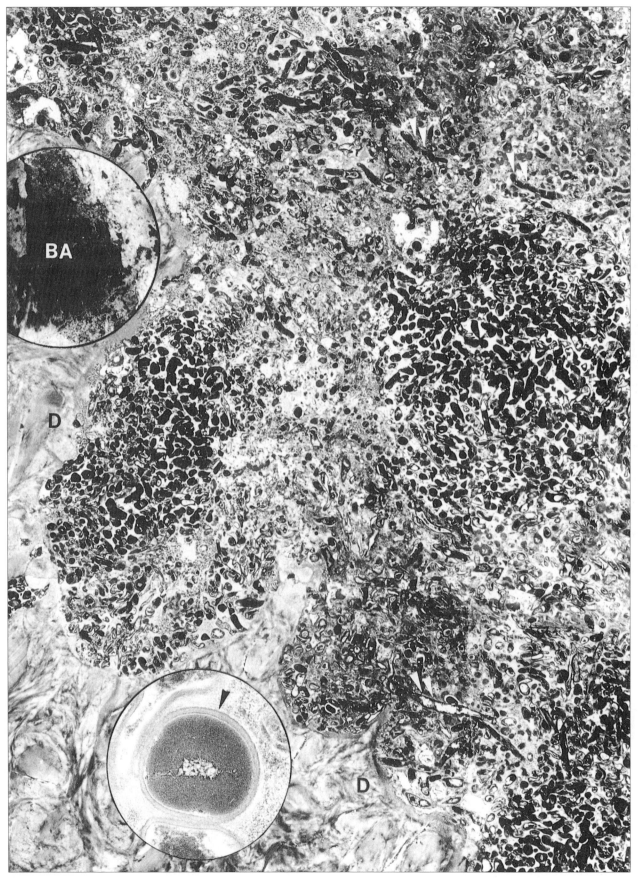

1.161 Transmission electron microscopic view of the bacterial mass (BA, upper inset) illustrated in **1.160a**. Morphologically the bacterial population appears to be composed only of Gram-positive, filamentous organisms (arrowhead). Note the distinct Gram-positive wall in the lower inset. The upper inset is a magnification of the bacterial cluster (BA) in **1.160a**. Original magnification: × 3400; upper inset × 132; lower inset × 21 300 (courtesy of Dr Ramachandran Nair)

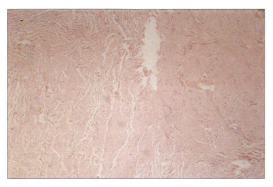
1.162 Fibrous healing (histological view)

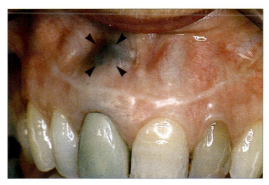
1.163 Bony defect following surgery

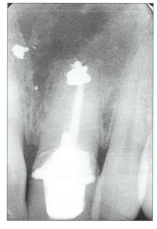
1.164 The bony defect in **1.163** appears as a radiolucency

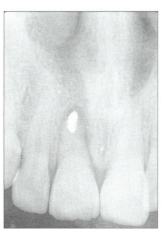
1.165

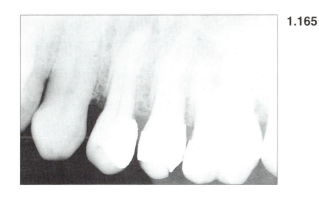
1.166

1.165, 1.166 Retrograde treatment without conventional root canal therapy is only occasionally successful

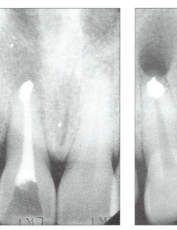
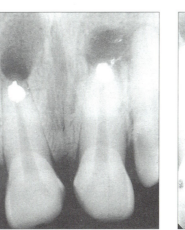
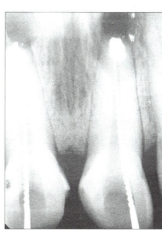

1.167 1.168 1.169 1.170

1.167–1.170 Retrograde treatment will fail if not preceded by root canal therapy

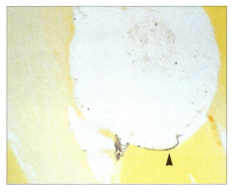
1.171 Low-power view of a plaque of bacteria between dentine and retrograde filling (courtesy of Dr T. Pitt Ford)

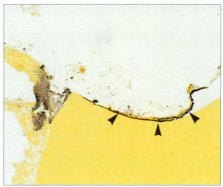
1.172 High-power view of plaque in **1.171**

face between the dentine and the glass ionomer retrograde filling, which has dissolved during histological processing. Conventional root canal treatment may be adequate to achieve healing (**1.173, 1.174**) but occasionally a reservoir of microorganisms may develop in the junction between retrograde filling and root and may sustain the periapical lesion. If this happens further periapical surgery may be necessary.

Mummification

Some operators feel that the anatomy of the root canal system is so complex that adequate biomechanical debridement is impossible, and advocate using chemical agents to destroy and fix the organic pulp tissue as well as the bacteria. A variety of materials, all containing formaldehyde as the fixative agent, have been recommended. Used with some degree of mechanical canal preparation, and if the material is confined within the root canal system, the technique may be successful but it is at best unpredictable. There is no evidence on the ability of the chemical to overcome bacterial contamination. Furthermore, fixing the pulp tissue alters it antigenically, making it able to stimulate an immune response: unfixed necrotic tissue cannot.

Evidence suggests that extrusion of the material, albeit inadvertently, may have serious consequences. The toxicity of the material can cause necrosis and alter nerve function, causing severe pain, paraesthesia or anaesthesia, especially if the material is extruded into the inferior dental canal (**1.175**). These symptoms also occur if other, less toxic, materials are extruded into the nerve canal; most will resolve spontaneously, but recovery is unlikely with formaldehyde-containing materials.

Assessing success of conventional root canal treatment

Clinical judgement of the outcome of treatment is based on signs of infection and inflammation (pain, tenderness to percussion of the tooth, tenderness to palpation of the related soft tissues), absence of swelling and sinus, radiographic demonstration of healing and a normal periodontal ligament space.

The absence of signs and symptoms of periapical disease with a persistent periapical radiolucency may indicate healing by fibrosis or persistent chronic inflammation. Only time and acute exacerbation will identify the latter; the former should remain asymptomatic.

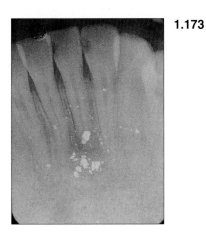
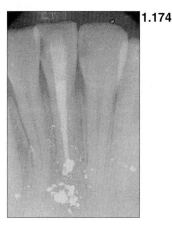
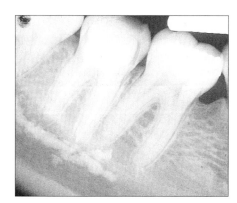

1.175 Extrusion of filling material into the inferior dental canal

1.173, 1.174 Healing following root canal treatment in a tooth previously treated by periapical surgery and retrograde filling

2 Patient assessment

At the first appointment the dentist must assess both the patient and the dental problem before commencing treatment because many factors affect the management of the patient and the method of treatment chosen. Accurate, clear records must be kept of all treatment undertaken and all relevant information taken from the patient. What is written on a patient's treatment card will be used as evidence in any legal disputes.

The operator will be examining the patient for a variety of disorders in an endodontic assessment. In many cases the patient seeks treatment because of pain, but many conditions are discovered only by clinical examination. Common disorders which may be revealed during an endodontic assessment include:

- inflamed pulp;
- concussed pulp;
- necrotic pulp;
- acute periapical inflammation;
- acute periapical abscess;
- chronic periapical inflammation;
- resorption of the tooth
    internal;
    external;
- fractured tooth
    crown (vital/non-vital pulp);
    root (vital/non-vital pulp);
    horizontal fracture;
    vertical fracture;
- periodontal disease;
- traumatic occlusion;
- iatrogenic problems (operator induced);
- local non-dental pathology
    soft tissues;
    hard tissues;
- systemic disease;
- atypical facial pain.

Health history

A medical history is taken to find whether the patient has any medical condition or is taking medication that could affect the treatment. The most convenient way of recording such information is to use a checklist that is kept in the patient's file, such as that shown in **Table 2.1**.

No medical conditions specifically contraindicate endodontic treatment, although patients with a history of infective endocarditis or prosthetic heart valves should be regarded as a special risk group and referred for specialist treatment. Rheumatic fever (particularly when there has been heart damage), insulin-controlled diabetes, anticoagulant therapy and sexually transmitted diseases may affect treatment, and if the practitioner is in any doubt, he or she should consult the patient's medical adviser before commencing treatment. Patients with cardiac abnormalities are usually administered prophylactic antibiotics to prevent infective endocarditis (see **Table 2.2**). The incidence of infective endocarditis in patients with cardiac abnormalities is increased with diabetes mellitus, immunosuppression, alcohol dependence, haemodialysis and intravenous drug abuse.

Any patient susceptible to infective endocarditis should use an oral antiseptic (chlorhexidine gel (1%) to the dry gingival margin, or a chlorhexidine mouthwash (0.2%)) 5 min before undergoing dental procedures. This should reduce the severity of any bacteraemia and may be used to supplement the antibiotic prophylaxis.

The initial consultation is most effectively carried out beside a desk with both patient and operator seated; patients find this less stressful than immediately being asked to sit in a dental chair (**2.1**).

The patient's attitudes to dental treatment must be assessed during the first appointment, and the dentist should consider the following questions: Has the patient received much previous dental treatment? Is the patient particularly nervous? Will he or she be able to tolerate endodontics? Should treatment be undertaken in short sessions? Is one particular time of day more suitable than others? Is cost of treatment important?

Table 2.1 Checklist for recording patient information

Rheumatic fever	Yes/no
Hypertension or cardiac disease	Yes/no
Bleeding disorders	Yes/no
Allergies	Yes/no
Hepatitis	Yes/no
Pregnant	Yes/no
Taking any drugs	Yes/no
Under treatment by GP or hospital	Yes/no
Serious illness in last 3 years	Yes/no
Upper respiratory tract infections	Yes/no

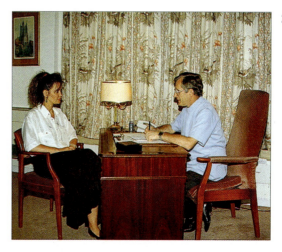

2.1 Consultation

Chief complaint

Listen carefully to the patient's explanation of his/her condition and use the patient's own words to record it. Obtain a detailed description of any pain: its nature (sharp, dull, throbbing, radiating); any initiating factors; duration; frequency; association with time of day; is relief obtained with analgesics?

Clinical examination

Extraoral

Extraoral examination is carried out for facial swelling, asymmetry and the presence of lymph nodes. Facial swelling is best viewed from above the patient (**2.2**, **2.3**).

Intraoral

The intraoral soft tissues, oral hygiene (**2.4**), general periodontal condition (**2.5**), incidence of caries (**2.6**), missing or unopposed

Table 2.2 Prophylactic antibiotic regimens

Procedures under local anaesthesia

Patients not allergic to penicillin who have not been prescribed penicillin more than once in the previous 4 weeks
Amoxycillin
    Adults: 3 g single oral dose under supervision 1 hour before procedure
    Children under 10 years: half adult dose
    Children under 5 years: quarter adult dose

Patients allergic to penicillin or who have had penicillin more than once in the previous 4 weeks
Clindamycin
    Adults: 600 mg single oral dose under supervision 1 hour before procedure
    Children 5–10 years: half adult dose
    Children under 5 years: quarter adult dose

Procedures under general anaesthesia

Patients not allergic to penicillin who have not been prescribed penicillin more than once in the previous 4 weeks
Amoxycillin
    Adults: 3 g oral dose 4 hours before anaesthesia followed by 3 g by mouth as soon as possible after operation
    Children under 10 years: half adult dose
    Children under 5 years: quarter adult dose

Patients allergic to penicillin or who have had more than one dose of penicillin in the previous 4 weeks
Teicoplanin and gentamicin
    Adults: intravenous teicoplanin 400 mg and gentamicin 120 mg just before induction of anaesthesia or 15 min before the procedure
    Children under 14 years: intravenous teicoplanin 6 mg/kg plus gentamicin 2 mg/kg

Advice on particular regimens is changing constantly: the operator should check with opinion that is current at the time of operation.

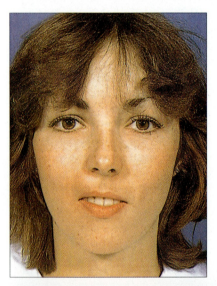

2.2 Any facial swelling should be noted

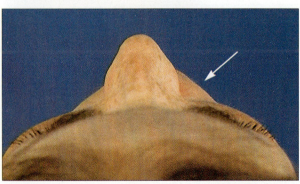

2.3 Facial swelling is most noticeable from above the patient

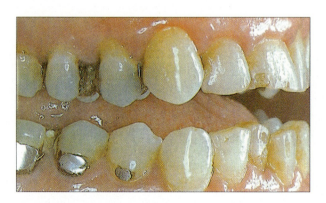

2.4 Poor oral hygiene

teeth (**2.7**), standard and amount of dental treatment (**2.8**), toothwear and faceting (**2.9**) should all be assessed.

Ease of access

An assessment should be made of the ease of access, particularly to the posterior part of the mouth. As a general guide, if a patient's mouth will not open wide enough to allow two fingers to pass between the incisors endodontic treatment of the molars is inadvisable (**2.10**).

Radiographic assessment

This is of the utmost importance. Preoperative periapical radographs should be taken using the paralleling technique (**2.11**). If a patent sinus is present preoperative radiographs may be taken with a size 20 or 25 gutta percha point in place. The point should be inserted into the sinus and gently teased by rolling the tip back

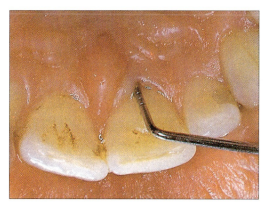

2.5 Periodontal condition

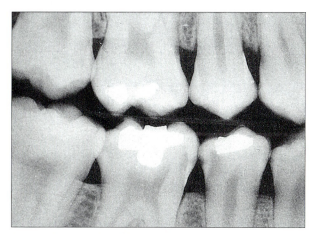

2.6 Incidence of caries

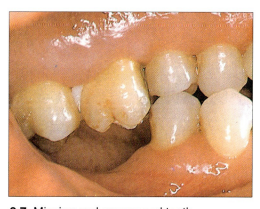

2.7 Missing and unapposed teeth

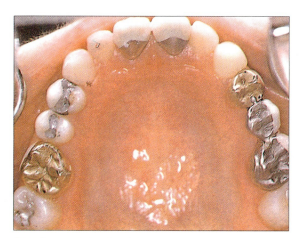

2.8 General dental state

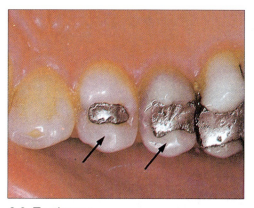

2.9 Toothwear

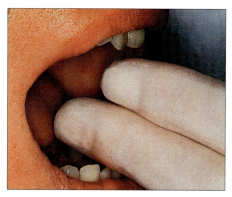

2.10 If it is not possible to insert two fingers between incisors endodontic treatment of the back teeth will be extremely difficult

and forth between the fingers until resistance or discomfort is encountered (**2.12–2.14**).

If endodontic treatment is being considered the following should be assessed on radiographs: shape, curvature and number of roots; presence and morphology of root canals; size of pulp chamber; type and size of coronal restoration; presence of peri-radicular pathology; periodontal bone loss, internal or external resorption; root fracture. If the tooth has been treated previously it should be possible to assess the type of root filling material used and the presence of any procedural errors such as perforation, untreated canals or a fractured instrument. The radiograph will often indicate to the operator the cause of the problem and the probable ease of treatment. Figure **2.15** shows a second molar tooth with external inflammatory resorption, distal caries and a fractured distal root: the tooth should be extracted. Figure **2.16** shows two maxillary premolars, the first of which has a periapical radiolucency and an inadequate paste root filling, the second showing gross caries in the coronal portion of the root canal. The first premolar was root filled (**2.17**) and the second extracted and replaced with bridgework.

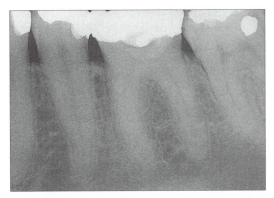

2.11 Radiograph taken using the parallel technique

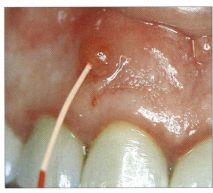

2.12 Gutta percha point in sinus tract

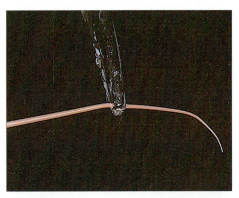

2.13 Depth of penetration of gutta percha point

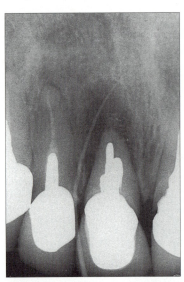

2.14 Gutta percha point visible on radiograph

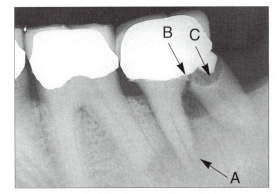

2.15 External inflammatory resorption (A), fracture (B), and distal caries (C)

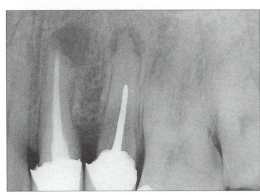

2.16 Inadequate root treatment and gross caries in the second premolar

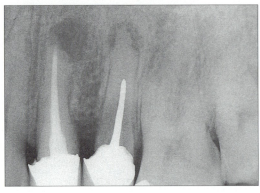

2.17 First premolar root treated; second premolar due for extraction

Clinical tests

Clinical tests are used for routine assessment or to locate and diagnose the source of pulpal pain. Many clinical tests are available but none is wholly reliable. It is not necessary to use all the tests in each case. The correlation between clinical symptoms and pulpal histology is poor; the operator faced with a case of pulpal pain must use his/her experience to decide whether the pulp is irreversibly damaged and has to be removed or whether removing the cause of the irritation will preserve the pulp. Correct diagnosis depends on tests and the operator's experience and acumen. As a guide, before a pulp cavity is accessed two independent indications for treatment should be established.

Palpation

The soft tissues overlying the apices of the teeth are palpated (**2.18**). The patient will report any tender area. Hard and soft swellings will be apparent: if hard, the site and size should be noted; if soft, the swelling should be palpated with two fingers to see if it is fluctuant. One finger is placed at either end of the swelling and pressure applied; if the swelling is fluctuant movement of the fluid beneath the oral mucosa will be apparent.

Percussion

Gentle tapping with a finger (both vertically and laterally) will locate a tender tooth (**2.19**). If ankylosis of a tooth is suspected tapping with a mirror handle in the long axis of the tooth will confirm the diagnosis: an ankylosed tooth has a distinctive solid ring.

Mobility

Mobility of a tooth is assessed by placing a finger on each side and pressing with one finger (**2.20**). The amount of movement is judged in relation to a proximal tooth.

Mobility may be graded as *slight* (mobility 1), which is considered normal, *moderate* (mobility 2), or *extensive* (mobility 3) in a lateral or mesiodistal direction, combined with vertical displacement in the alveolus.

Biting

Diagnosis of incompletely fractured teeth is one of the most difficult diagnoses in endodontics. A fracture is seldom visible in its early stages and may lie beneath a restoration. A patient presenting with pain related to chewing but with no evidence of periradicular inflammation may be suspected of having a fracture. Biting on a wooden stick or rubber wheel may elicit pain, usually on release of biting pressure (**2.21**).

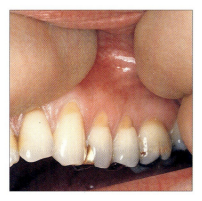

2.18 Palpation

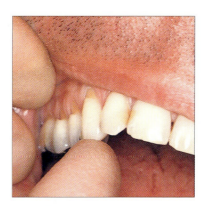

2.19 Percussion

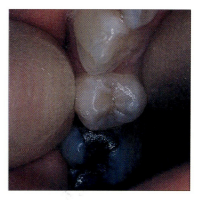

2.20 Mobility

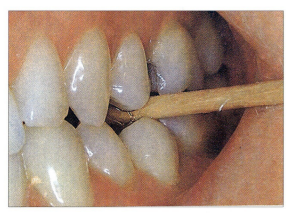

2.21 Wood stick test for fracture

Fibreoptic light

Transmission of a powerful light through teeth will show interproximal caries and (of particular interest in endodontics) a fracture. Extraneous light is reduced, the fibreoptic light placed next to the neck of the tooth and moved along its surface. The light will not pass across the fracture line, so the part of the tooth nearest to the light is bright and that beyond the fracture remains dark: **2.22** and **2.23** show this effect; the fracture is seen as a definite vertical line in **2.23**. Figure **2.24** shows a mandibular first molar with a coronal restoration removed – a fracture line is visible in the distal wall.

Pulp testing

This method is used only to decide whether the pulp is responsive; it tests the ability of the nerves within the pulp to conduct impulses but gives no indication of the state of the blood supply. Pulp testing neither quantifies disease nor measures health, and should not be used to judge the degree of pulpal disease. Pulp tests should be used only to assess vitality of the pulp.

Electric pulp tester

The electric pulp tester (EPT) uses gradations of electric current (alternating or direct) to excite a response from the nervous tissue within the pulp. Most modern pulp testers are monopolar.

An example of a pulp tester, the Analytic Technology pulp tester, is shown (**2.25**). The output stimulus is produced in bursts of ten high-frequency pulses of negative polarity. The power source is four 1.5 V AA batteries. The EPT is turned on automatically when the probe tip touches the tooth and turns off 15 sec after tooth contact is broken. The digital display reads from 0 to 80 and the only control possible is the rate of increase/decrease of the electrical stimulus.

Pulp testing technique

The teeth to be tested should be dried and isolated with cotton wool or rubber dam (**2.26**): note that the rubber dam is applied as small strips placed between the teeth. A conducting medium must be used – the one most readily available is toothpaste. The pulp tester is applied to the middle third of the tooth, avoiding

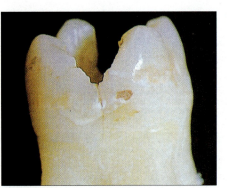
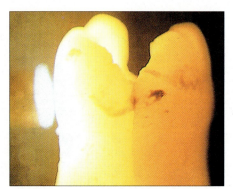
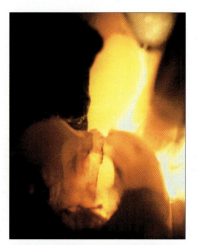

2.22, 2.23 Use of a fibreoptic light renders a fracture clearly visible

2.24 Mandibular molar with distal fracture

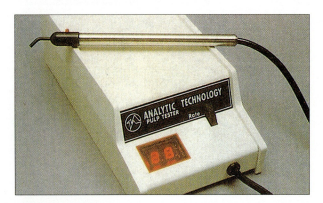
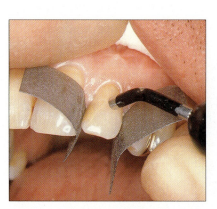

2.25 Pulp tester

2.26 Tooth isolated with rubber dam

contact with the soft tissues, and any restorations. Monopolar pulp testers require the circuit to be completed through the operator's hands, which is not possible if gloves are worn; this is easily overcome by asking the patient to hold the metal handle – as shown in **2.27**. As a general rule electric pulp testers should not be used on patients who have a cardiac pacemaker because of possible electrical interference; however, modern pacemakers are well shielded which will reduce the risk of interference.

Pulp testing of crowned teeth is possible, provided that a small area of dentine or enamel can be contacted without touching the gingival tissue. A special tip for the Analytic Technology EPT (**2.28**) is being used on the patient shown in **2.29**.

Disadvantages

Electric pulp testing has several disadvantages.

1. It gives no indication of the state of the vascular supply, which would give a more reliable measure of the vitality of the pulp.
2. False-positive readings may be obtained owing to stimulation of nerve fibres in the periodontium.
3. Readings taken from posterior teeth may be misleading because some combination of vital and non-vital root canal pulps may be present.

Thermal pulp testing

Thermal pulp testing involves either applying or removing heat from a tooth. Neither test is completely reliable, both producing false-positive and false-negative readings.

Heat

Dry heat

The last 3 mm of the end of a stick of gutta percha or composition is heated in a flame for 2 sec and applied to the suspect tooth (**2.30**). Two precautions are necessary to avoid the patient receiving sudden acute pain: (1) the tooth surface should be lightly coated with petroleum jelly to prevent the composition from sticking and care taken not to overheat the stick as it may stick to the tooth if overheated, despite the application of lubricant (2) local anaesthetic should be kept to hand. Another method is to use the heat generated from a rubber wheel in a standard handpiece.

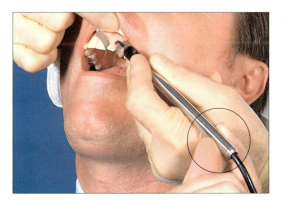

2.27 Patient holding pulp tester

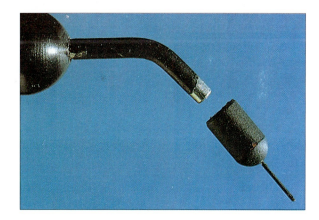

2.28 Pulp tester with removable tip

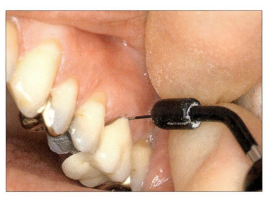

2.29 Pulp testing apical to margin of crown

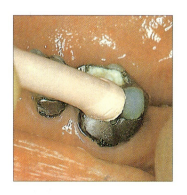

2.30 Hot gutta percha

Hot water

Some patients report pain with hot drinks, but do not react to heated gutta percha: this may be due to the presence of porcelain-bonded crowns or large restorations, which insulate the pulp. Hot water should be sipped and held in the mouth, first over the mandibular quadrant on the affected side and then over the maxillary quadrant if this does not elicit a response. An alternative method is to use a rubber dam to isolate each tooth in turn. If a response is noted, local anaesthetic is applied to the suspect tooth and the heat reapplied. No response means that the tooth with pulpitis has been identified.

Cold

Ice sticks may be made by filling the plastic protective covers for hypodermic needles with water and freezing them (**2.31**). To make them ready for use one end is removed by warming it slightly in the hand (**2.32**, **2.33**). An alternative method of pulp testing with cold is to soak a pledget of cotton wool with ethyl chloride and apply it to the tooth with tweezers. Some operators prefer to use a carbon dioxide probe (**2.34**, **2.35**) because it gives an intense reproducible response, and does not affect the adjacent teeth (which an air blast or ice stick may do).

Local analgesia

When the patient presents in pain or if the pain can be provoked by thermal testing, an infiltration injection of local analgesic may be used to identify the tooth. An intraligamental injection localizes the effect of the analgesic, although the proximal teeth may still be affected. Note that the bevel of the needle in **2.36** points away from the tooth to allow easier penetration into the periodontal ligament.

Caries removal and dressing

The first stage of treatment of a carious tooth is to remove the caries and establish whether pulp and/or tooth may be saved.

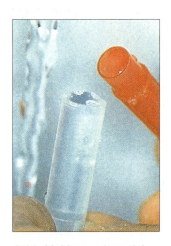

2.31 Making an ice stick

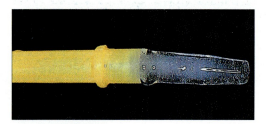

2.32 Ice stick

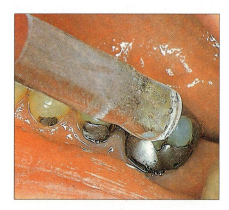

2.33 Applying ice stick

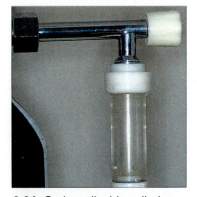

2.34 Carbon dioxide cylinder for pulp testing

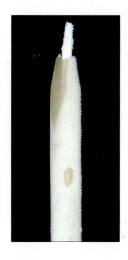

2.35 Carbon dioxide stick

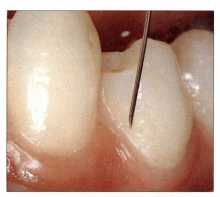

2.36 The bevel of the needle tip should point outwards during intraligamental injection

Cutting a test cavity

As a last resort a test cavity may be cut in a tooth which is believed to be pulpless. In the author's experience this test is not reliable because a positive response may be obtained from a tooth with a necrotic pulp.

Further tests

On occasion it may be necessary to carry out a preliminary procedure before the final treatment plan can be made. For example:

- Check crowns and bridge retainers to see if cementation has failed.
- Attempt to locate a sclerosed root canal.
- Remove a restoration to examine the floor of the cavity for a fracture.
- Attempt to remove a post to see if orthograde root canal treatment may be carried out.
- Fit a diagnostic occlusal splint to eliminate other sources of pain.

Future possibilities

More precise tests are required to assess the state of the pulp. Research has centred on a device that would assess the quantity of blood flow through the pulp, which would give a better indication of pulp vitality than the present method of testing for nerve response. Research is currently being carried out on the laser Doppler effect, pulse oximetry, dual-wave length spectrophotometry and infrared non-contact thermometry.

Diagnosis

Once the patient has been assessed and the clinical examination and tests completed diagnosis should be possible. The clinician should have a simple classification of pulpal disease and its possible sequelae that complements the rudimentary tests available. It must be emphasized that diseases of the pulp and periradicular tissues do not necessarily cause pain.

Normal pulp

This will be asymptomatic and give only a mild, transitory response to stimulation with thermal or electrical tests. Percussion and palpation do not cause pain. Radiographs show a definite pulp chamber and canal, which will be smaller and narrower in the older patient. The width of the periodontal ligament is normal, with no evidence of resorption.

Dentinal pain may be experienced when the dentine is exposed to the oral cavity, with thermal changes or exposure to sweet food or drink. The pulp is not normally affected.

Concussed pulp

The pulp may be concussed following trauma to the tooth and may not respond to thermal or electrical stimulation for a period of weeks or months. The tooth should be checked at regular intervals until the pulp tests return to normal or, if they do not, root canal treatment should be considered.

Reversible pulpitis

Heat or cold will cause a quick sharp pain, which subsides almost immediately once the stimulus is removed. The pain does not radiate and the tooth is otherwise symptomless. The radiograph shows no pathology.

Irreversible pulpitis

The pain encountered in this condition may vary – from none to spontaneous intermittent paroxysms or continuous pain – and may radiate from the maxilla to the mandible or *vice versa*. Pain commonly occurs at night, when it may be worse than during the day because lying down increases the intrapulpal pressure. In the early stages the patient is unable to locate the affected tooth but as pulpal inflammation spreads and toxins pass out through the apical foramen the tooth may become painful to touch. Application of heat or cold will generally start the pain, which gradually increases in intensity then slowly dies away and may last for a few minutes up to several hours. Radiographs will show changes associated with the root apex when pulpitis is well advanced, but occasionally apical rarefaction will occur at an earlier stage with pulpitis. **2.37** shows a mandibular second molar which has fractured. The patient was experiencing episodes of pain particularly at night and the tooth was tender: note the widened periodontal ligament space around the mesial root and a halo of condensing osteitis.

Pulpal necrosis

Necrosis may occur following irreversible pulpitis or as a result of trauma disrupting the blood supply to the pulp. Thermal and electrical pulp testing will produce no response, although in a

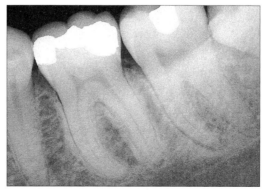

2.37 Fractured mandibular second molar

posterior tooth the pulp tissue in more than one of the canals may be vital, which makes tests inconclusive. In most cases a radiograph will show periradicular changes: in **2.38** a periapical radiolucent area is associated with the distal root of the distal molar. Provided that the pulpal disease has spread to the periradicular tissue palpation and percussion should give a positive response.

Acute periapical inflammation

Acute inflammation may be due to an extension of pulpal disease, trauma, a high restoration or endodontic treatment that has inadvertently been extended beyond the apical foramen. If the inflammation is caused by trauma the pulp may remain vital. The tooth is very tender to touch. Radiographic change will be minimal, but may show a little widening of the periodontal ligament. Figure **2.39** shows the posterior abutment tooth to a bridge which had become decemented and carious (**2.40**); the pulp is still vital (**2.41**). The pulp was extirpated and root canals prepared (**2.42**).

Acute apical abscess

An acute apical abscess implies the presence of purulent exudate around the apex. The tooth is extremely tender to touch and palpation of the overlying gingiva painful. Swelling develops in the later stages and the tooth becomes mobile. Pain usually abates when the swelling appears. In severe cases the patient is febrile. The patient in **2.43** has swelling and pyrexia, which has disappeared a week later (**2.44**). Radiographically the appearance is similar to acute periapical inflammation. A chronic lesion may flare up into an acute apical abscess – in such cases there will be a periradicular rarefaction.

Chronic apical periodontitis

This is a long-standing asymptomatic inflammation around the apex. From time to time the patient may become aware of the tooth. Radiolucency is apparent, although this varies from a

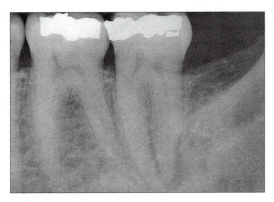

2.38 Distal root has periradicular area

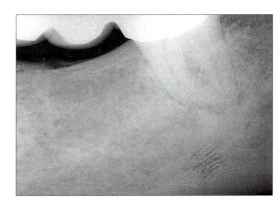

2.39 Bridge decemented from distal abutment tooth

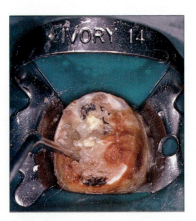

2.40 Gross caries

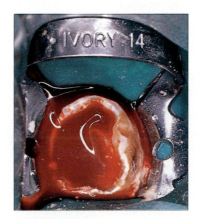

2.41 Carious exposure with hyperaemic pulp

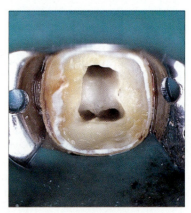

2.42 Pulp extirpated and canals prepared

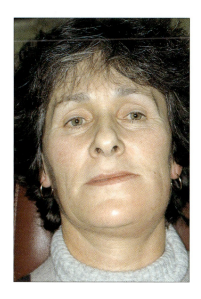

2.43 Patient with swelling and pyrexia

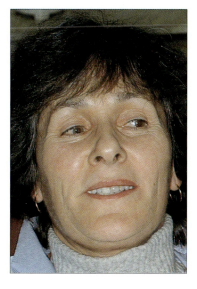

2.44 Patient in **2.43** 1 week later

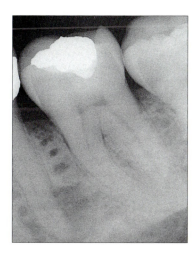

2.45 Periradicular area around distal root of first molar

widened periodontal ligament to a large area (**2.45**). There may be evidence of a sinus tract. The pulp will be non-vital.

Resorption

Internal

Internal resorption occurs as a result of chronic pulpitis. The tooth is usually symptomless. Diagnosis is made by the appearance of a smooth widening of the pulp on the radiograph. Root canal treatment should be carried out without delay (see Chapter 13).

External

External resorption may present in several forms (Chapter 15). It is important to identify the type of resorption so that appropriate treatment may be given. The main difficulty is in differentiating between internal and external resorption. Radiographs are invaluable in the diagnosis.

Fractured teeth

The obvious cause of tooth fracture is trauma but both restored and unrestored teeth with no history of trauma may fracture. Any restoration which acts as a wedge in the tooth, for example a cast inlay or a mesio-occlusal-distal amalgam, may cause the tooth to fracture. The incidence of tooth fracture is highest in the second mandibular molar (**2.37**, **2.38**), usually in the sagittal plane. Fractures can be difficult to diagnose and because both the pulp and the periodontium may be affected the range of symptoms is wide.

Fractured crown with vital pulp

This often presents as a non-localized pain associated with eating. There may be a history of trauma but more often the patient cannot remember any traumatic incident. The severity of the symptoms usually depends on the degree of bacterial contamination of the pulp. The patient may or may not be aware of pain during chewing. The fracture is extremely difficult to locate, particularly if it runs obliquely beneath the cusp of a molar. If not treated the pulp will become necrotic.

Fractured crown with non-vital pulp

This may be asymptomatic or may cause mild intermittent pain on chewing.

Fractured crown and root with vital pulp

Symptoms are similar to the crown-only fracture, except that the pain is more likely to occur during chewing – typically on release of the food bolus.

Fractured crown and root with a non-vital pulp

The fracture is usually long-standing and is easier to locate than in the case of vital pulp for two reasons: (1) the fracture line will have become stained and will show up with fibreoptic light; (2) the pain will be due mainly to stretching of the periodontal ligament as the fractured parts move during mastication. If the fracture has started from the apex of the root and the tooth has been root filled the fracture was probably caused by excessive use of force during treatment.

Atypical facial pain

This condition refers to apparent dental pain which has no organic cause. The patients are predominantly female and the range of symptoms diverse. The condition is difficult to diagnose and often the patient has been suffering pain for a considerable time. A thorough investigation must be carried out and any pathology treated. If symptoms persist the patient should be referred for specialist treatment. An example of atypical facial pain is given in **2.46**: a 43-year-old woman complained of pain in a maxillary right central tooth that had been root treated. The root treatment was redone (**2.47**) but her pain persisted. The patient was referred to a consultant who specialized in atypical facial pain and was successfully treated with antidepressants.

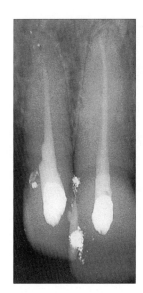

2.46 Atypical facial pain

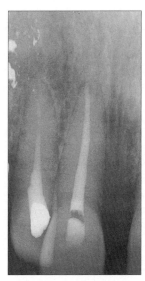

2.47 Root retreatment of central incisor

3 Radiography

Accurate dental radiographs are an essential requirement in the practice of endodontics. High-quality periapical radiographs improve initial diagnosis and assist greatly in success of treatment. Operators should endeavour to achieve high technical standards in order to minimize the number of film exposures needed to complete a clinical procedure. It is important to have a clear understanding of the materials, equipment, techniques and safety standards governing this discipline.

Radiographic equipment

The X-ray machine

The machine used (**3.1**) should conform with the requirements of the Ionising Radiations Regulations 1985. Its current and voltage influence the quantity and penetrating power, respectively, of the X-rays produced. The tube voltage should be no lower than 50 kV, and preferably about 70 kV for intraoral radiography.

The tube head

This houses the X-ray tube and transformer, and allows only the X-rays that form the beam (**3.2**) to pass through. The tube produces a divergent beam which is collimated by a diaphragm with a circular aperture to provide a parallel beam (**3.3**). The beam diameter should not exceed 60 mm in the area being radiographed. The filtration of the beam should be equivalent to no less than 1.5 mm aluminium for voltages up to and including 70 kV.

Density and contrast

Density is the degree of blackness of a film, *contrast* is the difference in the degrees of blackness between adjacent areas. The higher the voltage, the more shades of grey will be recorded (this is more likely to indicate early pathological changes in bone). The lower voltages show mainly black and white, with few shades of grey. A 65–70 kV machine suits most dental purposes.

The spacer cone

Field-defining spacer cones (**3.4**) are available in various lengths and should ensure a distance between focal spot and skin of no

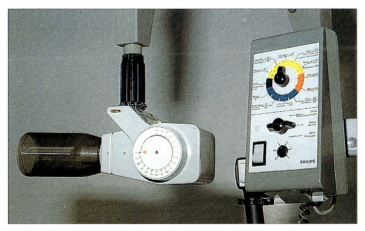

3.1 X-ray machine

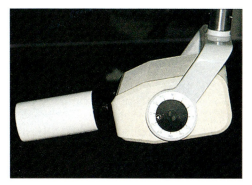

3.2 Tube head

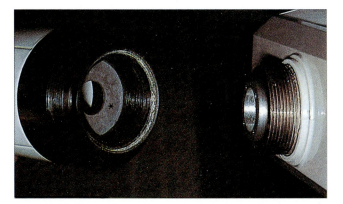

3.3 Collimator

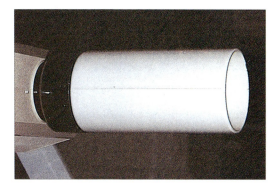

3.4 Spacer cone

less than 200 mm for equipment operating above 60 kV. The focal spot should be marked on the tube head. Modern machines are designed with the tube at the rear of the tube head to comply with the focal film distance (ffd) recommendations and allow the use of a 20- or 30-cm (8- or 12-inch) cone.

Warning lights

These lights must indicate 'mains-on' and exposure.

Films

The fastest films available, consistent with satisfactory diagnostic results, should be used: periapical D and E speed direct-action films are most often used in endodontics. Film speed depends on the number and size of the silver halide crystals in the emulsion; faster films have larger crystals but poorer image quality. Films suitable for children include DF-54 (34 × 22 mm), DF-57 and DF-58 (40 × 30 mm) for adults. The DF-54 films may also be used for anterior teeth or adults with small mouths.

Film holders

Film holders are beam-aiming devices, designed to hold the film at right angles to the X-ray beam to reduce distortion and produce a more exact image (**3.5**). Using these devices means that patients do not need to support the film with their fingers and the possibility of 'cone cutting' is reduced. Their use improves the diagnostic quality and allows the angle of radiographs to be similarly reproduced during recall assessment.

Simple beam-aiming film holders include:

- modified Spencer Wells;
- the Snap-a-Ray System (designed originally for the bisecting angle technique); and
- the Eggin holder.

More sophisticated holders include:

- Rinn XCP with anterior and posterior localizing rings (**3.6**);
- Dunvale Snapex System, a modification of the Snap-a-Ray System increasing the scope for use in general dentistry;
- the Masel precision paralleling instrument (**3.7**).

The Rinn EndoRay allows parallel radiographs to be taken in the presence of endodontic hand instruments. It is in two parts, the body (or film holder), and the handle (**3.8**). The film holder is placed over the tooth and the patient asked to bite lightly on it. The handle is then attached to the body to aid the operator in centring the film in the beam. More recent versions include a centring ring.

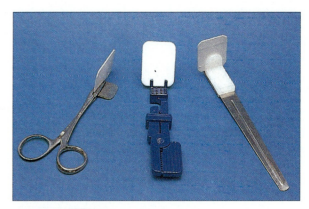

3.5 Film holders

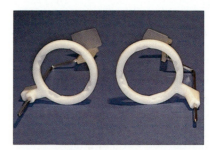

3.6 Rinn film holders

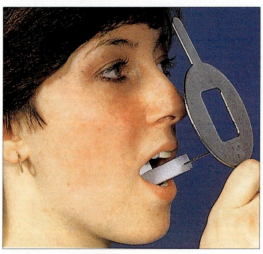

3.7 Masel precision paralleling instrument

3.8 The Rinn Endoray

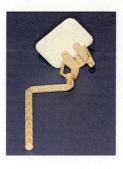

Processing equipment

A quick method of chairside film processing has always been desirable in endodontic radiography. In attempting to achieve a rapid result strict attention should be paid to producing consistently high-quality radiographs. Processing may be manual or automatic.

Manual

Films enclosed within a light-proof container, which also contains developer and fixer, are available: following exposure the processing fluids are released by pulling two tabs. The Super X-30 (**3.9**) is such a film type and takes approximately 80 s to process. The disadvantages of using film of this type include absence of a lead foil, rapid deterioration of image quality, and inability to use it with a paralleling device.

Manual processing may also be undertaken using a light-proof box (**3.10**) in which are four baths: one containing developer; one containing fixative; two containing water. The operator processes the film while looking through a light-safe viewing panel (**3.11**) and may complete the process within 50 s using high-speed chemicals. Further fixing and washing is required after examining the radiograph. The apparatus can be sited in the surgery because darkroom facilities are not needed.

Automatic

Automatic machines essentially consist of roller assemblies which transport and immerse films through developing, fixing, washing and drying stations. Processing time is usually 4–6 min. Automatic processors are expensive, require maintenance and occasionally break down. An example is the Velopex (**3.12**), which also contains a hot air unit that dries the films as they are

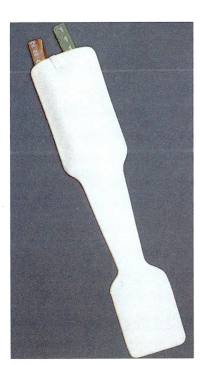

3.9 Super X-30 film

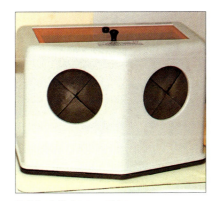

3.10 A light-proof box

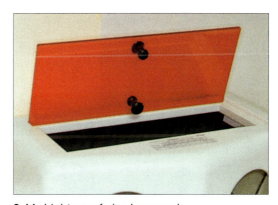

3.11 Light-proof viewing panel

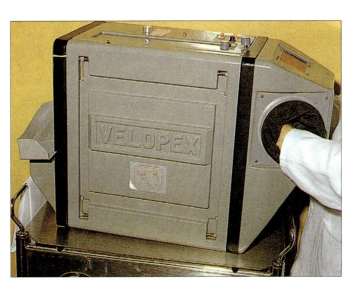

3.12 Velopex automatic processing machine

processed and enables the operator to place films directly into the patient's notes after viewing.

Viewing and storage equipment

Viewers

Optimum viewing of radiographs is accomplished using a clean viewbox and a magnification method that eliminates as much extraneous light as possible. A simple viewer which magnifies the image and cuts out glare is illustrated (**3.13**).

Mounts

Radiographs should be dated and mounted systematically. They may be stored in the patient's clinical records but should be protected for referral and examination without confusion. It is usual to place radiographs in labelled pouches or to laminate them between two sheets of acetate (**3.14**), either by stapling the sheets together or by using a heat-sealing machine (**3.15**). In practices where the turnover of radiographic work is high, lamination should be airtight.

Safety and regulations

The Ionising Radiation (protection of persons undergoing medical examination and treatment) Regulations 1988 lay down requirements relating to protection against radiation. It is the responsibility of all staff to be familiar with any legislation particularly relevant to them. The dangers of excessive radiation are minimal, provided simple precautions are observed. The first decision any practitioner should make is whether the use of X-rays is clinically necessary. Safety considerations of radiological techniques fall into three areas: the patient; the operator; and the equipment.

Patients

The radiation dose to the patient should be minimized. The cone should point away from the patient's body and gonads: this may be achieved quite readily by exposing films with the patient lying supine (**3.16**) and by using protective aprons, with a minimum lead equivalent of 0.25 mm (complying with British Standard 5783), as protection against scattered radiation. These aprons should not be folded and should be examined regularly to ensure that proper protection is still being afforded.

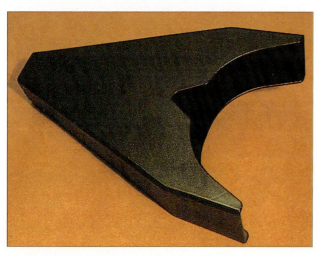

3.13 Simple magnifying viewer

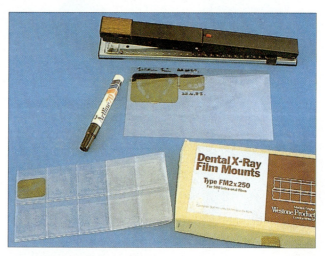

3.14 Film mounts

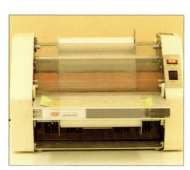

3.15 A laminating machine

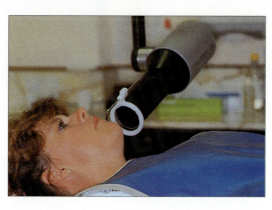

3.16 Radiography with the patient supine

Exposures need to be set to the minimum exposure time possible. Patients should not hold the film packet in position with their fingers: film holding devices and forceps (**3.17**) should be used (tongue spatulas (**3.18**) can also be conveniently used for this purpose). Anyone in the room who is not required for the examination should be excluded if possible.

Operators and other staff

All staff involved in dental radiography must understand the dangers of radiation and be conversant with the precautions necessary for proper handling of equipment and patients. Local rules relating to radiation protection in the practice should be conveniently displayed. No one under the age of 16 years should be allowed to work with ionizing radiations.

Several units are used for measuring radiation, distinguishing between exposure and dose.

Exposure is the amount of radiation in an area to which the patient is exposed. The roentgen (R) is a unit of exposure. One roentgen is the amount of X-rays needed to produce one electrostatic unit in one cubic centimetre of air in standard conditions.

Dose is the amount of radiation absorbed per unit mass of tissue at a particular site. The rad is a unit of radiation absorbed dose and is defined as 100 ergs of energy per gram absorber.

The rem (roentgen equivalent man) is the dose that will produce the same biological effects in humans as are produced by absorbing 1 roentgen of X-radiation or gamma radiation.

The SI unit of measurement for dose equivalent is the sievert (Sv: 1 Sv = 100 rem). The annual maximum permitted whole-body dose is 50 mSv.

Staff exposure to radiation should be closely monitored, using film badges and thermoluminescent dosimeters (**3.19**), if an individual's workload exceeds 150 intraoral films per week. Radiation dosage is reduced if the following precautions are observed:

- The operator must stand at least 2.0 m from the tube and the patient, and outside the primary beam.
- The operator should never hold the film, the tube housing or the patient during the exposure.
- When not in use the X-ray machine should be disconnected from the mains to prevent inadvertent exposure.
- If accidental over-exposure occurs, recommended procedures must be followed (EC Directives 80/836 and 84/467 Euratom). The incident must be fully investigated and the Health and Safety Executive informed. Chronic radiation effects have a long latency period, and records are therefore kept for 50 years.

Equipment

The equipment for taking dental radiographs must be installed in compliance with national standards and should be checked and maintained in accordance with the manufacturer's directions. A record of all maintenance and any defects should be kept. If any faults develop (e.g. faulty warning lights, timers or other electrical problems) the equipment should be disconnected from the mains supply and not used until it has been checked and repaired.

Radiographic techniques

Parallel periapical projections

Ideally, the part of the patient being radiographed is placed in the same plane as the film. The paralleling technique (**3.20**) is used

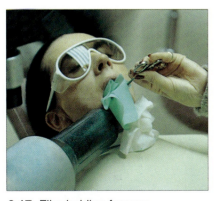

3.17 Film-holding forceps

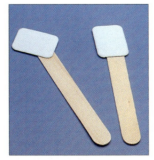

3.18 Film supported on a tongue spatula

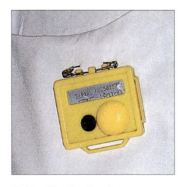

3.19 Film badge for measuring radiation dose

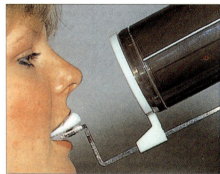

3.20 Paralleling technique

to position the film in the mouth parallel to the long axis of the tooth, and film-holding beam-aiming devices have been developed to facilitate film placement. The film tends to be held away from the tooth, except in the lower molar region. The poor definition and possibility of magnification using this technique are overcome by using a longer focal spot to object distance (ffd).

Figure **3.21** shows a paralleling periapical radiograph of the central incisors being taken using a Rinn holder and localizing ring. The resultant radiograph is also shown (**3.22**).

The reliability of the paralleling technique increases with practice. It is possible to obtain reproducible undistorted views, and by using localizing rings coning off can be avoided (**3.23**). The apices of maxillary molars tend to lie below the level of the zygomatic bone (**3.24**) unless the patient has a small mouth or a flattened palate. Taking paralleling radiographs with film holders may cause the patient discomfort, and is cumbersome with a rubber dam in place. Compromises involve the use of cotton wool rolls (**3.25**), tongue spatulas and forceps (**3.26**).

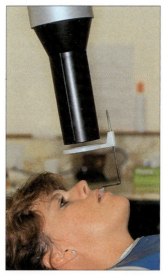

3.21 The Rinn paralleling technique

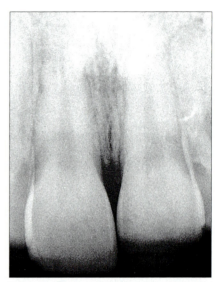

3.22 Radiograph achieved using the paralleling technique

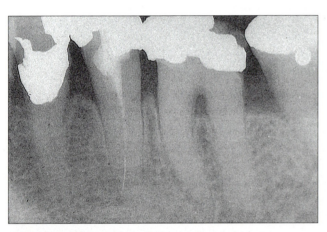

3.23 An undistorted paralleling radiograph

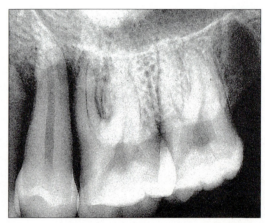

3.24 Roots of maxillary molars in relation to the zygoma

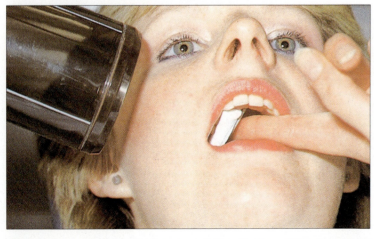

3.25 Use of cotton wool rolls necessitating the use of finger support

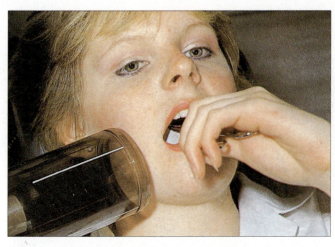

3.26 Use of forceps avoiding the use of finger support

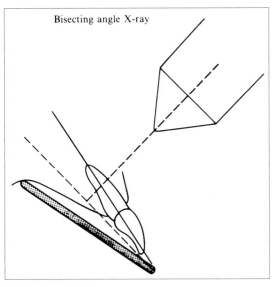

3.27 The bisecting angle technique

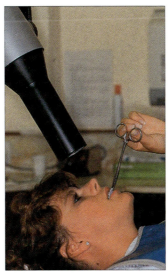

3.28 Forceps used in the bisecting angle technique

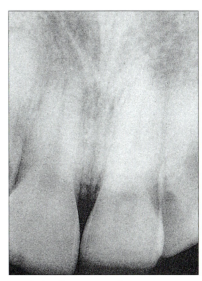

3.29 Radiograph achieved using the bisecting angle technique

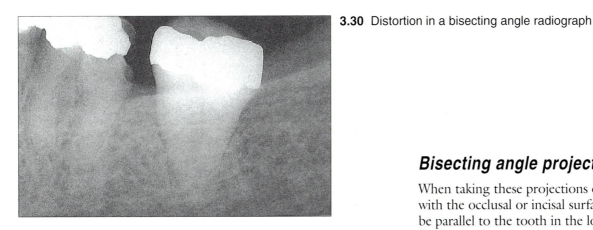

3.30 Distortion in a bisecting angle radiograph

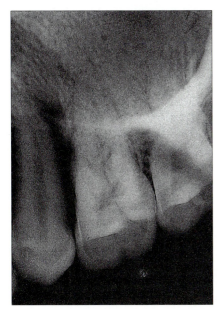

3.31 Superimposition of the zygoma

Bisecting angle projections

When taking these projections one edge of the film is placed level with the occlusal or incisal surface of the tooth. The film axis may be parallel to the tooth in the lower molar region but in the anterior regions a considerable angle may be produced between the axis of the tooth and the film (**3.27**). The main beam is directed at right angles to the plane bisecting the angle between the tooth and film. The dose of radiation used in these projections is very similar to that in parallel periapical radiographs.

In **3.28** a bisecting angle periapical is being taken: note the difference in tube angulation. A bisecting radiograph, corresponding to the paralleling radiograph in **3.22**, is shown in **3.29**.

The bisecting angle technique requires no additional equipment, is quick and easy to use with the rubber dam in place and is relatively comfortable for all patients, even those with small mouths. It does, however, tend to produce distorted and partial images, particularly if varying the angles or if the cone is incorrectly sited in relation to the film (**3.30**). Anatomical structures such as the zygomatic arch are frequently superimposed over the apices of teeth and it is not always possible to gauge the relationship between the roots, other anatomical structures and alveolar bone (**3.31**). It is also difficult to reproduce a radiographic view for review and recall purposes.

Parallax techniques

Horizontal and vertical parallax techniques are most useful in endodontics in the diagnostic and treatment phases. Radiographs taken from different horizontal angles can be used to indicate the position of intra dental structures in relation to the external surface of the tooth. This is most useful in the identification of perforations (**3.32–3.34**). Vertical parallax techniques can be performed to emphasise the radiographic appearance of selected roots in multirooted teeth (**3.35, 3.36**). A combination of the two can also be put to good effect.

Film processing

If high standards of image production are to be maintained the chemicals selected must be diluted accurately, temperature and immersion times controlled carefully, and contamination avoided.

Technical problems

Certain technical faults should be prevented:

- Bent film gives rise to dark lines (**3.37**).
- Distortion occurs when the film is curved under pressure, par-

3.32–3.34 Horizontal parallax in radiographic use

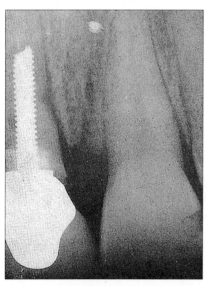

3.32

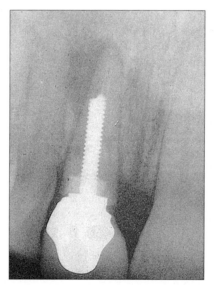

3.33

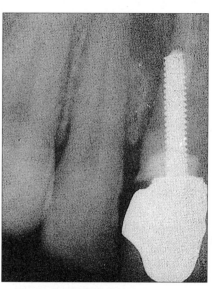

3.34

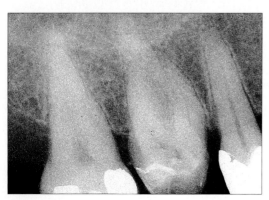

3.35

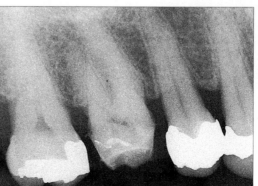

3.36

3.35, 3.36 Vertical parallax

ticularly when finger pressure is used to hold the film in place (**3.38**).
- When the film is still wet the emulsion is easily removed. Without this protective coat the film can be scratched, most commonly by fingernails (**3.39**).
- A partial image ('coning off') results from failure to aim the main beam at the centre of the film. This error leaves a white unexposed portion on the radiograph (**3.40**).
- If the patient, film or tubes moves during exposure the image will appear blurred (**3.41**).
- The image may be damaged if care is not taken to clip the film for processing in a position that will not interfere with essential parts of the image (**3.42**).

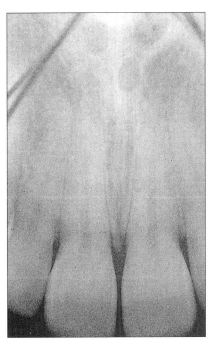

3.37 A bent film will cause dark lines on the radiograph

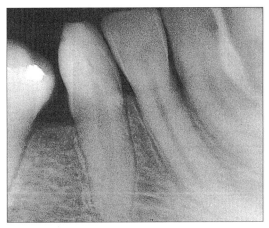

3.38 Distortion produced by a curved film

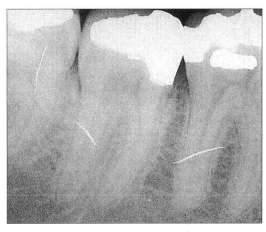

3.39 Scratched emulsion

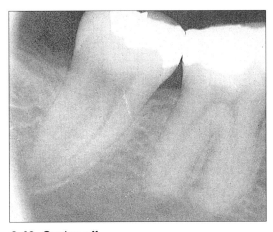

3.40 Coning off

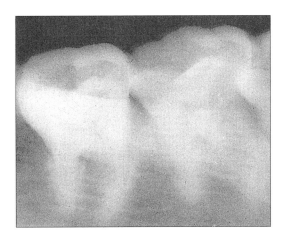

3.41 A blurred image

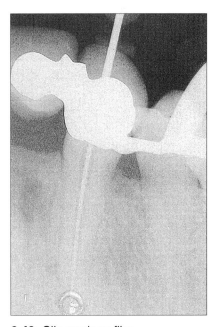

3.42 Clip mark on film

- Extraneous radio-opaque objects such as saliva ejectors (**3.43**), rubber dam frames (**3.44**) and clamps or spectacle frames with metal inserts may become interposed between the cone and film and obstruct the intended image.
- Prolonged exposure and development times, high processing temperatures or a high concentration of developer will produce dark films (**3.45**).
- Insufficient exposure or development time, exhausted developer, low processing temperatures or use of excessively diluted developer are likely to produce light films (**3.46**).
- If a film is placed with the wrong side pointing towards the tube the radiograph appears light and carries a pattern derived from the lead foil in the film packet (**3.47**).
- Fogging (**3.48**) occurs if the film has been stored incorrectly or for a long time, if additional exposure to light or radiation occurs, or if a faulty safe light is being used.
- Streaks, brown marks, spots and encrustations will occur on the film (**3.49**) unless meticulous attention is paid to clean processing, thorough fixing, and the film is washed in running water for an adequate period.
- Blank films will result if the X-ray machine is not switched on, if an unexposed film is inadvertently developed or if the film is placed in fixative instead of developer.

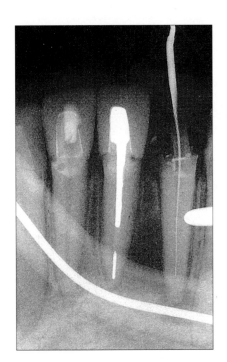

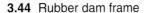

3.44 Rubber dam frame

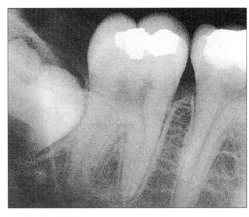

3.45 Dark film

3.43 Saliva ejector

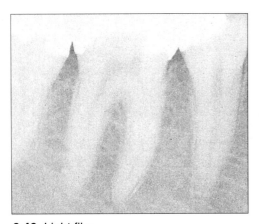

3.46 Light film

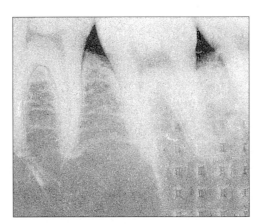

3.47 Reverse exposure of film

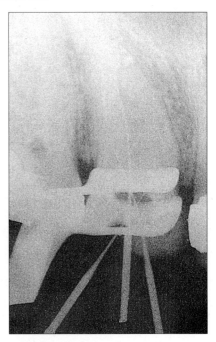

3.48 Fogging

Interpretation of radiographs

The interpretation of radiographs should be approached with a degree of caution and care because what might be considered abnormal radiographic areas in the maxilla and mandible could be due to artefact. Tube angulation can at times produce deceiving images: holes of graduated depth that have been burred into the cortical plate of the dried mandible in **3.50** take on different appearances depending on whether the radiograph is paralleled (**3.51**) or bisecting angle (**3.52**). Similarly, the radiographic appearance of a dried mandible changes little when cancellous bone is removed from the socket of a molar (**3.53**, **3.54**).

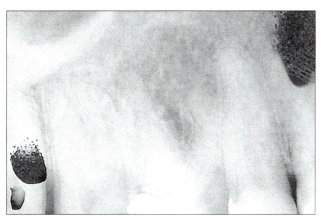

3.49 Marks on the film

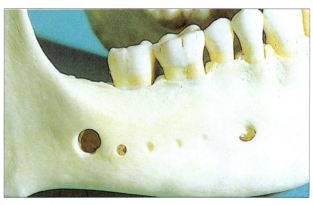

3.50 Drilled holes in a dried mandible

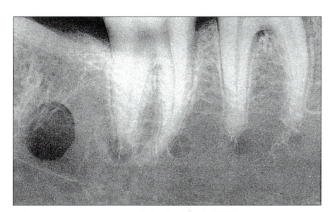

3.51 Paralleling view of the holes in **3.50**

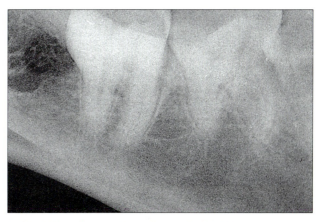

3.52 A bisecting angle radiograph of **3.50** gives a very different appearance

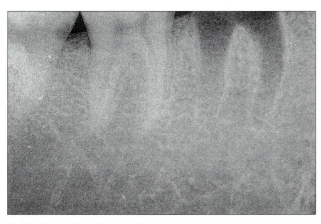

3.53 Normal molar socket

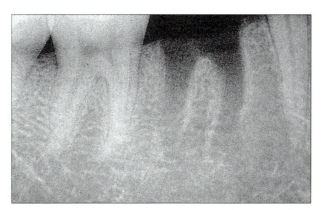

3.54 Appearance of socket after removal of cancellous bone

It is essential that the operator understands the normal radiographic appearance and landmarks of anatomical structures before attempting to identify what might be considered abnormal.

Normal radiographic landmarks

Enamel, dentine and cementum

Enamel is the most radio-opaque structure in the mouth. Dentine is darker and has a uniform density. Cementum cannot be seen radiographically. Radiographic 'burn out' occurs in the cervical region and may be confused with root caries (**3.55**).

Cancellous bone

The trabeculae have a coarser pattern in the mandible than in the maxilla, where they are finer and more lace-like (**3.56**). Trabeculae run in a horizontal direction.

Periodontal ligament

This appears as a narrow even radiolucent line around the root surface within the bone. It is also referred to as the periodontal ligament space. Widening of this space is indicative of pathological change.

Lamina dura

This is the name given to the white line forming the lining of the tooth socket seen on radiographs. This structure is not hypermineralized and is a radiographic artefact. It is unwise to place much diagnostic importance on any variations in the appearance of this line on radiographs.

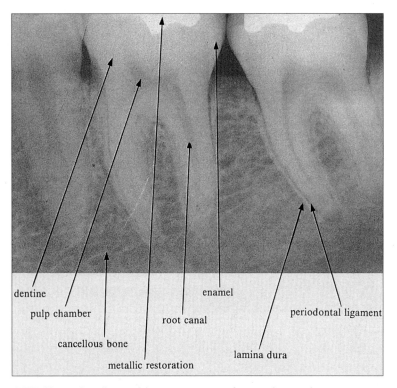

3.55 Normal radiographic appearance of posterior teeth

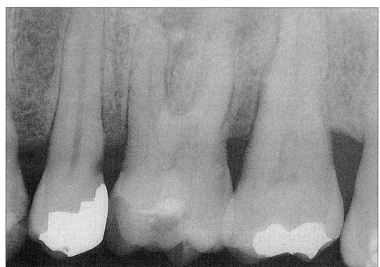

3.56 Radiographic appearance of maxillary cancellous bone

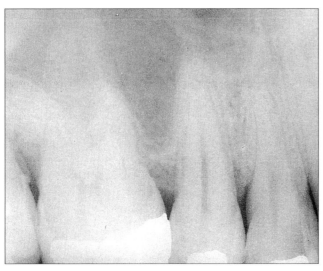
3.57 The floor of the antrum

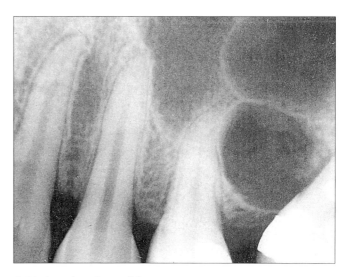
3.58 Loculated antral floor

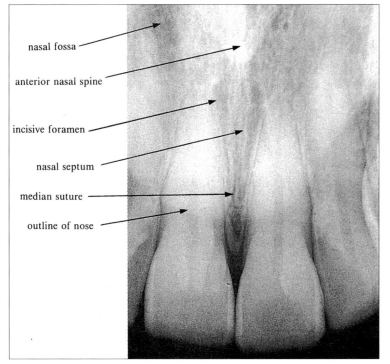
3.59 Radiographic appearance of the anterior maxillary region

Pulp system

The pulp chamber and larger root canals are usually readily visible on the radiograph, but finer canals may be more difficult to see. Root canals that appear to be completely sclerosed rarely are. Stones are common in the pulp and present as a problem only when they block root canals.

Maxillary antrum

This may extend from the premolar region in the maxilla to the tuberosity. The floor of the antrum may be closely associated with the roots of the premolars and molars and may dip between the roots (**3.57**). It may appear loculated and take on the appearance of a cyst (**3.58**). The floor of the antrum appears as a white line. The continuation of this line should be carefully traced when viewing teeth with possible periapical change.

Median suture

This appears as a radiolucent line between the central incisors (**3.59**).

Anterior nasal spine

This appears as a V-shaped radio-opacity above or superimposed on the incisive foramen.

Nasal septum

The nasal septum appears as a radio-opaque line separating the two nasal fossae.

Nose and lip line

The outline of the nose produces a definite line across the radiograph. A similar line may be formed by the lips.

Incisive foramen

The radiolucent circular shadow of the incisive foramen (**3.60**) may be superimposed over the apex of a central incisor and be mistaken for a periapical lesion (**3.61**).

Mandibular canal

The mandibular or inferior dental canal (**3.62**) runs from the mandibular foramen in the ramus of the mandible to the mental foramen in the premolar region. It is seen as a radiolucent band and may approximate the apices of the roots of the molar and premolar teeth; it may be mistaken for a lesion (**3.63**). Extrusion of irrigants, medicaments and filling materials beyond the apex may damage the inferior dental bundle.

Mental foramen

The mental foramen (**3.64**) is situated below and distal to the apex of the mandibular first premolar. Occasionally the angulation of a periapical radiograph may result in superimposition of the structure on the apex of one of the premolars (**3.65**). The foramen may then be confused with a periradicular lesion.

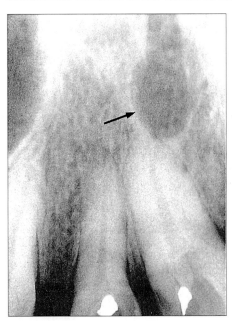

3.60 Incisive foramen

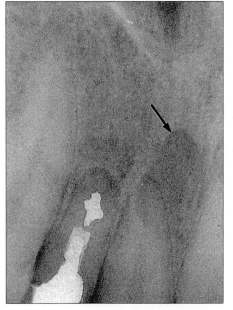

3.61 Incisive foramen

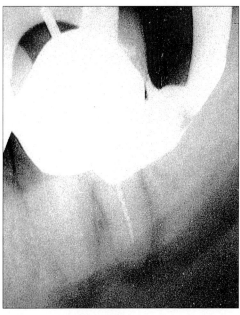

3.62 Mandibular canal

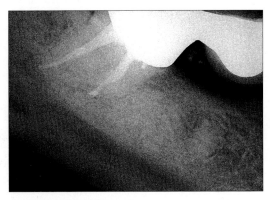

3.63 Mandibular canal

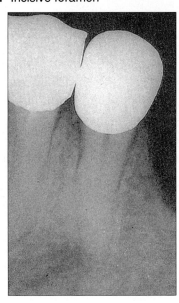

3.64 Mental foramen

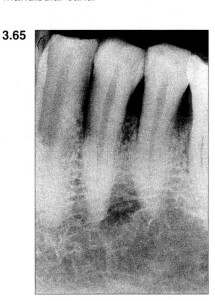

3.65

Lingual foramen

In radiographs of the mandibular incisors the lingual foramen (**3.66**) may be seen as a white radio-opaque area with a small central radiolucent dot.

Nutrient canals

These canals (**3.67**) contain blood vessels supplying both the mandible and the maxilla. They usually appear as vertical radiolucent lines.

Lesions of the periodontal ligament space

Periradicular lesions

These are the most common source of apical radiolucencies. The radiolucency usually has a definite outline (**3.68**) and in long-standing lesions the area may be surrounded by a radio-opaque line (**3.69**). Early lesions are identified by thickening of the periodontal ligament space (**3.70**) and discrete areas of radiolucency (**3.71**). Early periapical change may be noticed in the cancellous

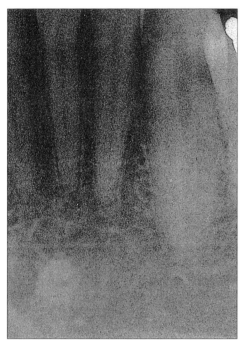

3.66 Lingual foramen

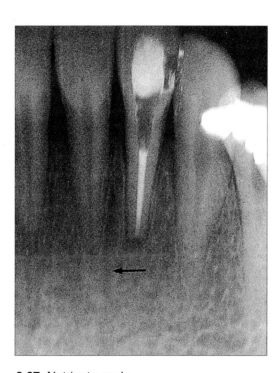

3.67 Nutrient canals

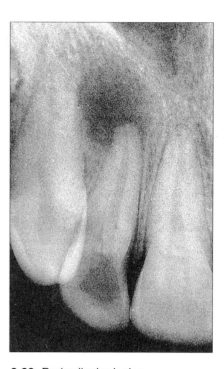

3.68 Periradicular lesion

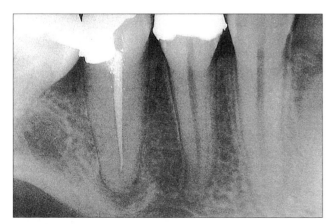

3.69 Periradicular lesion surrounded by a radio-opaque line

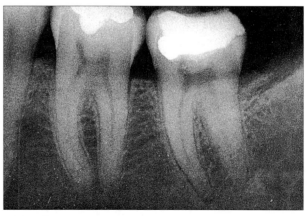

3.70 Thickened periodontal ligament space

bone in the form of changed trabecular pattern (**3.72**) or radio-opaque change (**3.73**). Some of these changes may be reversible and the vitality of the pulp may be maintained.

Lateral lesions

Widening of the periodontal ligament space (**3.74**) and formation of radiolucencies unrelated to the apex (**3.75**) are associated with pathology in the lateral canals. These canals may become visible only after canal obturation (**3.76**).

Fractured root lesions

Radiolucencies associated with the pathology of fractured roots are often of a diffuse nature (**3.77**). The ability to determine the presence of a fracture will depend upon the plane of the fracture in relation to the main X-ray beam (**3.78**): if the beam does not pass through the fracture it may well remain undetected.

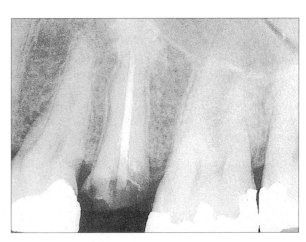

3.73 Alterations in radio-opacity also indicate periapical changes

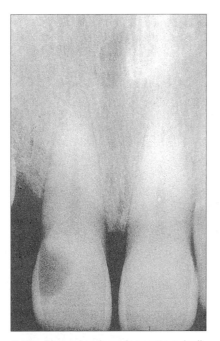

3.72 Altered trabecular pattern indicates periapical change

3.71 Discrete radiolucency

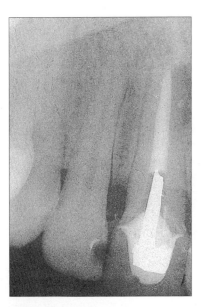

3.74 Widening of the periodontal ligament space

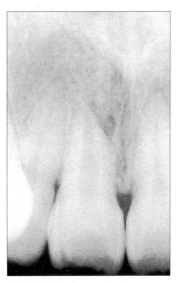

3.75 Radiolucency of the lateral canal

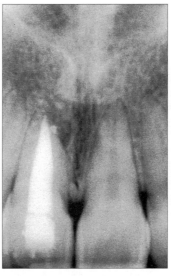

3.76 Obturation of the lateral canal

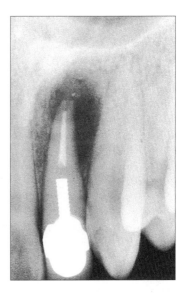

3.77 Diffuse fracture lesion

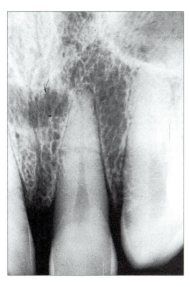

3.78 Fractures are not always detected on radiography

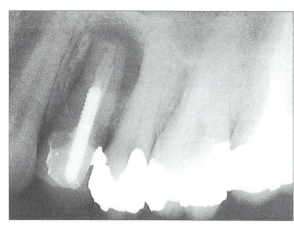

3.79 Diffuse radiolucency

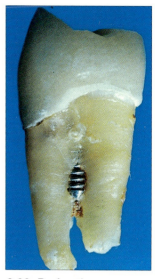

3.80 Perforation

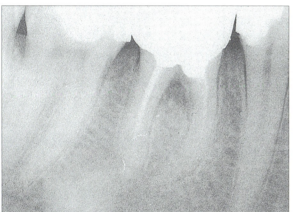

3.81 Condensing osteitis

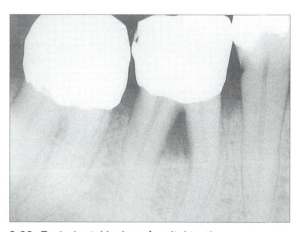

3.82 Periodontal lesion of a vital tooth

Perforation lesions

Perforations (**3.79**) can lead to rapid bone loss and the radiolucencies tend not to be discrete. The presence of a post-retained restoration in a tooth with a large diffuse lesion involving more than just the apical region should arouse suspicion of a perforation or fracture (**3.80**).

Condensing osteitis

This appears as a radio-opacity (**3.81**) and is indicative of a long-standing low grade infection which gives rise to a circumscribed proliferation of the periapical bone. It is usually related to a non-vital pulp or one which is in the process of degeneration. The condition is often symptomless.

Lesions not of dental origin

It is important to be able to distinguish lesions of endodontic origin from those arising from other disease processes.

Periodontal lesions

Periodontal lesions within bone can give rise to radiographic changes which can be confused with periradicular areas (**3.82**). The teeth usually remain vital despite the bone loss.

Osteosclerosis

This condition does not appear to be the result of an infectious process. It is thought to be a compensatory response to abnormal stress. The radiographic appearance closely resembles that of condensing osteitis; however, the tooth reacts normally to vitality testing.

Cemental dysplasia

Early cemental dysplasia or cementomas (**3.83**) present as radiolucent areas, most commonly in relation to the roots of mandibular incisors. These lesions progress to form radio-opaque areas during a period of 5–10 years. The teeth remain vital and endodontic treatment is not required.

Non-odontogenic lesions

A number of inflammatory, cystic and neoplastic lesions not of endodontic origin are capable of producing radiolucencies. The operator should always be alert to the possibility of non-dental causes of bone destruction (**3.84**).

Radiographic advances

Xeroradiography

Dental xeroradiography uses a rigid aluminium photoreceptor plate instead of an X-ray film. The plate is electrically charged, placed in a light-proof plastic cassette, positioned in the mouth and exposed to X-rays. This technique of image processing is fast, requiring only 25 secs for a dry permanent image. The plates may be reconditioned, recharged and used repeatedly.

The xeroradiograph may be viewed by reflected or transilluminated light. The image consists of a range of greys rather than the variation in optical densities from black through grey to white seen on conventional film. Xeroradiography has the property of edge enhancement of all imaged boundaries, giving an image that depicts small structures extremely well. The system provides better visualization of instrument tips and root apices, which may allow more accurate length measurement. At present, processors are very expensive and the use of the technique in endodontics has not been fully appreciated.

Radiovisiography

Radiovisiography systems (**3.85**) consist of an X-ray set, an intra-oral sensor (**3.86**) containing an image receptor, a display-processing unit and a printer. Images are shown on a television monitor in the display-processing unit, and may be 'enhanced' by increasing the contrast while decreasing the latitude of the system. This system has the capacity for image manipulation, and can be linked to a computer for image storage and retrieval. Hard copies of the various images (**3.87**) may be produced using a thermal heated video printer. Radiovisiography is a low-dose, rapid imaging system, but has a lower resolution than the conventional dental film.

Recent studies suggest that radiovisiography, when used with enhancement, is an adequate substitute for conventional film radiography in determination of root canal length. Clinical evaluation of this 'real time' diagnostic system is necessary to confirm its promising prospects for use in endodontics.

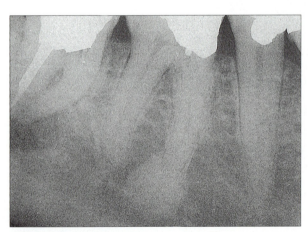

3.83 Cementoma

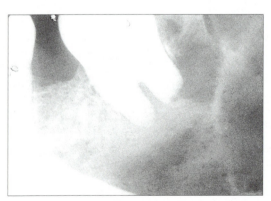

3.84 Non-dental lesion

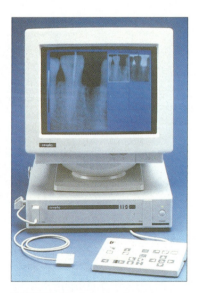

3.85 Radiovisiography equipment

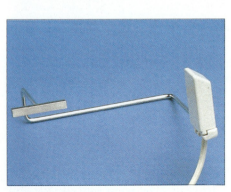

3.86 Sensor used for radiovisiography

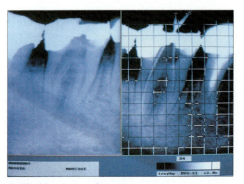

3.87 Hard copy/image

4 Treatment planning

Treatment planning involves the collation of all pertinent information gained from the history, examination and relevant tests performed for the patient. This information is used to formulate the treatment requirements for the patient, at that time, in those given circumstances.

The end point of history taking and examination is the establishment of a diagnosis, albeit tentative. Once the diagnosis has been made, the most appropriate and effective treatment plan must be drawn up for that particular patient. There are three stages in the planning process.

Planned initial treatment

Immediate relief of symptoms

The relief of pain is a valuable service and should precede other forms of treatment. The provision of emergency endodontic care for patients in pain of pulpal or periapical origin need not be anxiety-ridden or time-consuming, and can assist in building the reputation of a practitioner.

The treatment required for the immediate relief of pain may be obvious – for example, a very carious, unrestorable tooth (**4.1**) may be extracted.

Where the appropriate treatment is not so obvious it is possible to institute endodontic treatment for the relief of symptoms before making a definitive decision about the future of the tooth – e.g. endodontic treatment may be commenced in a tooth with a suspected fracture before undertaking further investigations to establish the true prognosis (**4.2**).

Stabilization

When disease is at an advanced stage and threatens the survival of a tooth or teeth, its progression may be controlled without delivering full effective, definitive treatment. The most easily understood example of this is the dressing of carious teeth (**4.3**) to arrest caries progression and protect the pulp.

The same principle may be applied to pulpally involved teeth. Endodontic treatment may be instituted and the canals in the teeth provisionally dressed to control the development of the pulpal disease without completing the definitive therapy (**4.4**). Endodontically speaking, the teeth are placed on 'hold' while other aspects of the patient's total care are being managed.

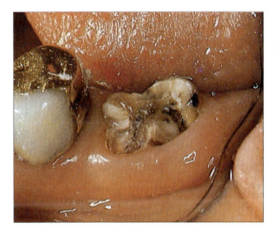

4.1 A carious unrestorable tooth

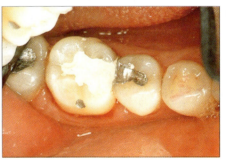

4.3 A dressed tooth

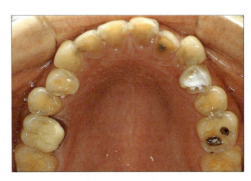

4.4 Endodontic stabilization

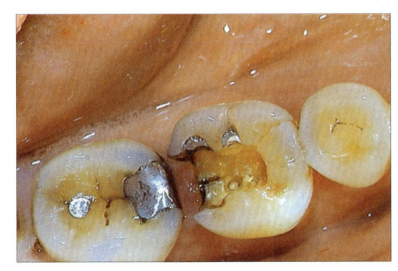

4.2 Fracture in molar tooth

Planned definitive treatment

The type of endodontic treatment planned for a particular patient should take into account the patient's general health and dental state. The choice of treatment may be influenced by a number of factors.

Overall restorative plan

Not all teeth with pulpal and periradicular pathology are candidates for endodontic treatment, and on occasions the retention of a pulpally compromised tooth should be questioned if it unnecessarily complicates the restorative plan. One such example is an endodontically compromised remaining incisor, where the restorative option is a removable prosthesis (**4.5**).

Sometimes teeth with perfectly normal pulps are judged to require endodontic treatment for restorative reasons, as in the case of the restorative re-alignment of teeth or overdenture construction (**4.6, 4.7**).

Endodontic treatment should also be considered for any tooth with low-grade symptoms, particularly if it is to receive an extensive restoration or is to be used as an abutment for a fixed prosthesis (**4.8, 4.9**). It is more difficult – and in the long term more expensive – to carry out the endodontic treatment of a tooth already restored with a large cast or ceramometal restoration. Following the root treatment the restoration may need to be remade.

Access and the final restoration

When planning the endodontic treatment of a tooth the physical demands of the final restoration should be borne in mind. Full consideration should be given to the way in which access and root canal preparation will influence the amount of available coronal tooth substance and canal space for post construction. Good access leads to success in endodontics, but access produced without thought may make the restoration of the tooth more difficult (**4.10**).

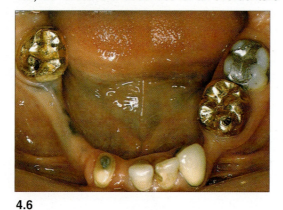

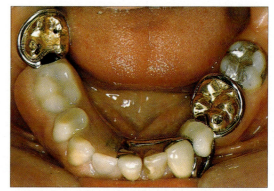

4.6, 4.7 Elective endodontics for an overdenture

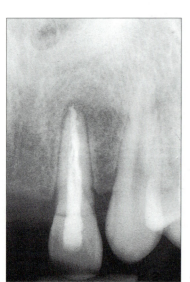

4.5 Endodontically unsound incisor

4.8, 4.9 Endodontic treatment for a molar with questionable vitality

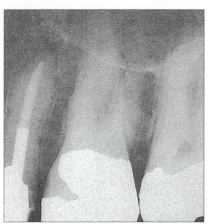

4.10 An over-prepared access cavity

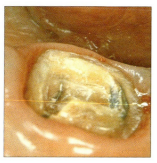

4.11 Root-filled tooth with subgingival margins

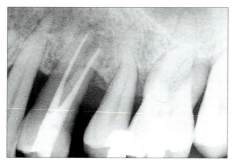

4.12 Root-filled tooth with loss of periodontal support

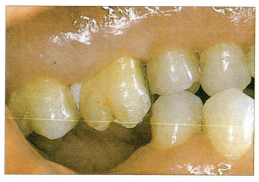

4.13 Unapposed molar

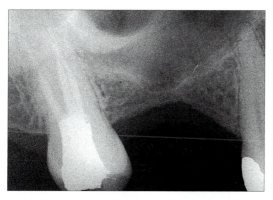

4.14 Tooth defending the need for a free end saddle

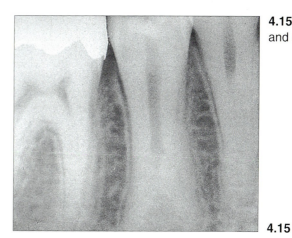

4.15–4.17 Bizarre root and canal forms

4.15

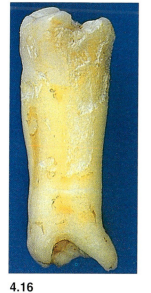

4.16   **4.17**

Restorability of teeth

Following endodontic treatment it should be possible to restore a tooth to function and health. Particular attention must be given to the support that can be provided for a coronal restoration and the position of finishing margins. Finishing margins benefit from being above the alveolar crest, and preferably supragingival. If the prospects of providing an adequate restoration seem remote, extraction should be considered as an alternative treatment. The example in **4.11** shows a well treated tooth which will require an innovative restoration, and possibly surgery, to satisfy the marginal needs of the final coronal restoration.

Periodontal support

Loss of periodontal attachment on its own is not a contraindication for endodontic treatment. Provided a tooth has, or can be made to have, a healthy periodontal apparatus, endodontic treatment may be carried out (**4.12**).

Strategic importance of teeth

The importance of a particular tooth in the dental arch should be considered before embarking on endodontic treatment. Clearly unapposed and functionless teeth (**4.13**) are strategically less important than single standing teeth which prevent the need for a free end saddle denture (**4.14**).

Canal anatomy

Bizarre root forms and root canal anatomy, congenital grooves and dilacerations may all present difficulties if endodontic treatment is attempted. These unusual forms may affect the outcome of treatment (**4.15–4.17**).

Root resorption

The loss of tooth tissue structure may lead to fracture. The prognosis for teeth affected by internal resorption is good (**4.18, 4.19**). The process may be arrested by pulp removal and, provided the remaining tooth substance is strong enough, the tooth can be retained. Treatment of resorption arising on the external surface of the root (**4.20**) is less predictable. External inflammatory resorption is treatable and responds to root canal treatment. The treatment of other types of external resorption is unpredictable. Defects can be repaired surgically and also made supragingival; there is, however, a tendency for this type of external resorption to continue.

Root fractures

Fractures which communicate with the oral environment (**4.21**) provide a route for infection. Vertically fractured teeth (**4.22, 4.23**) have a worse prognosis than those with horizontal fractures, which are also easier to detect radiographically (**4.24**). Crown–root fractures passing through the attachment apparatus and involving alveolar bone require careful assessment to establish accurately the endodontic and restorative needs of the remaining tooth substance. Posterior teeth with fractures involving the floor of the pulp chamber have poor long-term prospects.

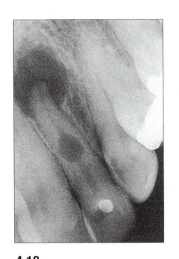

4.18

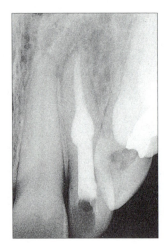

4.19

4.18, 4.19 Internal resorption

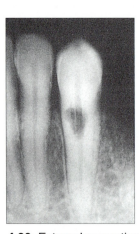

4.20 External resorption

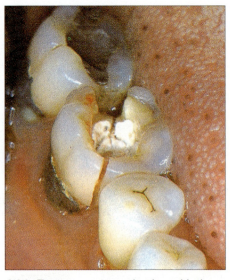

4.21 Fracture communicating with the oral cavity

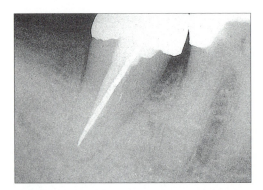

4.22

4.22, 4.23 Vertical fracture of a mandibular molar

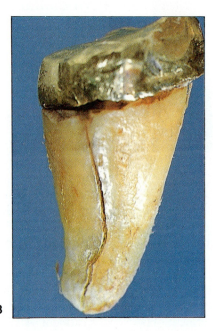

4.23

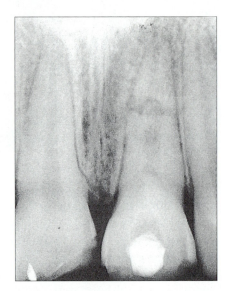

4.24 Horizontal fracture of a maxillary incisor

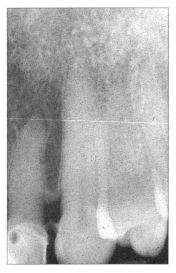
4.25 Sclerosed canal

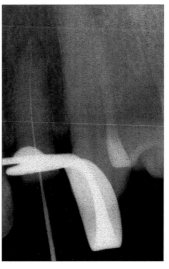
4.26 Located sclerosed canal

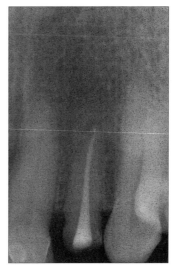
4.27 Treated sclerosed canal

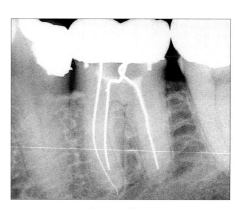
4.28 Previously root-filled tooth requiring retreatment

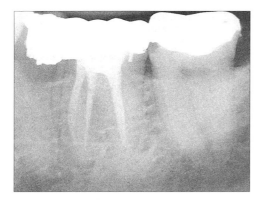
4.29 Retreated case

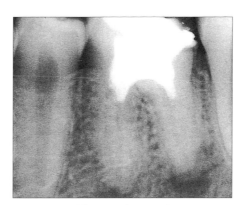
4.30 Root-filled tooth requiring new restoration

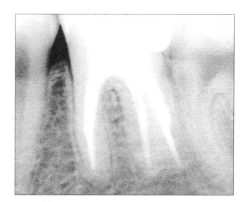
4.31 Tooth retreated and restored

Sclerosed canals

Root canals that are not visible radiographically (**4.25**) may be very difficult to locate and negotiate if endodontic treatment is necessary. However, in many cases they are possible to find and treat (**4.26**). It is impossible to predict the outcome of treatment until an attempt has been made to locate them (**4.27**).

Teeth with a history of trauma experience progressive narrowing of the pulp space. Such teeth should be reviewed radiographically and if there is evidence of sclerotic change endodontic treatment should not be contemplated until there are radiographic periradicular indications of necrotic change occurring within the canal.

Previous root treatment

The decision to retreat a previously root-filled tooth (**4.28**) should be based on clear criteria. If the treatment appears to be failing because it shows symptoms, sinus tracts, persistent or developing radiolucencies, separated instruments and iatrogenic perforations, retreatment should be considered (**4.29**).

The replacement of coronal restorations in endodontically treated teeth can give rise to symptoms, but why this should be so is not fully understood. It has been suggested that altered occlusal loading, the effects of post space preparation and restoration cementation hydrostatic pressures may account for the problems. Such problems are probably related to coronal reinfection of the canal system.

Previously treated teeth requiring new restorations (**4.30**) should be examined with care, and if the adequacy of the sealing of the pulp space is in doubt retreatment should be considered (**4.31**).

Where post-retained restorations exist in teeth requiring endodontic retreatment a choice has to be made regarding the approach to treatment. Conservative retreatment is likely to damage the restoration, and post removal may precipitate a root fracture. Conservative treatment gives a better opportunity to clean the canal system and eliminate coronal leakage as a possible cause for failure but does not treat extraradicular infection.

A surgical retrograde approach to retreatment preserves existing restorations but does not eliminate coronal leakage as a cause of

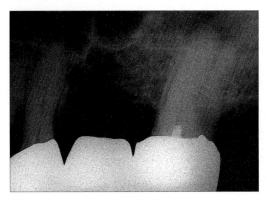
4.32 Radiograph of endodontic case

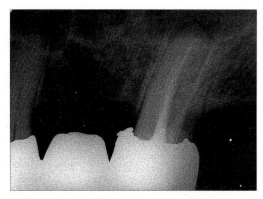
4.33 Radiograph, 1 year after treatment

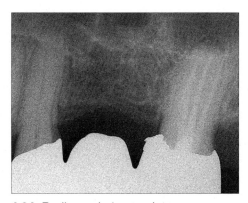
4.34 Radiograph 4 years later

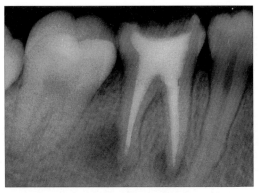
4.35 Postoperative radiograph of lesion

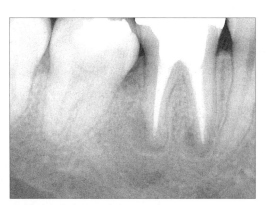
4.36 Lesion remaining static

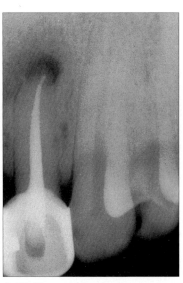
4.37 Pre-existing lesion

failure. It is difficult to clean the canal system thoroughly; however, a surgical approach offers an opportunity to eradicate extra radicular infection.

In cases involving retreatment of teeth with large and irregular looking lesions the use of decompression and biopsy techniques should be considered to establish a clear diagnosis.

Finally, the practitioner should always assess his or her ability to improve on the existing situation. If this ability is in doubt, referral to a colleague specializing in this area should be considered.

Planned review

Reassessment and re-evaluation of the status of dental health of patients is an integral part of the planning process. It involves examining the patient again, often taking elements of the history again, re-establishing a diagnosis, and formulating a new treatment plan for whatever new or residual problems are encountered.

Clinical and radiographic follow-up, at regular intervals for an indefinite period, are essential for the assessment of endodontic treatment. Observation periods of at least 4 years are desirable (**4.32**). Endodontic treatment should be assessed annually (**4.33**).

Indications of success are absence of pain, swelling and other symptoms, no sinus tract, no loss of function, and radiographic evidence of a normal periodontal ligament space around the root (**4.34**).

The outcome of treatment is considered uncertain if radiographs reveal that a lesion has remained the same size or has diminished in size, but total repair has not occurred (**4.35**, **4.36**).

Treatment is considered to have failed if radiographs reveal that a lesion has appeared following endodontic treatment or a pre-existing lesion has increased in size (**4.37**, **4.38**) or there is conflicting evidence with respect to symptoms and radiographic evaluation. For example, a tooth may have persistent low-grade symptoms and yet appear healthy on radiography.

Factors that may to lead to secondary failure of a previously successful endodontic treatment include recurrent caries and coronal leakage (**4.39**), caries extending into the root canal (**4.40**), or furcation, root fracture (**4.41**) or perforation (**4.42**).

In conclusion, all dental treatment should be undertaken applying the principle of continuous review. Endodontic treatment provides definite indications for scheduling review appointments and should be looked upon as an integral part of treatment planning.

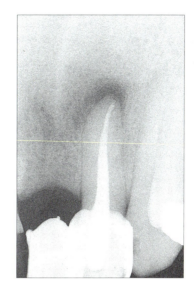

4.38 Lesion increasing in size

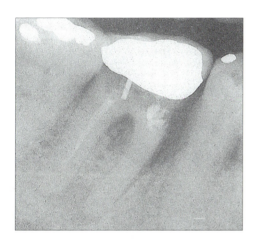

4.39 Caries leading to failure of restoration

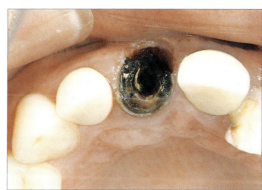

4.40 Caries in a root canal

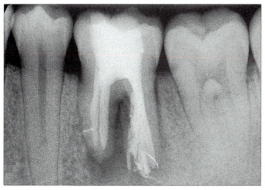

4.41 Postoperative root fracture

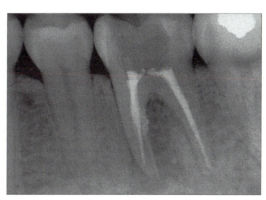

4.42 Postoperative root perforation

5 Pre-endodontic management

Endodontics can be one of the most satisfying aspects of dental practice, provided it is performed in a well managed working environment. Consideration should be given to specific organizational requirements which affect the operatory, the staff, the patient and ultimately the tooth to be treated.

The clinical area

The clinical area or 'operatory' benefits from having a fresh, bright, warm and welcoming atmosphere. The design, layout and decor does a great deal to enhance its image. An environment that has been constructed to allow staff to work efficiently, with comfort and ease, will decrease stress, encourage smooth relaxed working days, and increase job satisfaction. The operatory should be designed in an uncluttered fashion to facilitate movement to and from the working area.

Equipment location

The organization of endodontic equipment requires some thought and should be planned carefully to satisfy the needs of the operator's working methods.

Cabinetry and cupboards within the working area, whether they are placed in an L- or U-shaped configuration, should be within the reach of both operator and assistant.

The use and location of conventional rotary instrumentation are important for the preliminary access to the pulp canal systems but is probably secondary to the use of specific endodontic instrumentation. Work can often be simplified by considering the most useful positions to place the more commonly used instruments.

The distance that the hand instruments have to travel during procedures should be minimized – use of a cervical tray (**5.1**) may achieve this. Simple cervical trays without handpiece and 3 in 1 cord fittings allow instruments to be approximated to the tooth being treated.

Ultrasonic units are used regularly in root treatment; these units should be as easily accessible as conventional handpieces and not be seen as an *addition* to the usual dental equipment. Ultrasonic units may be mounted as a permanent fixture on the dental unit (**5.2**) or stored in an accessible position. Sliding shelves or drawers are most useful in this respect (**5.3**).

Radiographic viewers should also be sited within easy reach. The viewer may be placed on a nearby work surface or in a sliding drawer.

Work surface organization

The work surfaces of dental units and cupboards readily collect infected material and surfaces should be chosen that are easy to keep clean.

Between clinical sessions all work surfaces, including those which are apparently uncontaminated, should be cleaned with a detergent or a microbicidal disinfectant.

Contamination zones

Work surfaces should be defined as zones of high or low contamination.

Surfaces liable to become contaminated with body fluids or infected matter should be identified and designated high contamination zones. These areas benefit from impervious disposable coverings that can be changed and the surface beneath cleaned between patients. All disposable and sterilizable instruments and trays fall within this area.

Low contamination zones include all other areas which, during normal clinical procedures, would not be expected to become impregnated with infected material. In these areas procedures should be adopted to limit the surfaces touched each time a patient is treated.

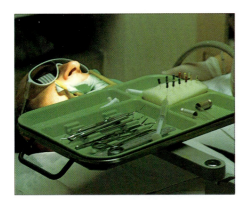

5.1 Cervical tray

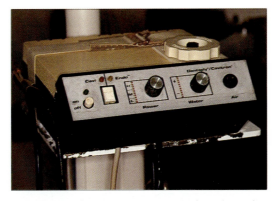

5.2 Ultrasonic apparatus mounted on the unit

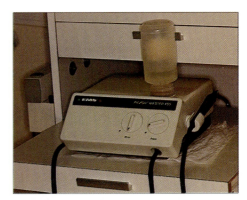

5.3 Ultrasonic apparatus on a sliding drawer

Instrumentation and storage

A very wide range of instruments designed specifically for endodontic treatment is available. Some of these instruments have been used for many years; others are new and, in some cases, highly technical. The instruments described in this book are readily available and commonly used.

Generally used instruments and materials include:

Basic instrument packs
Rotary instruments
    Friction grip burs
    Conventional burs
    Safe-ended burs
    Gates–Glidden burs
    Rotary fillers
    Peeso drills
Hand instruments
    Barbed broaches
    Reamers
    Files
    Other root canal instruments
Rubber dam and accessories
Power-assisted instruments
    Reciprocating
    Sonic
    Ultrasonic
    Others
Measuring devices
    Electronic
    Rules, gauges, stops, paste
Instrument and post retrieval kits
Irrigating syringes
Paper points
Gutta percha points
Instruments for lateral and vertical condensation of gutta percha
Instruments for thermomechanical compaction of gutta percha
Equipment for thermoplastic injection of gutta percha
Equipment for solid core gutta percha techniques

Consideration must be given to storing, cleaning and sterilizing all these items.

The basic instrument pack

A pre-sterilized basic pack (**5.4**) is required for all routine root canal procedures. The pack contains

Front surface mirror
Endodontic locking tweezers
Canal probe
Briault probe
Long-shanked excavator
Amalgam plugger
Flat plastic
Metal rule
Surgical haemostats
Sterile cotton pledgets and rolls

Use of the *front surface mirror* overcomes the problems associated with double images, which are produced when the reflecting surface is beneath a layer of glass. The *endodontic locking tweezers* (**5.5**) allow small items to be gripped safely and transferred between assistant and operator. They are particularly useful when handling gutta percha points, paper points and cotton wool pledgets. The tips of the beaks should be blunt and grooved. The *canal probe* should be long, fine, sharp and strong. It is used to feel the floor of the pulp chamber when locating canal orifices. A *Briault probe* is used to feel for overhangs when removing the roof of the pulp chamber. Two other probes, although not included in the basic kit, are useful in periodontal assessment and are worth mentioning here: the *curved American pattern probe No. 3* (**5.6**) (used to probe furcations in posterior teeth); and a

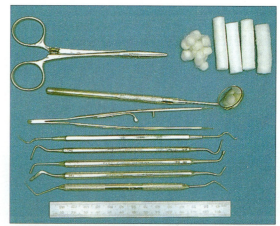

5.4 Basic pack

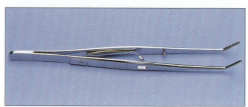

5.5 Endo locking tweezers

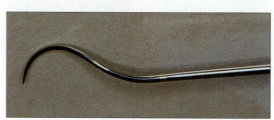

5.6 American probe No. 3

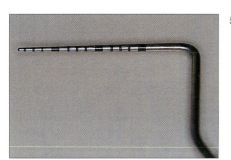

5.7 Periodontal probe

pocket measuring probe with a fine shank, blunt end, and millimetre markings (**5.7**). *Long-shanked excavators* come in a range of designs to allow access to the pulp chamber. These are used for scooping out the remains of the pulp and excess gutta percha; also for flicking away pulp stones. The *amalgam plugger* and *flat plastic* assist in placement of interappointment provisional restorations. The *haemostats* are used to grip radiographs and the *metal rule* to measure instrument lengths in calculating root canal length.

Storage

The most convenient storage systems for endodontic instruments involve the use of trays, boxes and test tubes.

The *RAF tray* (**5.8**) is made of aluminium and measures 28 × 18 × 3.5 cm. The tray has a separate metal lid, is divided into four compartments and contains a stand for the hand instruments. Any *plastic tray* may be adapted to achieve the same function. The tray in **5.9** has no lid and measures 38.3 × 26.6 cm. A removable sterile sponge is cut to fit one of the compartments and is retained by pins or screws. The sponge provides an ideal site for placement of ready-use hand instruments and burs.

Metal containers (**5.10**) are available in many forms. Most of these boxes have lids and magazines for instruments, and are designed to be sterilized in a hot-air oven. Sterile instruments are taken from one box and are placed in a second box after use. At the end of the working day the box is replenished and sterilized for use the next day. Using this process means that many instruments are sterilized several times without being used, which may reduce the cutting efficiency of the hand instruments.

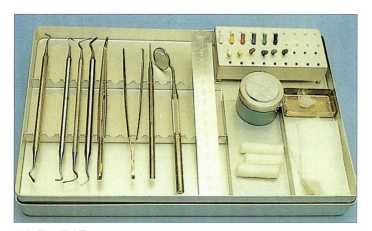

5.8 The RAF tray

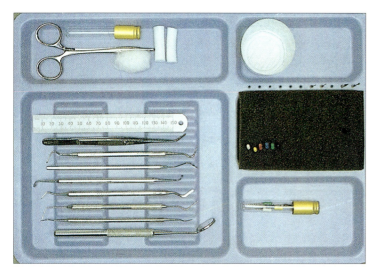

5.9 Plastic tray

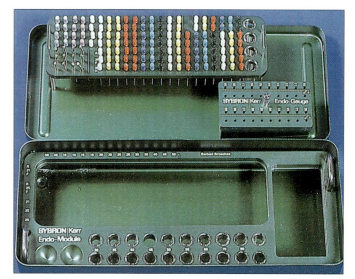

5.10 Instrument box

Standard 11 mm wide Pyrex test tubes with colour-coded caps are convenient receptacles for sets of six hand instruments (**5.11**). The instruments are sterilized in an autoclave within the test tube. The test tubes may be stored in racks (**5.12**) or drawer compartments (**5.13**). Selected instruments are removed from the test tube and placed in a stand or sterile sponge (sponge squares and blocks are inexpensive and may be sterilized in the autoclave). Sponges may also be used to rationalize drawer storage, allowing instruments to be grouped according to size and length (**5.14**).

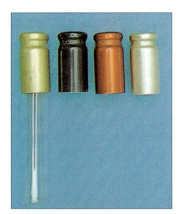

5.11 Pyrex test tube

Cleaning and sterilization

All instruments should be cleaned and sterilized after use.

Removal of gross debris

All debris, which harbours and protects micro-organisms, should be removed as soon as possible. Instruments are cleaned by scrubbing in soap or detergent in warm water; gross debris is removed from small files by stabbing them into sponges impregnated with detergent. Ultrasonic baths (**5.15**) are the most reliable way of eliminating gross debris. The person cleaning instruments should always wear protective gloves to avoid inoculation with debris.

Sterilization

Chemical methods

Chemical disinfection should be reserved only for items that may not be sterilized by conventional methods. Chemicals have variable effects on different micro-organisms, a reduced efficiency in the presence of organic matter, tend to deteriorate with storage

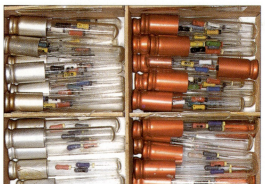

5.13 Pyrex tubes in a drawer

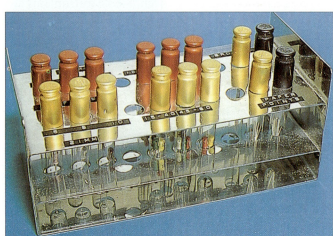

5.12 Pyrex tubes in rack

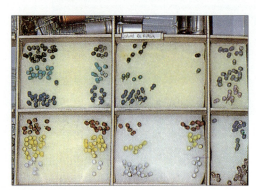

5.14 Sponges in a drawer

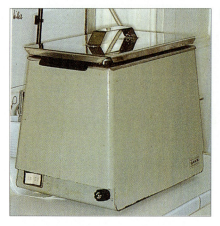

5.15 Ultrasonic bath

and may be toxic. Of the solutions available, those containing glutaraldehyde seem to be the most effective against hepatitis B and HIV. Sterilizing solutions should be kept in a closed container at all times. Certain patients may become sensitized to the chemicals used in sterilizing instruments, and other methods are preferred.

Dry heat

Dry heat is widely used in sterilization – a temperature of 160 °C is recommended for at least 60 min. Hot air sterilizers (**5.16**) tend to use a long cycle (at least 90 min) and the high temperatures reached may damage some instruments. This form of sterilization is most useful for paper points, cotton wool, oils and powders.

Bead sterilizers

Salt (**5.17**) and glass bead sterilizers are useful for treating small instruments at the chairside. The temperature gauge allows the operator to check that the working temperature (218 °C) has been reached (sterilization time is 10 s). Bead sterilizers have been criticized because it is relatively easy to introduce beads into the root canal and create an obstruction; salt sterilizers are now preferred because they give a favourable temperature gradient.

Pressure steam (autoclave)

This method of sterilization is effective and has a reasonably short cycle (3 min at 134°C). The effectiveness of autoclaving wrapped instruments in sterilizing chambers that are not evacuated has been called into question and steam sterilizers with a vacuum phase (**5.18**) are generally recommended. However, this type of sterilization has the disadvantage of causing corrosion and dulling of sharp instruments and is unsuitable for sterilizing cotton wool and paper products.

Checking temperatures

Two simple methods of checking that sterilizing temperatures have been reached are available. Browne's tubes (**5.19**) change colour from red to green, and certain sterilization bags have vertical pale brown stripes which turn dark brown when the correct temperature is reached (**5.20**).

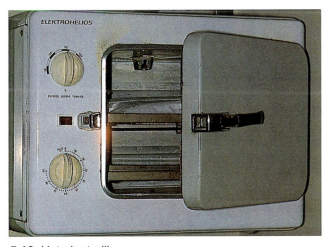

5.16 Hot air sterilizer

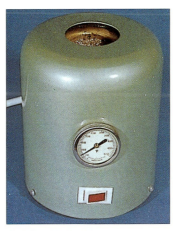

5.17 Salt sterilizer

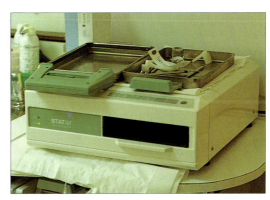

5.18 Steam sterilizer

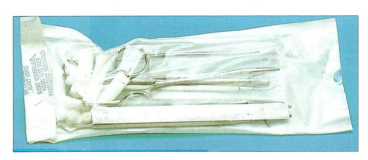

5.19 Browne's tubes

5.20 Sterilization bag

Infection control

Implementation of a cross-infection control protocol requires a thorough knowledge of the risks and the practical measures needed. To minimize the risk of transmission between patients and between patients and clinical staff, a sensible and practical routine for the prevention of infection and cross-infection should be followed with every patient treated. Clinical staff should ensure that their immunization against hepatitis B (HBV) and other infectious diseases (e.g. tuberculosis) is up to date.

During the history taking, patients might disclose that they are HIV or HBV carriers. HBV carriers and patients with HIV who are otherwise well may be treated routinely in dental practice, but patients with HIV in ill health or with oral manifestations of the disease should be referred for expert advice. Confidentiality should always be preserved and the obligation to provide care realized. Refusal to treat these patients is illogical – undiagnosed carriers of infectious disease pass undetected through practices every day. Operators who are HBV- or HIV-positive should seek appropriate advice.

All staff should understand the modes of transmission of infections, sterilization and infection-control requirements, the proper use of protective clothing and equipment, the remedial actions to be taken in the event of accidents, the importance of general hygiene and of keeping immunizations up to date.

Inoculation injuries are the most common route for transmission of blood-borne viral and other infections in dentistry. Great care should be taken when handling all sharps and specially designated bins should be used in their disposal. Needle protection devices are available and should be used for resheathing.

The dental nurse

The dental nurse should be well trained and hold a relevant qualification. In a specialized field such as endodontics in-house training is also necessary to ensure that the nurse understands fully the various techniques employed. Emergency and resuscitation training requirements should also be met.

Anticipation

One of the greatest assets a dental nurse can have is the ability to anticipate the needs of patient and operator. The nurse should be aware of the aspects of care that optimize a patient's comfort, safety and protection. Dental nurses should be encouraged not to adjust the patient's chair until the medical history has been established – and certainly not before explaining what is about to happen – because sudden chair movements may frighten patients unnecessarily. Particular attention should be paid to the angulation of the chair and the head position. It is wise to ask the patient if they are comfortable.

The patient must wear spectacles, to protect their eyes, and a waterproof bib (**5.21**). These items protect against dropped instruments and spilled sodium hypochlorite.

With the patient supine the assistant should sit slightly higher than the operator to allow adequate visibility (**5.22**). Adjustment of the light is the nurse's responsibility.

If patients spend long periods lying supine, the chair should be returned to the upright position slowly on completion of treatment, and the patient asked to sit for a moment or two before leaving the chair – this will prevent problems arising from postural hypotension.

In order to provide effective operator support the nurse must anticipate the actions of the operator. Clinical procedures should be understood and learned thoroughly and a rationalized work sequence developed between the operator and nurse. Use of arranged spoken and unspoken signals will improve the efficiency and flow of working movements.

A dental nurse can be of considerable help during the placement of the rubber dam (**5.23**), instrument transfer, irrigation and suction procedures (**5.24**), and handling paper and gutta percha points (**5.25**).

The nurse should also be able to judge the length of hand instruments required and set working lengths when instructed (**5.26**).

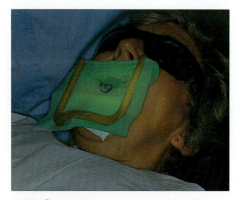

5.21 Spectacles and protective bib

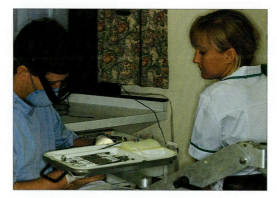

5.22 Operator and seated nurse

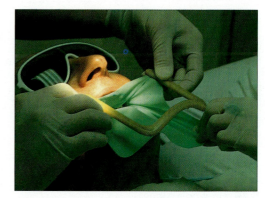

5.23 Rubber dam placement

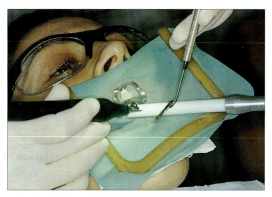
5.24 Irrigation and suction procedures

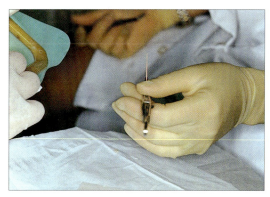
5.25 Gutta percha point transfer

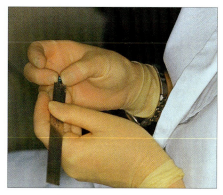
5.26 Setting working length of instruments

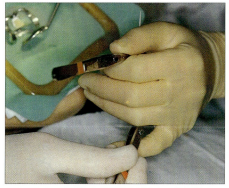
5.27 Instrument transfer

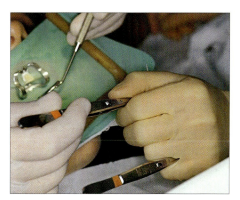
5.28 The transfer zone

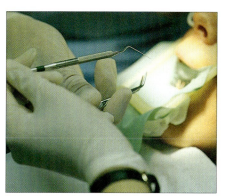
5.29 Parallel transfer

Close support

The specific operations involved in endodontics are generally delicate and require a high level of concentration on the part of the operator. Control of the operating field is one of the main aims of close support. The operator and nurse control visibility, soft tissues, moisture and saliva, instruments, water coolants and contaminants.

In endodontics the greatest aid in achieving this degree of control is a rubber dam. Isolation using a rubber dam can greatly improve efficiency by gaining time normally lost by patients rinsing, dentists continually changing wet cotton rolls and assistants struggling with saliva ejectors.

Instrument transfer

This should be smooth, safe, unobtrusive and require a minimum amount of movement on the part of the operator (**5.27**). Transfer of instruments should take place in the so-called transfer zones. Most instruments may be transferred in the region of the patient's chin (**5.28**). Instrument exchange becomes important during the obturation phase of root canal treatment, when the system of parallel transfer can be employed to advantage (**5.29**), as it allows the alternate exchange of spreading instrument and accessory cones to be accomplished speedily.

The patient

Education and information

All treatment should be fully explained to the patient before any is carried out. Patients who understand the treatment that they are about to undergo will be less anxious, easier to handle and more appreciative. Information may be made available in the waiting room – patients are most receptive in the few minutes before their appointment – in the form of leaflets produced by the practice or commercially available (**5.30**). In the clinical area the dentist should use models which make the procedures easier to explain: a patient will understand the radiographs better if he or she is given a basic knowledge of anatomy.

Most (if not all) patients attending the dental practice for the first time will be nervous. A calm, pleasant manner, showing that you are concerned about the patient's welfare, will make treatment easier for both patient and operator.

Anaesthesia and analgesia

Pain control is a most important aspect of endodontic procedures: the patient's confidence will be gained if they undergo a painless procedure. *Analgesia* removes pain sensation without

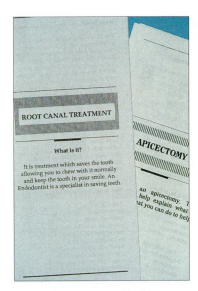

5.30 Sample patient education leaflets

loss of tactile sense. *Anaesthesia* results in complete loss of all sensation, and may be induced locally or generally (when the patient will lose consciousness). In dentistry analgesia is usually all that is required because we wish merely to remove pain; occasionally, with an injection, we may achieve anaesthesia but this is surplus to requirements. Local anaesthesia is more accurately described as local analgesia.

Before treatment begins the type of analgesia or anaesthesia must be decided. Guidelines for this decision are given below.

Routine root canal treatment

Regional or infiltration local analgesia is all that is necessary.

Acute hyperaemic pulp

Regional or infiltration analgesia, followed by additional local analgesic (for details see Chapter 13).

Anxious patient

General anaesthesia in the dental chair is governed by strict regulations (Poswillo report, 1992), which have restricted its use in general dental practice. However, the vast majority of anxious patients may be managed satisfactorily by one or more of the following methods.

Oral sedation

A suitable benzodiazepine may be prescribed for the night before and/or one hour preoperatively. Many drugs are available for this purpose and the operator is advised to consult the relevant text books for correct dosage, contraindications, precautions and other important data. For all types of sedation male operators must be accompanied by an escort when treating female patients, and all patients must be accompanied home by a responsible adult.

Intravenous sedation

This is usually administered by an anaesthetist. The technique involves using various drugs – most common among which are the benzodiazepines such as diazepam and midazolam – to produce a state of quiet calm tranquillity. Analgesics are occasionally given in addition to a benzodiazepine to produce a finer quality of sedation and to raise the pain threshold; this is particularly useful in patients in whom inferior dental blocks do not 'take' very well. Patients with medical conditions such as Parkinson's disease or epilepsy can be controlled well with this technique. Antisialogogues such as atropine may be added to the sedation to produce a dry field.

Intravenous sedation, which may be used for any endodontic procedure, has a far quicker recovery time than general anaesthesia and is more suitable for the ambulatory patient.

Relative analgesia

This is a safe, easy technique using varying quantities of a mixture of nitrous oxide (N_2O) and oxygen (O_2) administered via a nasal mask. However, difficulties may arise in that the nose piece may hinder the operator in root treatment and endodontic surgery in the maxillary incisal region.

Gag reflex

In mild cases once the rubber dam is applied treatment may be carried out routinely with local analgesia as the patient has an effective barrier and is unaware of instruments or fingers in his or her mouth. In the more severe cases intravenous sedation or relative analgesia will control the reflex.

Endodontic surgery

If more than two teeth are to be apicected intravenous sedation may be necessary.

Medication

Following treatment the patient should be advised to take a suitable analgesic for any postoperative pain. There is some evidence to show that postoperative pain can be reduced by taking a non-steroidal anti-inflammatory drug 1 hour *before* treatment.

Patients who are already on medication must be advised of any change during the endodontic treatment. The patient's medical adviser should be contacted if it is thought necessary to alter the dosage or to stop a drug that has been prescribed (for example warfarin or steroid therapy).

Patients requiring antibiotic cover

Patients at risk from infective endocarditis (**Table 5.1**) should be given antibiotic cover (see also Chapter 2). Some patients (those who have already suffered an attack of infective endocarditis or require a general anaesthetic and are either allergic to penicillin or have already had more than one course of penicillin in the previous month) are at special risk and must be referred to hospital for endodontic treatment.

All patients at risk should be encouraged to maintain a high degree of oral health to reduce the severity of possible bacteraemias. Patients who require endodontic surgery should be advised to take a chlorhexidine mouthwash, starting 24 hours before surgery and continuing for 4–5 days afterwards.

Patients with HIV/HBV

Every patient must be considered a possible source of infection from herpes simplex 1 and 2, HBV and HIV. Barrier protection, gloves, mask and protective spectacles should always be worn by the operator during treatment and gloves should be changed after each patient. The risks of transmission of HBV during dental treatment are well known, but HIV is less easily transmitted. By providing a physical barrier between the operating site and the patient's saliva, a rubber dam reduces the contaminated aerosol effect and therefore the risk of infection. All health workers should receive regular vaccination against hepatitis B. Well HIV-positive patients may be treated in general dental practice, but if they show evidence of ill health or oral manifestations of disease then they should be referred to special units for advice or treatment.

The tooth

Removal of caries/restorations

Any carious, leaking or suspect restorations must be removed. The amalgam illustrated (**5.31**) is obviously leaking and should be removed. When a bridge abutment requires root canal treatment the bridge should always be checked to see if it has been decemented by hooking a Briault probe under the pontic, near the retainer, and applying pressure to remove the bridge: bubbles around the retainer margins and a slight sucking noise indicate decementation. In the case illustrated (**5.32**, **5.33**) the bridge must be removed.

Table 5.1 Infective endocarditis: symtoms seen in patients at risk

History of infective endocarditis
Ventricular septal defect
Patent ductus arteriosus
Coarctation of the aorta
Prosthetic heart valve
Rheumatic heart disease
Degenerative valve disease
Persistent heart murmur
Atrial septal defect repaired with a patch

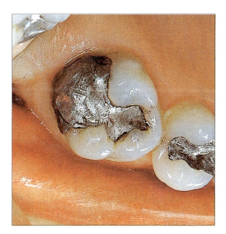

5.31 Leaking amalgam

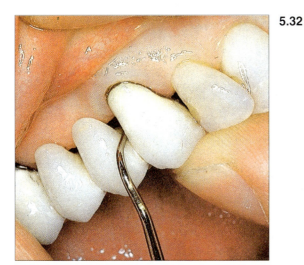

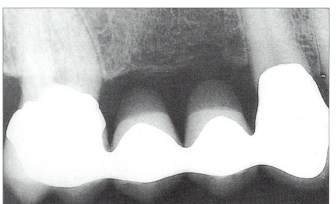

5.32, 5.33 Decemented bridge

Provisional restoration of broken-down teeth

Broken-down teeth should be restored sufficiently to allow the placement of a rubber dam but complete restoration of the tooth before root treatment is unnecessary, time consuming, and may jeopardize the final restoration. The best possible view of the floor of the pulp chamber is seen in severely broken-down teeth (**5.34**).

It is usually possible to place a clamp on a broken-down tooth but on rare occasions some build-up or a crown lengthening procedure is required to remove excess tissue and expose the margins of the tooth. Figure **5.35** shows proliferative gingival tissue around the root face of a lateral incisor. Electrosurgery (**5.36**) was used in this case to remove the tissue so that the clamp could be placed (**5.37, 5.38**). Figure **5.39** shows the electrosurgical tip used.

If a clamp cannot be placed because of the loss of tooth substance the tooth may be built up with a restorative material such as a light-cured composite to allow clamp placement and temporary filling. Another option is to fit and cement a copper band or steel orthodontic band around the tooth but this has the disadvantage that the band must fit accurately or the attachment apparatus may be damaged. Where possible, the band must be left clear of the gingival margin (**5.40, 5.41**). The case illustrated (**5.42**) shows a first mandibular molar with a fracture line in both the distal and buccal walls of the crown. A copper band was selected and trimmed with a stone to fit (**5.43, 5.44**), cotton wool placed in the pulp chamber with softened stick gutta percha over the top, and the band cemented.

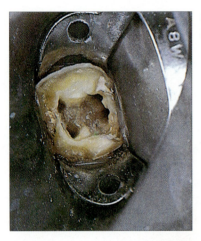

5.34 Best possible access

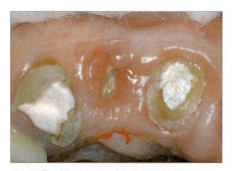

5.35 Proliferative gingival tissue

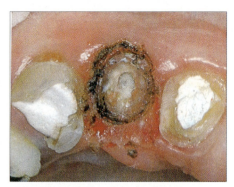

5.36 Electrosurgery completed

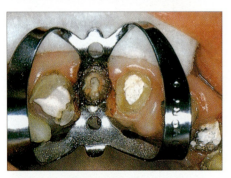

5.37 Clamp in position

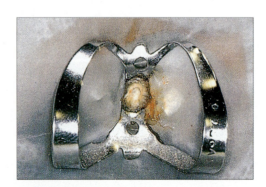

5.38 Rubber dam in place

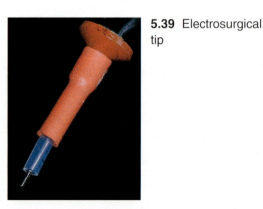

5.39 Electrosurgical tip

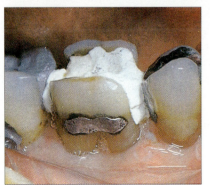

5.40

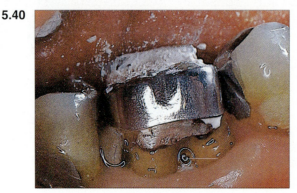

5.41

5.40, 5.41 Band left clear of gingival margin

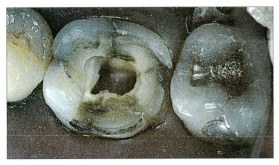

5.42 Fractured tooth

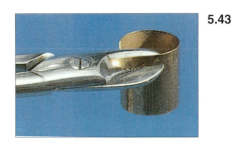 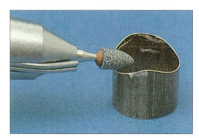

5.43, 5.44 Trimming a copper band

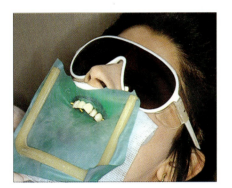

5.45 Rubber dam and protective spectacles

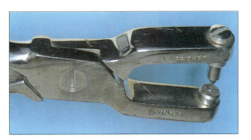

5.46 Rubber dam punch

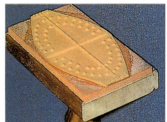

5.47, 5.48 Rubber dam stamp

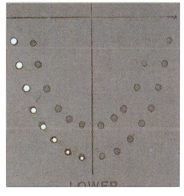

Tissue management

There are several reasons why the periodontal tissues should receive attention before root treatment, including removing excess tissue to allow the placement of a rubber dam. The periodontal health around the tooth margin is examined, any inflammation pointed out to the patient and oral hygiene instruction given. Root canal treatment will be followed by a permanent restoration, often a crown, and it is important to establish good gingival health. Sometimes the contact between a restoration in the tooth and the proximal tooth is poor, and it may be necessary to change the restoration to prevent periodontal breakdown in susceptible patients. Pockets around the tooth should be measured and noted; in molars the furcation area should be probed for defects.

Isolation using a rubber dam and other devices

A rubber dam provides the best protection of the oropharynx and should be used for root canal treatment (**5.45**). The use of a rubber dam also makes root canal treatment easier and quicker, allows better visual access, prevents irrigating fluids from entering the mouth and prevents the patient's tongue and saliva from contaminating the canal system.

Rubber dam kit

The rubber dam is manufactured in squares of two sizes: 130 and 150 mm. The larger square is the most convenient for endodontics. A variety of thicknesses are available; heavy (0.25 mm) or extra heavy (0.3 mm) are the least likely to tear.

The *punch* (**5.46**) may be used to make several differently sized holes in the dam but only one medium-sized hole is necessary. If several teeth need to be isolated a *rubber stamp* can be used to locate the holes precisely (**5.47, 5.48**).

Forceps (**5.49**) allow clamps to be placed and removed from teeth. The beaks should be deep enough to allow the clamp to be fitted around the gingival margin in a small mouth.

Frames (**5.50**) should be wide enough to provide good access with good retaining spikes for the dam.

Clamps are manufactured in a wide variety of shapes and sizes to suit different teeth and situations. The choice of which one to select depends largely on personal preference. Root canal treatment requires only a small number of clamps. The four Ivory clamps shown in **5.51** are sufficient to cover most situations.

Applying the dam

Root canal treatment usually requires isolation of a single tooth. Two methods are established for placing the dam. The first of these is to fit the clamp so that all four jaws are in contact with the tooth (**5.52**, **5.53**), punch one or two holes together, then stretch the dam over the clamp bow and the tooth (**5.54**). The second method is to insert the wings of the clamp into a hole punched in the dam, then to carry the dam and clamp to the mouth and place them over the tooth (**5.55**); the dam is then slipped off the wings so that it lies around the neck of the tooth.

In the anterior part of the mouth the dam may be fitted without clamps (**5.56**) using rubber or wooden wedges.

Other devices

Many other devices are used to protect the oropharynx but none is as effective as the rubber dam. One of the most popular is the parachute chain (**5.57**) but this method is cumbersome and wastes time because it necessitates application of the chain each time the instrument is changed. A handle called the Endogrip is also used: it has a similar attachment device at one end for the hand file but is also awkward to use. The safest alternative to a rubber dam is to place the file in a handpiece (see Chapter 7) but even using cotton wool rolls in the buccal and lingual sulci it is difficult to prevent saliva from contaminating the canal system. In addition, the benefit of the rubber dam retracting the soft tissues is lost, which means that visual access is poor.

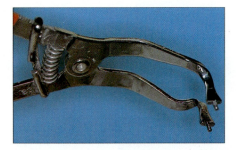

5.49 Rubber dam forceps

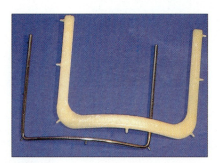

5.50 Rubber dam frames

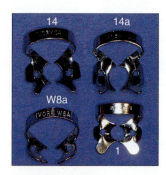

5.51 Ivory clamps, clockwise from top left: 14 (small and medium-sized molars), 14a (large molars), 1 (premolars), W8a (broken-down molars)

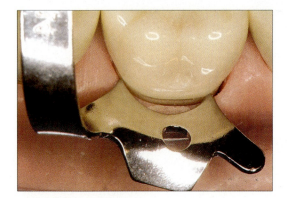

5.52 Clamp placed onto tooth

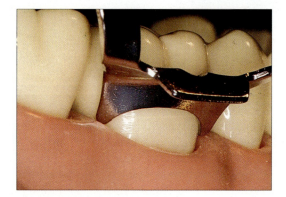

5.53 Clamp in position

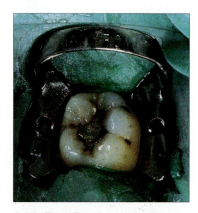

5.54 Dam fitted over tooth

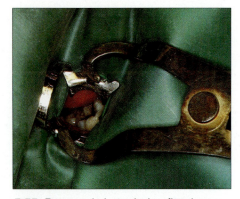

5.55 Dam and clamp being fitted over tooth together

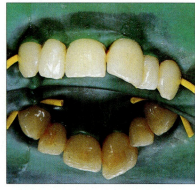

5.56 Dam retained with rubber wedges

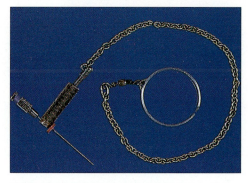

5.57 Safety chain (parachute)

6 Root canal morphology

Canal configurations

Many of the problems encountered in root treatment may be directly attributed to an inadequate understanding of the canal morphology of teeth. It is important to try to develop a visual picture of the expected locations and numbers of canals in a particular tooth before treatment and it may be necessary to take more than one preoperative paralleling radiograph to gain as much information as possible.

The pulp canal system is complex and canals may branch, divide and rejoin and present forms that are considerably more involved than many textbooks of anatomy would lead us to believe. Vertucci (1984)[1] identified eight separate pulp space configurations (**6.1**) for any single root and further configurations have been added to the complexities since then. The complex nature of the gross morphology of pulp is typified by the example of a cleared molar specimen (**6.2**).

Pulp space

A number of general comments, which have a significant bearing on the practice of endodontics, can be made about pulp canals.

Roots and root canals are rarely straight even when they appear so radiographically (**6.3–6.5**). The buccal view of the lateral incisor does not indicate the degree of curvature evident when the tooth is viewed in a mesiodistal direction.

Because roots tend to be broader buccolingually than they are mesiodistally, pulps follow the same proportions and tend to take on the outline of the root (**6.6**). The volume occupied by the pulp is also much greater than the normal buccal view might suggest (**6.7**). Fanibunda (1986)[2] calculated the mean volumes of ten teeth of each tooth type, the results of which (**Table 6.1**) illustrate the large volumes occupied by dental pulps, particularly in molar teeth.

Table 6.1 Mean volume and standard deviation (SD) of dental pulp cavities

Tooth type	Maxillary		Mandibular	
	Mean vol (mm³)	SD	Mean vol. (mm³)	SD
Central incisor	12.4	3.3	6.1	2.5
Lateral incisor	11.4	4.6	7.1	2.1
Canine	14.7	4.8	14.2	5.4
First premolar	18.2	5.1	14.9	5.7
Second premolar	16.5	4.2	14.9	6.3
First molar	68.2	21.4	52.5	8.5
Second molar	44.3	29.7	32.9	8.4
Third molar	22.6	3.3	31.1	11.2

Some canals become completely separated to form two distinct canals (**6.8**); others have fin-like grooves in their walls (**6.9**).

The diameter of the root canal decreases towards the apex and is narrowest 0–1.5 mm from the apical foramen. This point is called the *apical constriction*, and may be round, oval or serrated. From this point the canal widens out into the apical foramen, which may open onto the root surface anywhere between 0 and 3 mm from the root apex (**6.10**).

Lateral and accessory canals

These occur in the middle and coronal thirds of 59–76% of molars.[3,4] They occur anywhere along the length of any root and vary in size from a few microns in width to the size of a main canal. These canals are demonstrated in histological sections (**6.11**), cleared teeth (**6.12, 6.13**) and clinical radiographs (**6.14**). The blood vessels passing through these canals contribute to the vascular system of the pulp and allow interchange of inflammatory breakdown products between the pulp and the

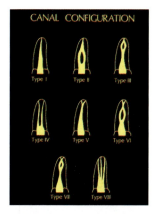

6.1 Pulp space configurations

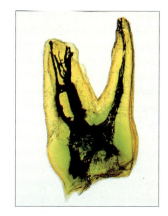

6.2 Cleared molar

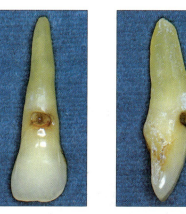

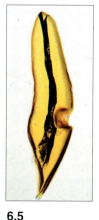

6.3   6.4   6.5

6.3–6.5 Buccal and approximal views of an incisor

periodontal tissues – which influences the outcome of endodontic treatment and the maintenance of periodontal health.

Sclerosed canals

The dental pulp reacts to injury by laying down secondary or irritational dentine, reducing the volume of the pulp space and leading to an apparent lack of canals (**6.15**). Canals gradually decrease in size with age. Pulps age, not only with the passage of time, but also under the stimulus of function and chronic irritation. The rate at which pulps lay down secondary dentine and decrease in volume varies among teeth and patients. No canal becomes completely sclerosed, but pulp chambers and the coronal portions of root canals often become obliterated, leaving a patent apical portion within which the remaining pulp becomes necrotic or infected. Such canals are difficult to locate and treat (**6.16**).

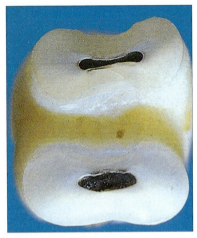

6.6 Root in cross-section

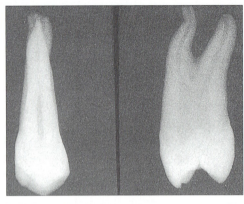

6.7 Buccal and approximal views of a pulp space

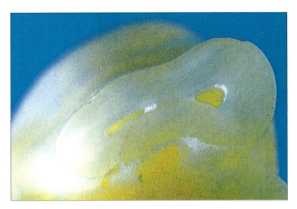

6.8 Cross-section of two canals

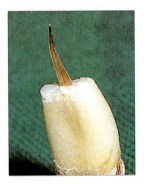

6.9 Pulp fin

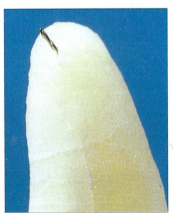

6.10 Instrument piercing apical foramen

6.11 Histological section, showing lateral canal

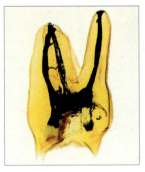

6.12

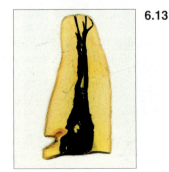

6.13

6.12, 6.13 Cleared teeth demonstrating lateral canals

Average values

A knowledge of the average lengths of teeth will help determine the depth of insertion of working length instruments (**Table 6.2**). A working understanding of the percentage of teeth that might contain two canals in one root also helps to establish the possible configurations of teeth requiring treatment (**Table 6.3**). However, the information presented may not be wholly applicable to teeth in patients of non-Caucasian origin: practitioners who treat negroid and mongoloid populations are aware that these values do not coincide with their own clinical experiences.

Anatomical variations of individual teeth

Maxillary incisors

It is extremely rare for these teeth to have more than one root or root canal. The canal is tapering in shape, with an irregular triangular or oval cross-section cervically which gradually becomes round towards the apex. Generally there is very little apical curvature in central incisors, and where it is present it is either distal or labial (**6.17**). The apex of lateral incisors is often curved, generally in a distopalatal direction (**6.18**).

Table 6.2 Average lengths of teeth (mm)

	Maxillary	Mandibular
Central incisor	22.5	20.7
Lateral incisor	22.0	21.1
Canine	26.5	25.6
First premolar	20.6	21.6
Second premolar	21.5	22.3
First molar	20.8	21.0
Second molar	20.0	19.8

From Black[5]

Table 6.3 Root configuration frequencies. Percentage of teeth containing two canals in one root.

	Mandible	Maxilla
Central and lateral incisors	40	Rare
Canine	18	Rare
First premolar	23	84*
Second premolar	6	40
First molar		
Mesial root	87	Mesiobuccal root 1st and 2nd molars 60
Distal root	30	
Second molar		
Mesial root	87	
Distal root	5	

*62% have two separate roots

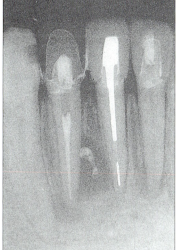

6.14 Lateral canal in a filled tooth

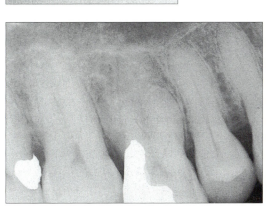

6.15 Sclerosed tooth

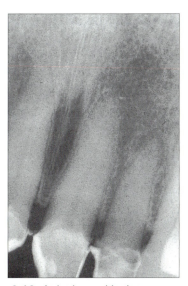

6.16 Apical canal lesion

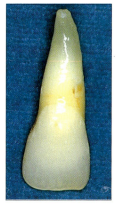

6.17 Apical curvature in a central incisor

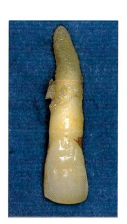

6.18 Apical curvature in a lateral incisor

Maxillary canines

The root is wide labiopalatally and the canal does not begin to become round in cross-section until the apical third, where there may be a distal curve (**6.19**). The apical constriction is not as well defined as in the incisors. The canal in the coronal third often has a bulge (**6.20**).

Maxillary first premolars

The tooth is generally considered to be two-rooted with two canals (**6.21, 6.22**): they are single-rooted in less than 40% of teeth of Caucasians, but in more than 60% of teeth of mongoloid origin. Irrespective of race the teeth tend to have two canals. Occasionally these teeth have three roots and three root canals, two buccal and one palatal (**6.23**).

Maxillary second premolars

These tend to be single-rooted with a single canal, which is wide in a buccolingual direction (**6.24, 6.25**). Two canals occur in 25% of cases, when the floor of the pulp chamber extends well below the cervical level.

Maxillary first molars

These teeth are generally three-rooted with four root canals, the additional canal being located in the mesiobuccal root (**6.26**) in over 60% of cases. The minor mesiobuccal canal lies on a line joining the major mesiobuccal and palatal canal orifices (**6.27**). As both mesiobuccal canals lie in a buccopalatal plane they are often superimposed on the preoperative radiograph. The mesiobuccal root often curves distopalatally in the apical third of the root

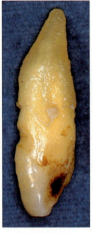

6.19 Maxillary canine

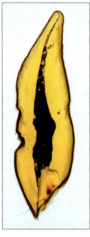

6.20 Maxillary canine bulge

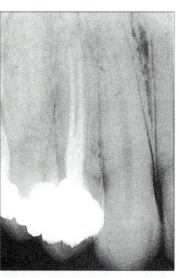

6.21 Radiograph of maxillary first premolar

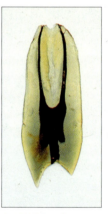

6.22 Maxillary first premolar

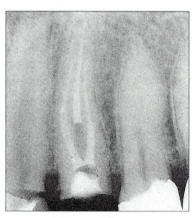

6.23 Maxillary first premolar with three canals

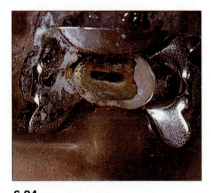

6.24

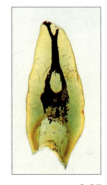

6.25

6.24, 6.25 Maxillary second premolar

6.26 Maxillary first molar with a second mesiobuccal canal

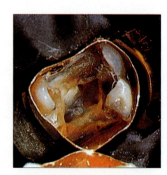

6.27 Mesiobuccal canal viewed from the pulp floor

(**6.28**). The distobuccal canal is the shortest of the three canals and leaves the pulp chamber in a distal direction but may curve mesially in the apical half of the root. The palatal canal is the largest and longest of the canals and tends to curve buccally in the apical 4–5 mm (**6.29**). This curvature is not apparent on the radiograph. The variable anatomy of this tooth extends to extra roots (**6.30**) as well as extra canals.

Maxillary second molars

The situation in these teeth is a small replica of the first molar. The roots are less divergent and root fusion is much more frequent than in the maxillary first molar (**6.31**), and the buccal canal orifices tend to be closer together. Teeth with three roots and three canals are prevalent.

Maxillary third molars

The root form and canal anatomy is highly variable. It may possess three roots but more often fusion occurs and only one or two canals are evident (**6.32, 6.33**).

Mandibular incisors

Over 40% of these teeth have two canals, which usually join in the apical third (**6.34**). The highest recorded figure for two separate apical foramina is 5.5%. In teeth with a single root canal the canal is usually straight but may curve to the distal (and less often to the labial) side. The grooving present on the mesial and distal aspects of the roots of these teeth (**6.35**) makes them susceptible to perforation if over-instrumented.

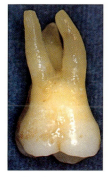

6.28 Curved mesiobuccal root

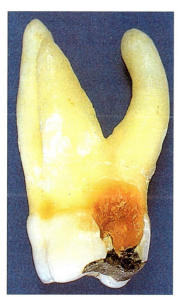

6.29 Curved palatal root

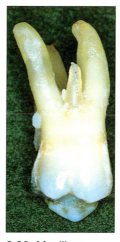

6.30 Maxillary molar with an extra root

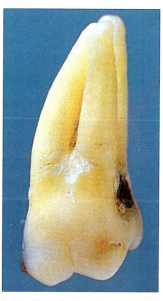

6.31 Root fusion in a maxillary second molar

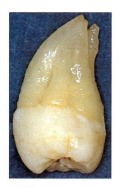

6.32

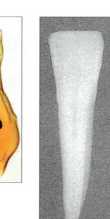

6.33

6.32, 6.33 Cleared maxillary third molar

6.34 Mandibular incisor with two canals

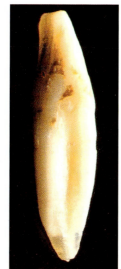

6.35 Approximal groove in a mandibular incisor

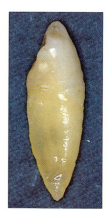

6.36 Mandibular canine

Mandibular canines

The mandibular canine resembles the maxillary canine, although its dimensions are smaller (**6.36**). It rarely has two roots and the mean frequency of two canals is in the order of 14% (**6.37**); only 6% have two separate apical foramina.

Mandibular first premolars

These teeth occasionally present with a division of roots in the apical half (**6.38**). Up to one-third of these teeth demonstrate division of canals in the apical half of the root, where the canals tend to remain separate and produce separate apical foramina. Three canals appear in less than 2% of these teeth.

Mandibular second premolars

The frequency of second canals in these teeth (**6.39**) is much lower than in the first premolars. The single canal is wide in a buccolingual direction, with a tendency to curve to the distal. There is a clinical impression of a high frequency of lateral canals (**6.40**).

Mandibular first molars

These teeth usually have two roots (**6.41**): in a mongoloid variation (which may occur in over 40% of such teeth) a supernumerary distolingual root is present (**6.42, 6.43**). The two-rooted molar usually has a canal configuration of three canals; two canals in the mesial root and one in the distal root (**6.44**). There is only one apical foramen in the mesial root in 45% of cases. The single distal canal is usually larger and more oval in cross-section and has a tendency to emerge on the distal side of the root surface short of the anatomical apex (**6.45**). More than 25% of the distal roots have two canals, half of which have two separate apical foramina (**6.46**). The frequency of second distal canals is higher in mongoloid teeth, and specimens with five canals have been observed (**6.47**). The mesiobuccal canal is the most difficult canal to instrument because of its tortuous path. It leaves the pulp chamber in a mesial direction, which alters to a distal direction in the middle of the root. When a second distolingual canal is present it has a tendency to curve towards the buccal.

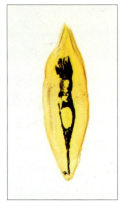

6.37 Mandibular canine with two canals

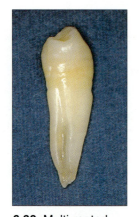

6.38 Multi-rooted mandibular first premolar

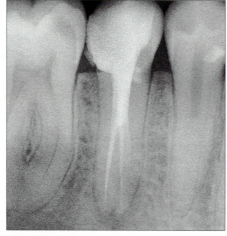

6.39 Root-filled mandibular second premolar with multiple canals

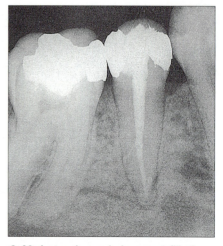

6.40 Lateral canals in a root-filled mandibular second premolar

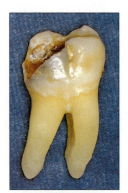

6.41 Mandibular first molar

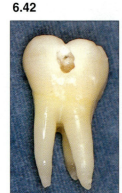 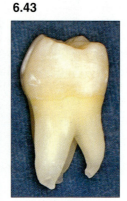

6.42, 6.43 Three-rooted mandibular first molar

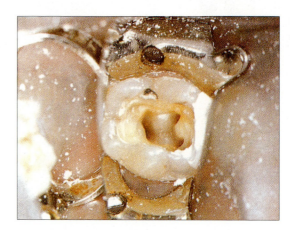

6.44 The pulpal floor of a mandibular first molar

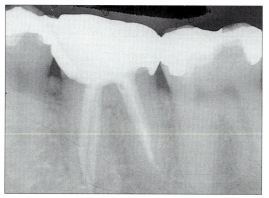

6.45 Apical foramen exiting from the distal root surface

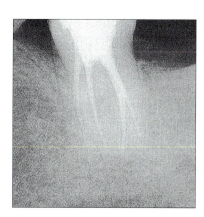

6.46 Mandibular first molar with four canals and apical foramina

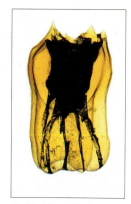

6.47 Mandibular first molar with five canals

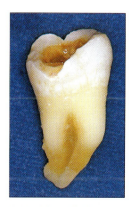

6.48 Mandibular second molar with fused roots

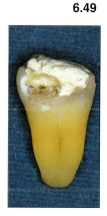

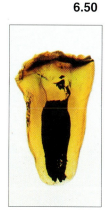

6.49, 6.50 Mandibular second molar with one canal

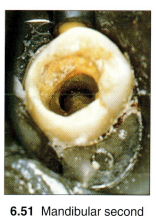

6.51 Mandibular second molar with a C-shaped canal

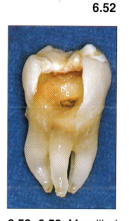

6.52, 6.53 Mandibular third molar with three roots

6.54, 6.55 Mandibular third molar with root fusion

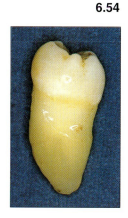

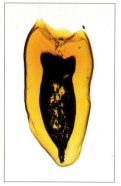

Mandibular second molars

In caucasoid teeth the mesial root has two (occasionally one) canals and the distal root usually has only one canal. The roots tend to be close together or even fused (**6.48**). Rarely only one canal is present when both roots are fused (**6.49, 6.50**). In mongoloid teeth the fusion of roots is common and where roots are incompletely separated interconnections are likely, giving rise to the C-shaped canal (**6.51**).

Mandibular third molars

The roots and pulp canals of these teeth tend to be short and poorly developed (**6.52, 6.53**). The anatomy tends to vary, and where root fusion exists the canals also fuse (**6.54, 6.55**).

7 Preparation of the root canal

Principles of canal preparation

In Chapter 1 it was concluded that the treatment of choice for periapical disease is elimination of microorganisms and their products from the root canal system. Micro-organisms may be found in suspension in the root canal or colonizing canal walls and dentinal tubules to a variable degree up to the apical foramen.

The complexity of root canal systems makes it impossible to sterilize them. Fortunately, in most cases of root canal treatment a reduction in the microbial content of canal systems is sufficient to promote periradicular healing; in other cases healing may be due to an altered and less pathogenic residual flora. Microbes and their products may be removed by mechanical or chemical means.

In the mechanical method, metallic instruments of graded sizes are used to remove intracanal dentine together with micro-organisms. The method largely relies on the ability to plane a significant surface area of the walls of the root canal system. This requires removal of a substantial amount of dentine and could weaken the root (7.1).

Micro-organisms may also be destroyed by antibacterial fluids or irrigants. The problems of this approach are twofold: (1) it may be difficult to ensure the irrigant penetrates to the narrow apical end and ramifications of the root canal system; (2) even if penetration is achieved, the multilayered, three-dimensional nature of microbial colonies and their polysaccharide matrix may protect the deeper layers of organisms (7.2). The first problem can be overcome by enlarging the root canal sufficiently to allow the irrigant to the apical end using a large narrow gauge hypodermic needle or endosonics. The second problem may be overcome by using a high enough concentration and volume of irrigant to prevent it becoming spent by chemical reaction with organic debris and organisms. This effect is enhanced by mechanical agitation of the irrigant with a file and frequent replenishment with fresh solution. In wide straight canals, minimal filing of canal walls is required, as the irrigant will reach most aspects (7.3).

The combined action of mechanical and chemical cleaning is more efficient than either method alone, and allows a more conservative canal preparation as reliance on dentine removal for decontamination is reduced. This is the chemomechanical method of canal preparation.

Canal preparation in teeth with vital pulps has similar but not identical aims. The concern in such teeth is to remove not micro-organisms but pulp tissue, which may become necrotic and infected (7.4). In the case shown, the uninstrumented apical portion of the distal canal has resulted in a periapical radiolucency. It is therefore useful if the selected irrigant both dissolves organic tissue and destroys microorganisms.

This chapter deals with the stages and attention to detail necessary to meet the desired objectives of canal preparation and reviews the advantages and disadvantages inherent in different techniques and instruments available.

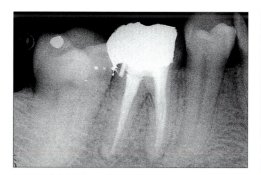

7.1 Widely flared canals

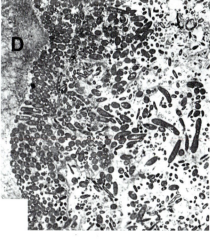

7.2 Multilayered nature of microbial colonies on root canal wall: D = dentine

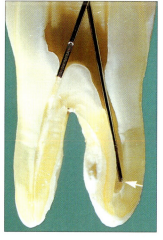

7.3 Deep penetration of irrigant needle in wide unprepared canal

7.4A & 7.4B Development of periradicular area around distal root following vital extirpation

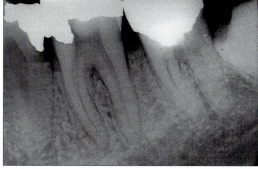

7.4A

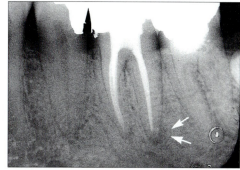

7.4B

Access cavities

Principles of cutting an access cavity

- To remove the roof of the pulp chamber so that the pulpal remnants can be removed and the canal entrances exposed (7.5, 7.6).
- To provide straight-line access to the first curve in the root canal (7.7).
- To avoid damage to the floor of the pulp chamber. This will avoid perforation of the pulp chamber floor and make it easier to locate the canal entrances (7.8, 7.9). The natural floor tends to guide an instrument into the canal orifice.
- To conserve as much tooth substance as possible to prevent weakening and fracture of the remaining enamel and dentine (7.10).
- To provide resistance form so that the temporary access cavity seal remains intact until the final restoration is placed (7.11, 7.12).

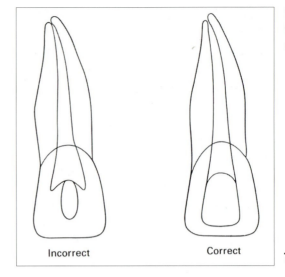

7.5, 7.6 Removing the roof of the pulp chamber

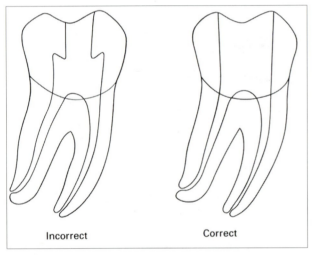

7.6

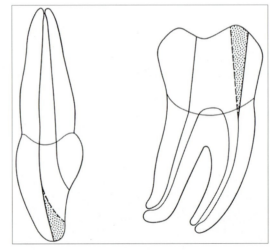

7.7 Straight line access

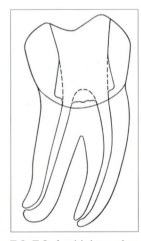

7.8, 7.9 Avoid damaging the pulp chamber floor

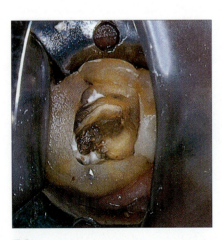

7.9

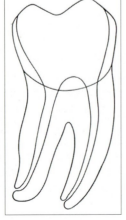

7.10 Conserve tooth substance (over prepared access shown)

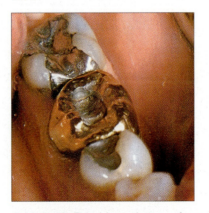

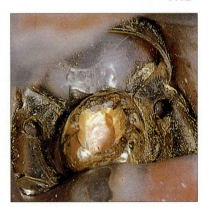

7.11, 7.12 Provide resistance form. In this case the amalgam has been depressed into the cavity

Cutting the cavity

Initial penetration is made with a tapered fissure tungsten-carbide bur aimed towards the largest part of the pulp chamber. When a porcelain crown is present a round diamond is used followed by a tungsten-carbide bur to cut through the metal beneath (7.13). Once the roof of the pulp chamber has been penetrated a safe-ended tapered diamond bur is used to reduce the risk of damaging the pulpal floor while the roof is removed. The depth of penetration is judged by holding the handpiece containing the bur against the preoperative radiograph (7.14). Older teeth have smaller pulp chambers and therefore require a smaller access cavity. Thought must be given to the type of permanent restoration that will be used afterwards as this will alter the shape and approach to cutting the access cavity; for example, in the case of an onlay the walls of the access may be reduced before the root treatment is carried out, or in the case of an anterior tooth which is to be crowned and is lingually inclined consider access from the buccal (7.15, 7.16). Figure 7.17 shows that straight-line access can be just as effective from the buccal aspect as from the lingual.

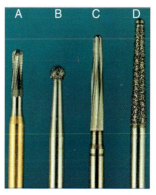

7.13 Diamond and tungsten access burs. A = Tungsten carbide dome fissure crosscut FG; B = round diamond FG; C = tungsten carbide tapered non-end cutting FG; D = tapered diamond non-end cutting FG

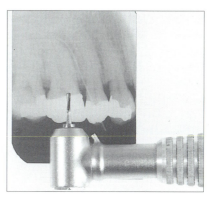

7.14 Judging access cavity depth

7.15, 7.16 Access cavities cut in buccal aspect of mandibular incisors

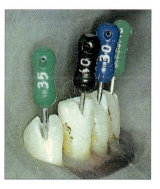

7.15

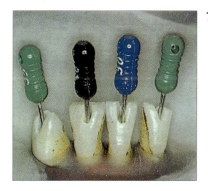

7.16

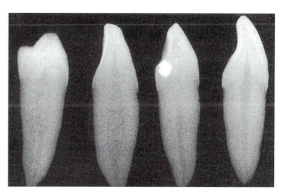

7.17 Access from either buccal or lingual aspect

7.18, 7.19 Maxillary central incisor

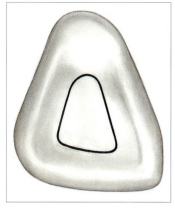

7.18

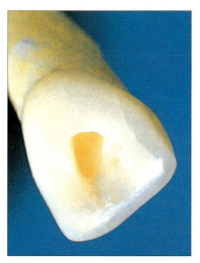

7.19

Outline shape

The outline shape of the access cavities are given in **7.18–7.37**. The size of the cavity is dictated by the size of the pulp chamber and will therefore tend to become smaller in older patients.

In anterior teeth straight-line access into the canals of incisors and canines means that the cavity must be cut high up on the tooth near the incisal edge. This type of access cavity will leave the cingulum intact, which provides the maximum retention for a full crown.

The shape of the pulp chamber, and therefore the access cavity, of the maxillary first molar is rhomboid due to a widening over the palatal canal orifice. The second and third molars show a mesiodistal flattening of the pulp chamber which also lies nearer the mesial aspect of the tooth.

The access to the mandibular first molar is also rhomboid in shape because the distal canal is either broad buccolingually or because there are two separate canals. The second and third molar access cavity is more triangular as there is usually only one distal canal

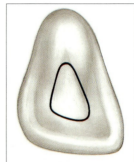

7.20 Maxillary lateral incisor

7.21

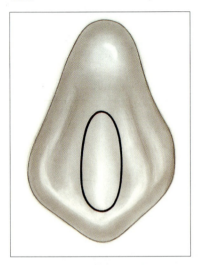

7.22

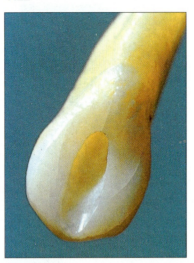

7.21, 7.22 Maxillary canine

7.23

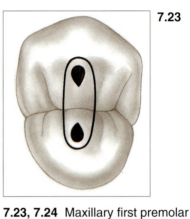

7.24

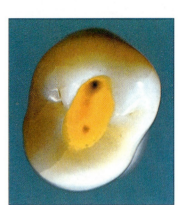

7.23, 7.24 Maxillary first premolar

7.25

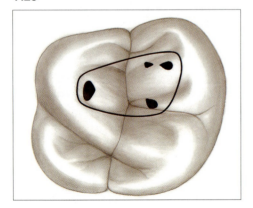

7.26

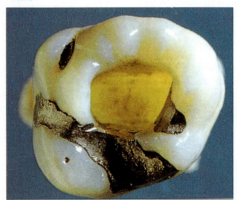

7.25, 7.26 Maxillary first molar

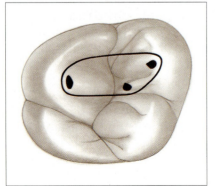

7.27 Maxillary second molar

7.28

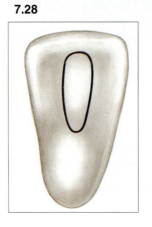

7.29

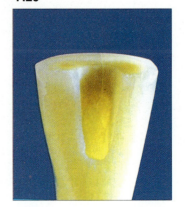

7.28, 7.29 Mandibular incisor

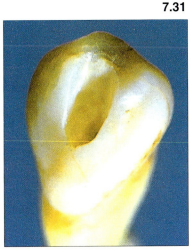

7.30, 7.31 Mandibular canine

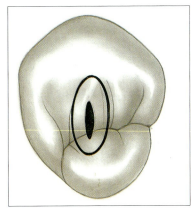

7.32 Mandibular first premolar

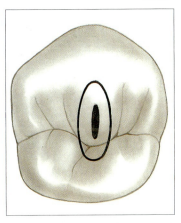

7.33, 7.34 Mandibular second premolar

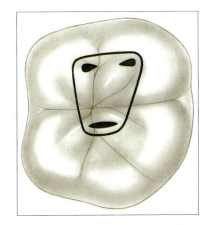

7.35 Mandibular first molar

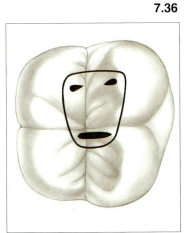

7.36, 7.37 Mandibular second molar

Determination of working length

Point of termination of canal preparation

Micro-organisms in a root canal system may extend to the apical foramen or constriction, where defence mechanisms of periapical tissues stem their progress. It is impossible to determine the extent of contamination of a root canal clinically; it is best to assume contamination up to the apical foramen in all cases with necrotic pulps and to clean the canal to this point (see **1.141**). It is safest to clean to the apical termination of root canals even in cases where the tooth is vital.

Clinical determination of position of apical constriction/foramen

This is not easy, but one approach is favoured. First, an estimate of the average length of tooth is made from a parallel preoperative periapical radiograph (**7.38**). A file is placed in the root canal 1–2 mm short of this estimated length, ensuring that a coronal reference point is selected that is reproducible and not part of a portion of tooth or restorative material (which is likely to break off). The file should be large enough to be visible on a radiograph (e.g. size 10). A parallel view radiograph is then taken (**7.39**). In teeth with multiple canals, diagnostic files should be placed in all canals and a single, angled view taken to minimize radiation (7.40). Canals may exit on the root surface at a variable distance and position from the root tip and it is impossible to judge the position of apical foramina satisfactorily from radiographs (7.41, 7.42). This pair of photographs shows three roots, with files which appear flush with the radiographic root tip but which are actually extended past the apical foramina. Figures 7.43 and 7.44 show a case taken from a clinical study in which a cemented file that is apparently flush with the root tip is actually extended well beyond the apical foramen. An average distance of 1 mm short of the radiographic apex is widely accepted as a reasonable estimate of the terminal position of the canal, but this may be inaccurate by up to 3.0 mm (7.45). Some clinicians believe that working length estimation can be aided by feeling an apical constriction using a file; however, this is a subjective assessment.

Although the working length is often taken to be 1 mm short of the radiographic apex, it should be shortened if there is apical root resorption or if the root tip is very narrow. In the case of resorption this is because the canal exit may be 'blunderbuss'

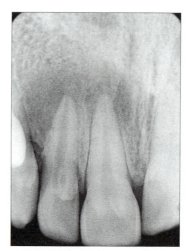

7.38 Preoperative parallel view radiograph

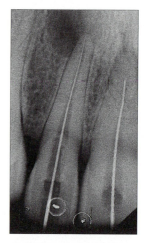

7.39 Periapical radiograph with diagnostic files

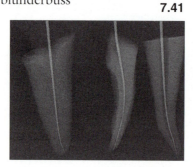

7.40 Angled periapical radiograph with diagnostic files

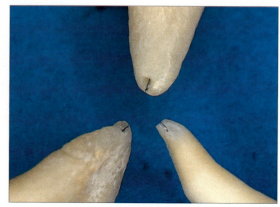

7.41, 7.42 Discrepancy between radiographic images of files and reality in relation to the root apex

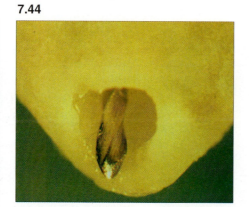

7.43, 7.44 Discrepancy between radiographic images and reality (taken from a clinical study)

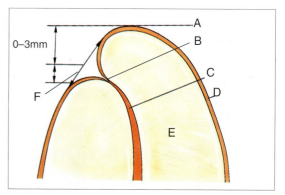

7.45 Relationship between root tip, apical foramen and apical constriction: A = root apex; B = apical constriction; C = root canal; D = cementum; E = dentine; F = apical foramen

shaped and allow extrusion of endodontic materials (**7.46, 7.47**); in a narrow root tip it is because perforation may occur if the root is prepared to a significant diameter (**7.48, 7.49**), especially in roots with a sudden apical curve (**7.50, 7.51**). In these cases, small flexible files may be used to the normal working length but any above size 25 should be used shorter.

Once a parallel radiograph of the tooth with diagnostic file(s) in the canal has been obtained, working length is calculated.

1. If the above sequence has been followed, in most cases the tip of the file will be short of the radiographic apex. This length is accepted as the working length if the distance is within 1 mm (as in the lateral incisor: **7.52**). If the distance is greater than 1 mm, then the distance between the file tip and the radiographic apex should be measured and 1 mm subtracted from this measurement (as in the central incisor: **7.52**). This figure is added to the length of the diagnostic file to give the working length (**7.53, 7.54**).

2. In some cases the file may be longer than the radiographic apex, in which case the distance between the file tip and a point 1 mm short of the radiographic apex should be measured (**7.55, 7.56**). Subtracting this figure from the length of the diagnostic file will give the working length.

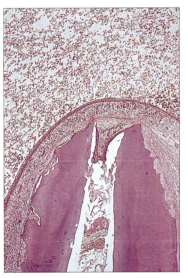

7.46 Apical root resorption: histological view

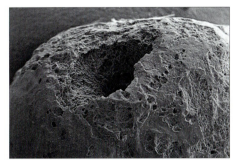

7.47 Apical root resorption: SEM view

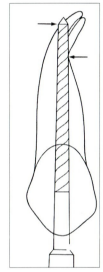

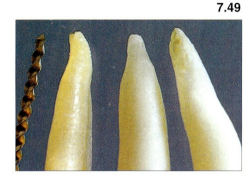

7.48, 7.49 Risk of apical perforation in narrow root tips

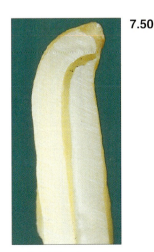

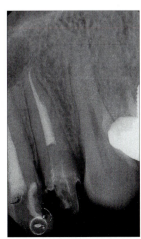

7.50, 7.51 Sudden apical curve in root canal

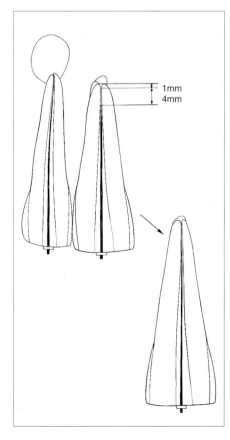

7.52 Diagram reproduced from **7.39**. Correct length in 2| accepted. Short length in is 1| corrected

Other methods have been recommended to estimate 'the required correction' if the file is not already within 1 mm of the apex. These include

1. using the formula

$$\frac{\text{length of file(real)}}{\text{length of file(apparent)}} = \frac{\text{length of canal(real)}}{\text{length of canal(apparent)}}$$

which makes the erroneous assumption that the image distortion is uniform.

2. A simpler method is to superimpose a millimetre grid on the radiograph (7.57), which overcomes the need for calculation, but is inaccurate if the radiograph has been bent during exposure. In addition, the grid may not be correctly oriented to the file for easy measurement and may obscure the tip (7.57).

3. Another method, which applies the same principle as in (2) but eliminates some of its disadvantages, uses graduations on the diagnostic file that are visible on a radiograph, for example the Endometric probe (7.58–7.60). This method gives accurate results but unfortunately the smallest file size available is No. 25.

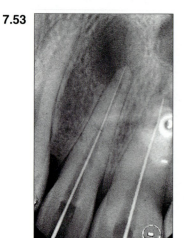
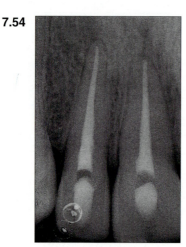
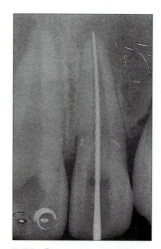
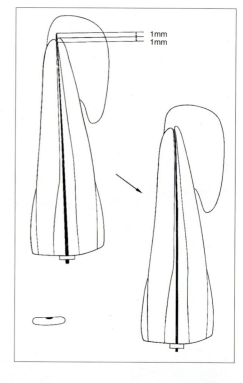

7.53, 7.54 Adjusted diagnostic files and final root fillings

7.55 Overextended file

7.56 Diagram reproduced from 7.55 shows corrected length

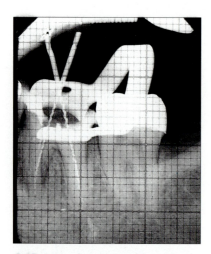
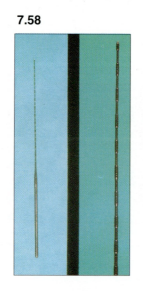
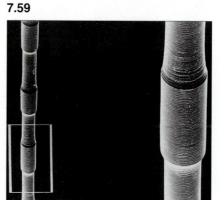
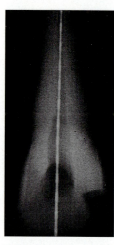

7.57 Use of radiographic grid

7.58, 59 Endometric probe at different magnifications (courtesy of Dr P. Dummer)

7.60 Radiograph of probe in tooth

Electronic apex locators

Electronic apex locators (7.61) enable indication of the true position of apical constriction/foramen, utilizing the fact that root canals, in common with other tubes with one end immersed in an electrolyte solution, exhibit certain electrical characteristics that are relatively constant.

The parameter of importance is the impedance of the root canal measured between a point along its length and the oral mucosa (7.62). Addition of electrolytes causes the impedance to drop and the gradient along the canal to decrease. The impedance value at the apical foramen under relatively dry conditions is taken as the impedance between the periodontal ligament and the oral mucosa measured via the root canal. This value (or an approximation) is used to calibrate commercial apex locators, but the impedance characteristics coronal to the apical foramen are not strictly calibrated. It is important therefore to note this terminal reading, and not one which indicates the file to be short of the apical foramen.

Apex locators work by applying an alternating current between two electrodes, one of which is attached to the file and the other via a clip to the lip or cheek mucosa (7.63, 7.64). The frequency of this current, which also influences impedance, is usually fixed in a given make of instrument but differs between makes. As the file is passed down the canal the apex locator measures the impedance and compares the value with its calibrated standard. A countdown scale indicates a 'zero' or 'apex' reading when the calibrated value is matched (7.65, 7.66). All currently available conventional apex locators use this principle but display the information differently (7.65–7.67).

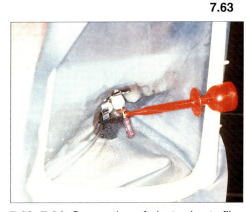

7.63, 7.64 Connection of electrodes to file and cheek

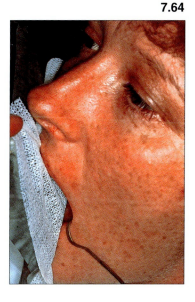

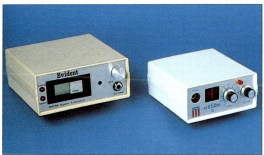

7.61 Electronic apex locators

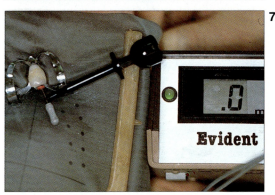

7.62 Electrical impedance of root canals at different distances from the apical foramen with water-filled and dry canals. Also shown is the average calibration of a typical apex locator

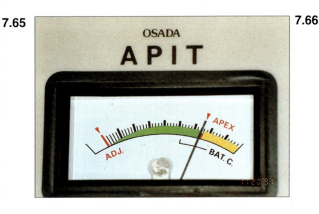

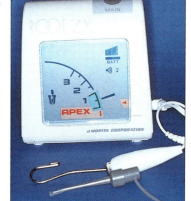

7.65–7.67 Apex indication in different electronic apex locators

The accuracy of different models of apex locators has been tested clinically and shows slightly variable results for the same apex locator in different studies and for different apex locators in the same study (**Table 7.1**). These differences may be attributed to many factors, including conditions of use and calibration of the instrument. Apex locators are reliable but not to the extent that they can be considered a substitute for radiographs. They help to reduce the number of radiographs necessary if there is uncertainty about the length but most cause problems in use, including short-circuiting if the file touches a metal restoration or if the canal contains excessive moisture or other electrolyte such as sodium hypochlorite. Manufacturers of the new generation of apex locators claim to have overcome the problem with electrolytes by measuring the impedance at two different current frequencies. One of these, the Apit (also known as Endex: **7.66**), uses the difference in impedance at two frequencies to calculate the position of the apical foramen: another (the Root ZX: **7.67**) compares the ratio of impedance at two frequencies to make a similar calculation. Initial studies appear to support the claims made for these instruments.

A diagnostic file is placed to the length indicated by the apex locator and a radiograph taken (**7.68**). The working length is then decided on the basis of the electrical, radiographic and tactile guidelines collectively.

Table 7.1 Accuracy of apex locators

Study	Locator used	Accuracy to foramen	Percentage accuracy
Inoue (1977)[1]	Sono Explorer	Foramen	92.9
		± 0.5	97.6
O'Neill (1974)[2]	Sono Explorer	Foramen	83.0
Blank et al. (1975)[3]	Sono Explorer	± 0.2	89.0
Bal and Chaudhary (1989)[4]	Neosono-D	Constriction	60
Stein et al. (1990)[5]	Neosono-D	± 0.5	57.5
Fouad et al. (1990)[6]	Neosono-D	± 0.5	70.0
	Exactapex	± 0.5	55.0
	Endocater	± 0.5	75.0
McDonald and Hovland (1990)[7]	Endocater	± 0.5	93.4
Keller et al. (1991)[8]	Endocater	± 0.5	51.5
Blank et al (1975)[3]	Endometer	± 0.2	85.0
Chanan et al. (1992)[9]	Endometer	± 0.5	92.0
Ferrand (1990)[10]	RCM	± 0.5	85.0
Ducoin (1991)[11]	RCM	± 0.5	62.0
Ricard et al (1991)[12]	RCM Mark II	± 0.5	86.5

Keeping instrumentation to the predetermined length

Two factors other than manual dexterity mitigate against instrumentation to the correct length: displacement of the stops on the files which designate length and loss of the reference point (either because of lack of care in noting it or because the original reference has been lost due to breakage of tooth or restoration). Some stops are more susceptible to displacement than others (**7.69–7.70**).

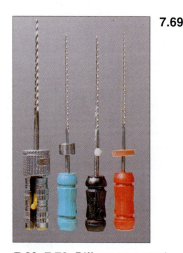

7.68 File placed to length indicated at 'zero' by apex locator

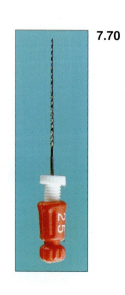

7.69, 7.70 Different types of stops

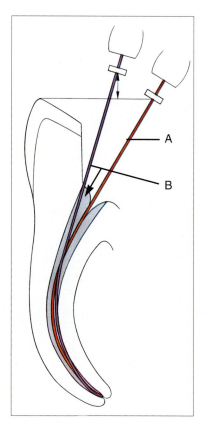

7.71 Change in length of canal as it is prepared: A = file before instrumentation; B = file after instrumentation

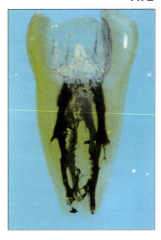

7.72 Cleared molar tooth showing complex canal system

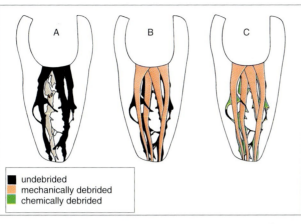

7.72, 7.73 Effect of original canal anatomy and canal preparation on the final shape of the root canal system. A = before preparation; B = after mechanical preparation; C = after chemical debridement

Legend: ■ undebrided; ▨ mechanically debrided; ▨ chemically debrided

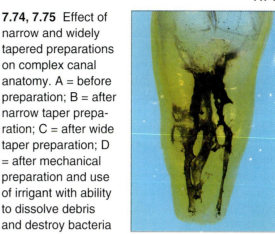

7.74, 7.75 Effect of narrow and widely tapered preparations on complex canal anatomy. A = before preparation; B = after narrow taper preparation; C = after wide taper preparation; D = after mechanical preparation and use of irrigant with ability to dissolve debris and destroy bacteria

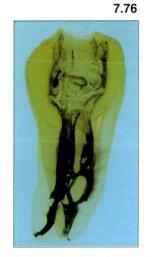

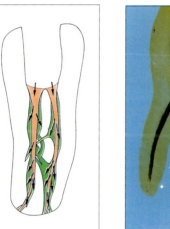

7.76, 7.77 Canal preparation as a radicular access

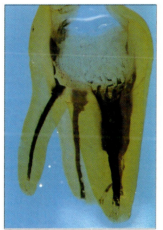

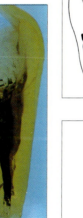

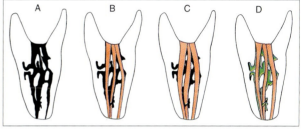

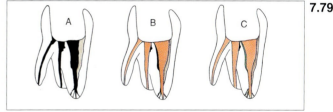

7.78, 7.79 Simple tubular canals encompassed by tapered canal preparation. A = before preparation; B = after mechanical preparation; C = after chemical irrigation with sodium hypochlorite

Changes in canal length during instrumentation

Canal length is often determined before preparation is commenced, but as a curved canal is prepared its effective length generally shortens (7.71). Most of the interferences that cause this change are confined to the coronal portion of the canal and it is possible to reduce this change in length by determining the definitive working length *after* coronal preparation has been completed.

Relationship between canal anatomy, its mechanically prepared shape and cleaning

It has traditionally been held that canals should be prepared by controlled dentine removal so as to produce a regular taper with the minimum diameter at the apical constriction and the maximum diameter at the coronal end, at the same time maintaining the original shape of the main canal as far as possible to preserve the strength and integrity of the root. The overall shape of the prepared canal is also dictated by its original shape (7.72, 7.73).

The width of the taper to which the canal should be prepared has been the subject of some debate. The choice is usually based on personal preference and individual clinical experience rather than on sound scientific rationale. Widely tapered canals may allow better irrigant penetration, better debridement and probably better obturation if using the cold lateral condensation technique (7.74, 7.75), but these benefits are achieved at the expense of root strength and possibly long-term survival of the tooth. Advocates of narrowly tapered canals argue that a taper that allows irrigant penetration using narrow needles is sufficient for debridement and that obturation of such canals can be satisfactorily achieved with the new thermoplasticized gutta percha techniques. Narrowly tapered preparations, if they allow adequate cleaning and obturation are more desirable as they do not compromise root strength.

The choice of irrigant and its mode of apical transport also influence the design of the canal preparation. Use of an irrigant that is unable to destroy micro-organisms and dissolve organic tissue would place greater reliance on mechanical removal of dentine for debridement, whereas one with the desired properties would reduce the need for excessive dentine removal during canal preparation. Selecting an obturation technique that does not require a predetermined canal shape allows the preparation to be influenced solely by the method of irrigant placement. The canal preparation may therefore be viewed as a *radicular access* to the canal system or simply as an *irrigation channel* (7.76, 7.77). In a new innovation, the Hydrodynamic method,[13] the irrigant is carried apically by a pulsed pressure change and no mechanical preparation is required but this system needs to be further researched and refined before clinical application.

The anatomy of root canal systems varies considerably (Chapter 6) and, although the width of the main canals is clinically determinable, their complexity is not predictable. In this section a series of canal systems has been selected to show the relationship between original shape, the mechanically prepared shape and the possible contributions of mechanical shaping and irrigation to cleaning.

Simple systems

When the canal system is simple, consisting of narrow main canals, preparation to a regular taper may entirely (or almost entirely) encompass the original canal system (7.78, 7.79). Figure 7.80 shows a root-filled tooth with regularly tapered canals completely encompassing the original canal anatomy. In such cases, cleaning may be achieved almost wholly by mechanical preparation with little reliance on the irrigant. The use of neutral irrigants such as water, saline or local anaesthetic will not compromise the outcome in such teeth.

In contrast, simple canal systems with irregular wide shapes such as canines, premolars (7.81) or incompletely formed roots (7.82), may not allow complete debridement solely by mechanical preparation. The lack of direct access for instrumentation places greater reliance on use of irrigants for cleaning. Access for irrigation is excellent in such teeth and therefore only minimal filing of the canal walls is necessary.

Mechanical debridement of teeth containing simple main canals with fins and ramifications extending off them would remove most microbes and organic tissue, but not from the accessory anatomy (7.83–7.86). Figure 7.87 shows a root-filled tooth in which the main canals have been prepared to a taper and filled, however, the accessory anatomy has not been debrided, and could be a source of problems in the long term. Some of this residual material may be eradicated using an irrigant active against it (chemomechanical preparation).

Complex systems

In teeth with more complex, irregular canal systems, the prepared taper is encompassed by the original canal system and may not be 'visible' (7.93, 7.94). Its preparation nevertheless helps to facilitate canal cleaning. This series of figures (7.72, 7.73, 7.88–7.92) shows canal systems with the relative proportions that might be

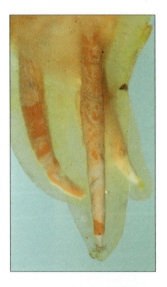

7.80 Root-filled tooth with tapered canal preparations completely encompassing the root canal system

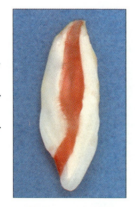

7.81 Irregular wide root canal in a maxillary canine

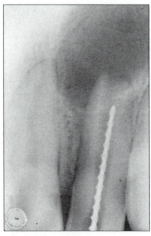

7.83

7.82 Wide, 'blunderbuss' canal in an incompletely formed root

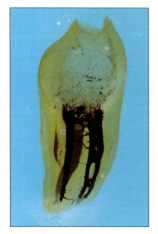

7.84

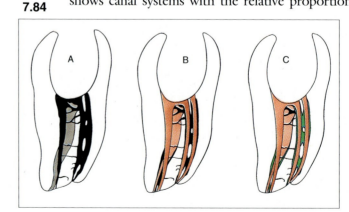

7.83–7.86 Simple main canals with complex intercommunications. A = before preparation; B = after mechanical preparation; C = after chemomechanical preparation

7.85

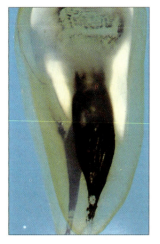

7.86

A   B   C

7.87 Root-filled tooth with tapered main canals but undebrided accessory anatomy

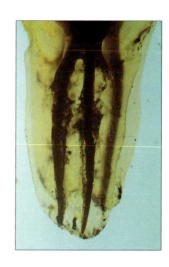

7.88

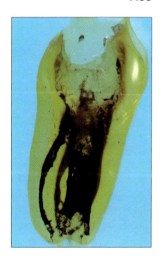

7.89

A   B   C

7.88–7.92 Effect of mechanical and chemical cleaning on complex irregular canal systems.

■ undebrided
■ mechanically debrided
■ chemically debrided

A = before preparation
B = after mechanical preparation
C = after mechanical preparation and sodium

7.90

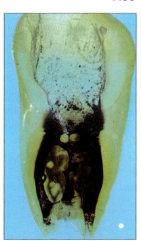

7.91   **7.92**

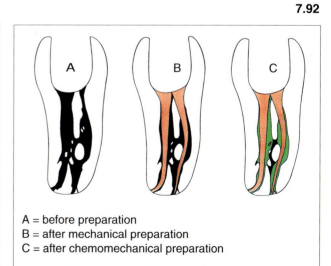

A = before preparation
B = after mechanical preparation
C = after mechanical preparation and sodium hypochlorite irrigation

A = before preparation
B = after mechanical preparation
C = after chemomechanical preparation

7.92 These diagrams are reproduced from cleared tooth shown in **7.76**

cleaned purely by mechanical preparations and by chemomechanical preparation. Figures **7.93** and **7.94** depict root-filled teeth with the tapered preparation encompassed by the original canal shape.

Canal preparation using hand instruments (shaping)

Mechanical preparation refers to controlled removal of dentine by manipulating root canal instruments. The amount and pattern of dentine removal is influenced by the design and sharpness of the cutting edges, the way in which it is manipulated and the force applied. The influence of the operator's skill, which is an intangible quantity, has not been studied but is clearly of extreme importance. It is probably influenced by the ability to discriminate tactile feedback from the instrument and the ability to manipulate instruments in a controlled way according to a mental image of the three-dimensional shape of the root canal system. This mental image is synthesised from knowledge of canal anatomy, radiographs and tactile feedback from root canal instruments. The design of instruments and their properties also dictate the manner and efficacy of their use.

Root canal instruments may be rotated (clockwise or anticlockwise) or used in a push-pull filing motion to effect dentine removal. The two modes may also be combined, e.g. 'ream and file' describes the 45–90° clockwise movement to engage dentine and straight pull withdrawal to cut the engaged dentine. The amplitude of motion and length/area of file engaged in cutting may also be varied. The design of cutting edges and rake angle determine the most efficient movement for a given instrument. In the rotary or reaming mode of action the blade engages dentine and force is exerted until the compressive strength of the dentine is exceeded, at which point a crack propagates through the weakened dentine and causes a chip. The cutting action of the filing or push-pull motion is similar to that of planing. The size and shape of dentine chips produced depend on the rake angle, sharpness of blade and force applied.

If root canal systems were straight tubular structures, their preparation would be a matter of following prescribed movements with a series of instruments of graded sizes, requiring relatively little skill. Unfortunately, root canal systems are irregular in shape, so it is important first to use a small instrument to explore the curves and other anatomical features. The mesiobuccal canal shown in **7.95** is seen to be curved in two planes at right angles when the file (**7.96**, **7.97**) is removed. Division of a canal at an apical level may also be detected using a precurved file as an explorer (**7.98**). Very few root canals are absolutely straight, so it is best to assume that they are curved. Knowledge of the curvature of a canal is the first step in preparing it without deviating significantly from the original curvature.

Errors in preparation

A number of canal preparation errors are recognized: ledging (**7.99**); zipping; transportation of apical foramen (**7.100**,

7.93, 7.94 Root-filled teeth in which the tapered canal preparation is encompassed by the original canal shape and is not 'visible'

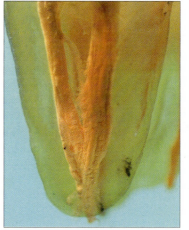
7.93

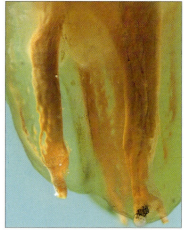
7.94

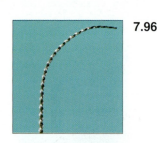
7.95 Use of small file as explorer

7.96

7.97

7.96, 7.97 Curvature (in two planes) of file removed from the mesiobuccal canal in **7.95**

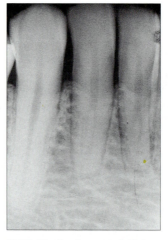
7.98 Radicular canal division should be detected using a precurved file

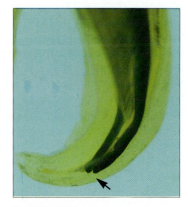
7.99 Ledging

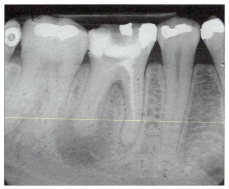
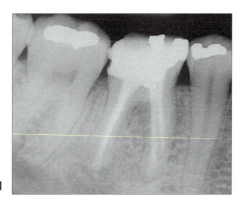
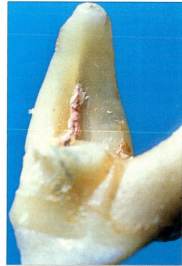

7.100, 7.101 Transportation of apical foramen

7.102–7.104 Perforation

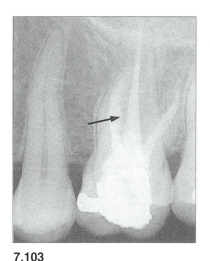

7.103

7.104

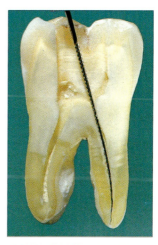

7.105 File fitting tightly in canal

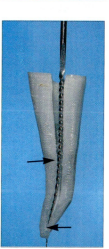

7.106 File fitting loosely in canal

7.101); perforation (7.102–7.104). These procedural errors result from uncontrolled dentine removal and may be caused by

1. *the force exerted by files on the dentine walls as a result of their tendency to straighten to their normal shape; and*
2. *unintentional removal of dentine from sites of preferential contact because the area of instrument capable of cutting is too large.*

These problems may be overcome by

1. *reducing the restoring force of straight rigid instruments on canal walls;*
2. *reducing the area of canal instrument actively engaged in cutting.*

A straight, rigid instrument placed in a curved canal and moved in a push-pull filing motion removes dentine preferentially where it makes contact with the necessary force. If the file fits tightly in the canal, dentine will be removed around the whole circumference (7.105) but if it fits loosely then removal will usually occur only on the inner aspect of the height of the curve and on the outer aspect of the curve at the apex (7.106). Rotation of the instrument will also preferentially remove dentine, depending on the rigidity of the instrument, pattern of flutes and direction of rotation.

Reducing uncontrolled forces on canal walls

Precurving the file

Uncontrolled forces may be reduced by precurving the file to reduce the mismatch between curvature of file and canal. This also helps negotiation of the canal. Closer approximation of curvature of the file to that of the canal reduces the number of preferential binding areas in the canal (**7.107**). However, there is a limit to the benefit of precurving: the curvature of file and canal can only match in one position and mismatch occurs at extremes of the filing stroke (**7.108**). It is therefore better to reduce the amplitude of filing strokes in severely curved canals (**7.109**).

Files may be precurved in a number of ways such as by using a cotton wool roll (**7.110, 7.111**) or using commercial devices (**7.112, 7.113**). The curve is estimated from the radiograph, the curvature of the initial explorer file and tactile feedback on placement of a precurved instrument in the canal. Files that are to be used at different lengths in the canal relative to the curvature should be appropriately precurved (**7.114**).

Use of smaller files

Smaller instruments (No. 20 or smaller) are used until the larger sizes pass in the canal without force. The temptation to speed the process by forcing large instruments into canals too early cause procedural errors often resulting in loss of length (**7.115, 7.116**).

Use of intermediate files

The temptation to force larger instruments into canals may be avoided, and a smoother progress through file sizes achieved, by creating intermediate files as described by Weine,[14] who suggest-

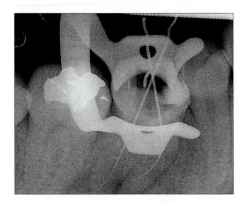

7.107 Precuring files to match canal curvature

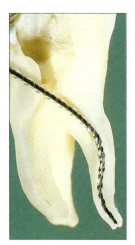

7.108 Files match canals in only one position

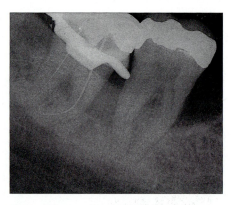

7.109 Reduce the amplitude of filing in severely curved canals

7.110

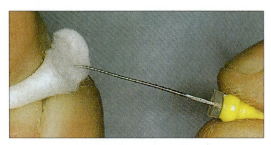

7.111

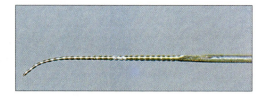

7.110, 7.111 Use of cotton wool roll to precurve file

7.112

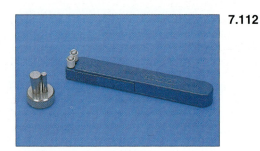

7.113

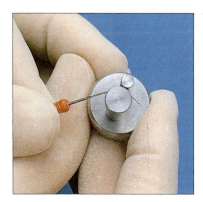

7.112, 7.113 Commercially available devices for precurving files

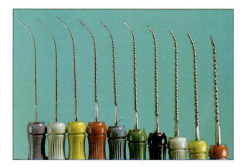

7.114 Files are precurved at different levels depending on the depth of insertion into canal

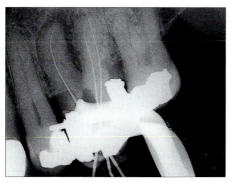 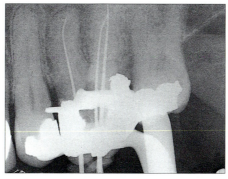 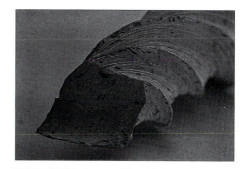

7.115, 7.116 Loss of length caused by forcing large instruments in canals too early

7.117 SEM view of file with tip clipped

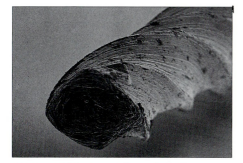 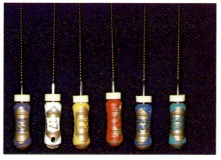

7.118 SEM view of file in **7.117** smoothed

7.119 'Golden medium' intermediate files (12, 17, 22, 27, 32, 37)

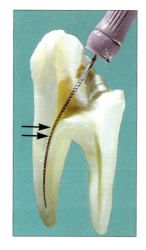 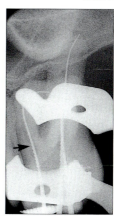

7.120, 7.121 Preflaring allows more direct apical access

ed trimming 1 mm from the tip of the file (**7.117**) and rounding off sharp edges on a diamond nail file (**7.118**). In this way, files sizes 10, 15, 20 and 25 may be converted to 12, 17, 22 and 27. The disadvantages of this technique are that the files are made disposable and the edges may be difficult to smooth, which therefore creates ledges during filing. A recent innovation by Maillefer overcomes these problems using the intermediate files 'Golden Mediums' (**7.119**).

Use of flexible files

Another way to reduce uncontrolled forces is to use flexible files (such as Flex-R, Flexo-file, nickel–titanium files). However, a file which is too flexible would be inefficient as adequate interfacial force cannot be placed on the instrument.

Reducing the area of canal instrument actively engaged in cutting

Modified canal preparation techniques

Preflaring or coronal–apical techniques, in which the coronal portion of the canal is flared first to eliminate or reduce coronal binding, may be used. This also helps to reduce uncontrolled forces (**7.120, 7.121**).

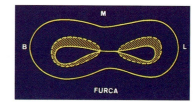

7.122 Cross section of a mesial root. Ideal removal of dentine during preparation (shaded area): B = buccal; M = mesial; L = lingual

Modified manipulation of instruments

Anticurvature filing

Anticurvature filing denotes filing preferentially away from the inner curve or furcal aspect, the site of potential perforation (**7.102, 7.122**). This method, which involves filing the buccal, mesial and lingual walls of the root canal with more strokes than the furcal wall by a ratio of 3:1 is effective (**7.123**). However simply following the prescription without regard for tactile feedback, flexibility and controlled manipulation of file will render it ineffective. A degree of straightening is occasionally inevitable (**7.124**).

Modified use of files

Files may be used in such a way as to reduce their area of contact. For example, in the crown-down pressureless technique only the tips of the instruments are used for cutting. The file is placed in the canal until it binds (**7.125**) and is then rotated twice without apical pressure to remove dentine at this point.

Modified instruments

Dentine removal may be limited by modifying instruments. Weine[14] has suggested blunting the cutting flutes with a diamond nail file where unwanted dentine removal would occur. This is effective but requires a unidirectional stop to help maintain the file in its correct orientation to the plane of curve of the canal. A recently introduced file has preblunted cutting edges and a facet on the handle to help correct orientation (**7.126–7.128**). Cooperation with manufacturers of root canal instruments has resulted in design of instruments with safe-ended non-cutting tips (Flex-R (**7.169–7.171**), Canal master (**7.175–7.177**) and Flexo-file (**7.147–7.149**). In addition to this, instruments have been modified so that they only have a short cutting zone apically (Canal master (**7.175–7.177**), Flexogates (**7.178–7.180**) and Heliapical (**7.172–7.174**)).

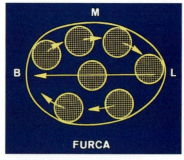

7.123 Anticurvature filing: 3x on B, M, L: 1 x furca

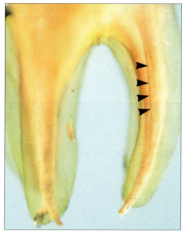

7.124 Mild straightening despite anticurvature filing

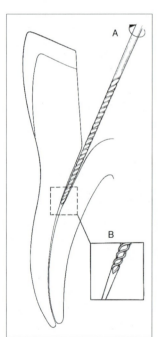

7.125 Modified use of files; A = circular movement of file; B = only the tip of the instrument engages and cuts dentine

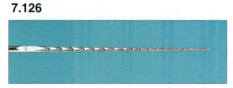

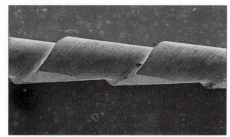

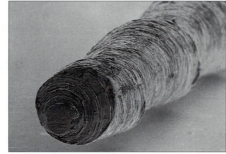

7.126–7.128 Preblunted safety Hedstroem file (Kerr's)

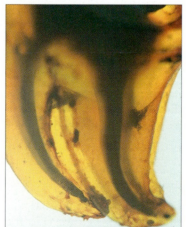

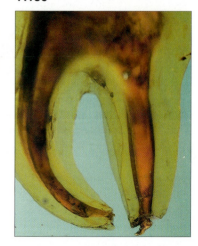

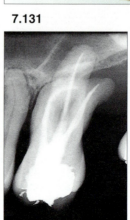

7.129–7.131 Prepared and filled root canals with curvatures maintained

A combination of these measures may be used to control root canal preparation in curved roots (**7.129–7.131**). In some cases, the canals curve in opposite directions in the same plane. The preparation of such canals is challenging but achievable in some cases (**7.132**): in other cases one of the curves may be straightened by preparing the coronal curve first and the apical curve second (**7.133, 7.134**). In some instances it is impossible to control instrumentation of the apical curve which may be straightened (**7.135, 7.136**).

Design of instruments

The large number of root canal instruments available are manufactured from metal wires of different alloys (stainless steel, carbon steel, titanium, nickel–titanium), cross-sectional shapes and diameters. These alloys have different physical properties: carbon steel is the most brittle, stainless steel more resilient, titanium more flexible and nickel–titanium is the most flexible. The cross-sectional shapes may be square (K file), triangular (Flexofile), rhomboid (K flex file), circular (Hedstroem file) or S-shaped (Unifile), and the shape will affect the physical properties of the instrument. The cutting edges may be generated by twisting the metal shaft along its long axis or by machining it. When twisted, the square blank produces the most rigid instrument, the triangular shape is more flexible and the rhomboid more flexible still. When machined, the depth of cut used to produce the flutes dictates the flexibility and strength of the instrument. The rake angle thus produced influences the optimal mode of use (rotational or push-pull). Machined instruments generally tend to be more susceptible to fracture.

Twisted instruments

These instruments are designed to meet the requirements of the American National Standards Institute (ANSI) for endodontic K-type files and reamers, which lay down the dimensional formulas for size, taper, length of cutting blade and tip angle (**7.137**). A number of companies manufacture instruments to these specifications, but only selected examples are shown here.

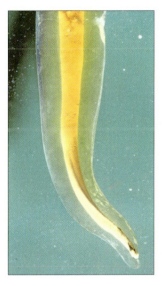

7.132 Curvature in opposite directions in the same plane

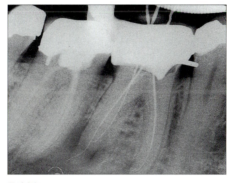

7.133

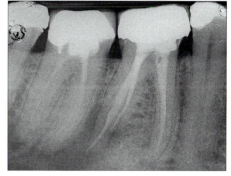

7.134

7.133, 7.134 Straightening coronal curve in the distal root

7.135, 7.136 Straightening apical curve in the mesial root

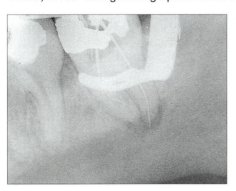

7.135

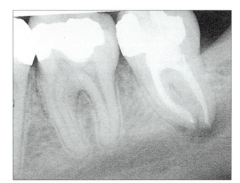

7.136

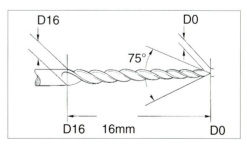

7.137 Dimensional formula of files and reamers: D = diameter

K-File

This instrument (**7.138–7.140**) is produced by twisting a four-sided pyramidal blank, i.e. a square cross-section. Some manufacturers use a triangular cross-section from size 35 upwards to reduce rigidity. The instruments have between one-quarter and just over one-half spiral per millimetre length. The resulting blade angle makes them best suited for cutting dentine using a push-pull filing motion.

K-Reamer

This instrument (**7.141–7.143**) is produced by twisting a three-sided pyramidal blank, i.e. a triangular cross-section, which makes reamers more flexible than K-files. These instruments have between less than one-tenth and one-quarter of a spiral per millimetre of length, giving a rake angle which cuts most efficiently using a rotary motion; hence reaming.

K-Flex file

This instrument (**7.144–7.146**) is twisted from a tapered blank with a rhombic cross-section. This shape results in alternating deep and shallow flute depth, which not only increases flexibility but is also said to facilitate removal of debris.

Flexofile

This is a flexible instrument twisted from a stainless steel blank of triangular cross-section (**7.147–7.149**) with 1.81 flutes per millimetre length. The tip is modified to be non-cutting. A recent addition, the so-called 'Golden Medium', is of similar design but provides a range of intermediate sizes (12, 17, 22, 27 and 32): size 27 is shown in Figures **7.150–7.152**.

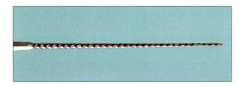

7.138

7.138–7.140 Kerr K-file No. 25

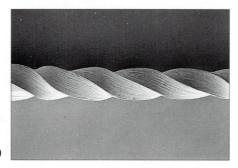

7.139

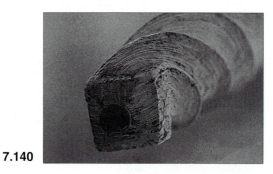

7.140

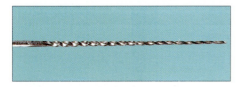

7.141

7.141–7.143 Kerr K-reamer No. 25

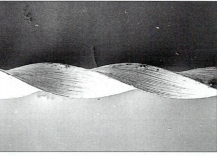

7.142

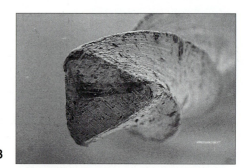

7.143

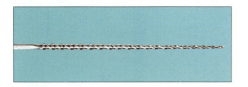

7.144

7.144–7.146 Kerr K-Flex file No. 25

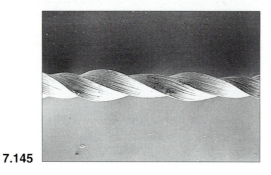

7.145

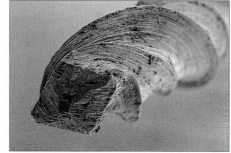

7.146

Zipperer Flexicut

This instrument is produced by twisting a triangular shank made from SCS spacecraft steel (**7.153–7.155**). It is a high-vaccum-fired chrome nickel steel which is claimed to give uniform structure. Its claimed advantages are its flexibility and non-aggressive tip.

Machined instruments

Hedstroem file

The dimensions of H-type or Hedstroem instruments are given by the ANSI specification No. 58 shown in **7.156**. Several com-

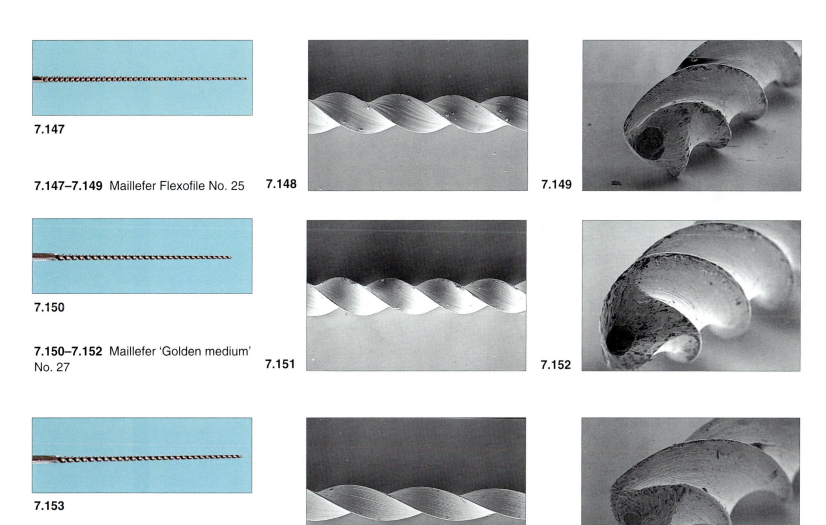

7.147

7.147–7.149 Maillefer Flexofile No. 25   **7.148**   **7.149**

7.150

7.150–7.152 Maillefer 'Golden medium' No. 27   **7.151**   **7.152**

7.153

7.153–7.155 Anteos Flexicut No. 25   **7.154**   **7.155**

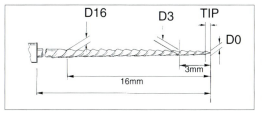

7.156 Dimensional formula of an H-type instrument (ANSI specification No. 58: D = diameter)

panies manufacture H-files, all with different designs and properties (**7.157–7.168**).

The H-file is machined from a blank of circular cross-section. The flutes are produced by machining a single helix into the metal stock, producing a series of intersecting cones which increase in size from tip to handle. The strength and flexibility of the instrument is determined by the depth of flute or the residual bulk of metal in the central portion of the file. The blades thus formed are virtually at right angles to the dentine surface and so the most efficient cutting motion is a pulling stroke; no dentine will be removed by the push stroke. Rotating the instrument with the tip of the file engaged in dentine is a common cause of fracture.

The latest modification to this type of instrument includes blunting one side to reduce the risk of uncontrolled dentine removal (**7.126–7.128**).

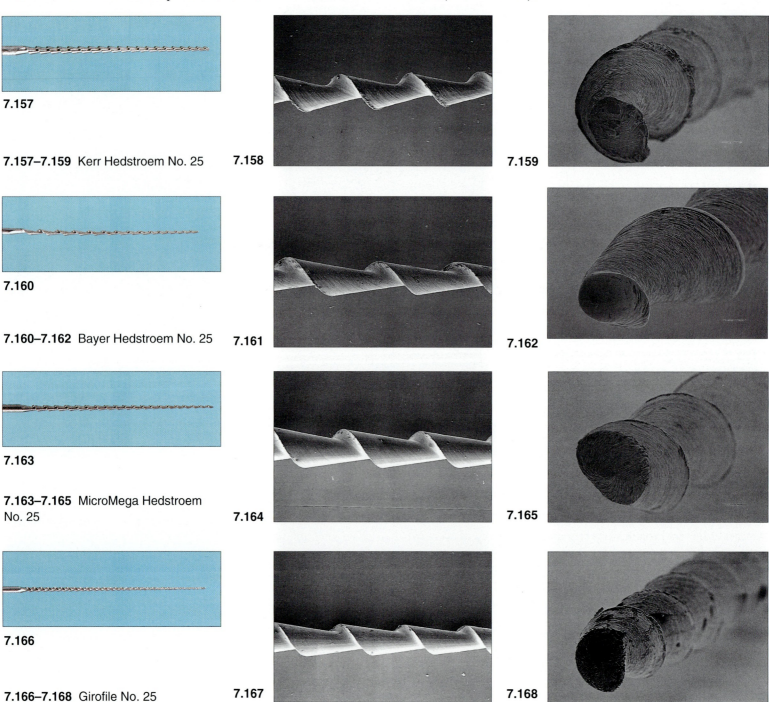

7.157

7.157–7.159 Kerr Hedstroem No. 25   **7.158**   **7.159**

7.160

7.160–7.162 Bayer Hedstroem No. 25   **7.161**   **7.162**

7.163

7.163–7.165 MicroMega Hedstroem No. 25   **7.164**   **7.165**

7.166

7.166–7.168 Girofile No. 25   **7.167**   **7.168**

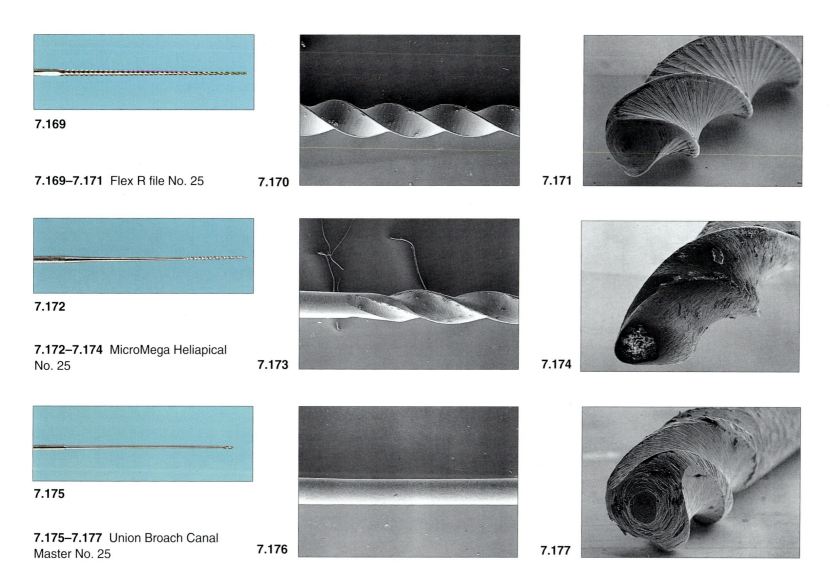

7.169–7.171 Flex R file No. 25

7.172–7.174 MicroMega Heliapical No. 25

7.175–7.177 Union Broach Canal Master No. 25

Flex-R file

This instrument (7.169–7.171) was designed to be used in the 'balanced forces technique'. Machined from a blank of triangular cross-section, it resembles a twisted instrument. The method of manufacture is said to allow greater control of strength and flexibility by controlling the angle of cutting edges and cross-sectional area of residual metal bulk. Thus, increased stiffness and strength may be achieved in smaller sizes and increased flexibility in larger sizes. This instrument is designed to cut most efficiently in anti-clockwise rotary motion but will remove dentine in a conventional filing mode. An important feature of this instrument is its modified safe-ended tip. In common with other machined instruments it has a tendency to fracture.

Several instruments that reduce the cutting ability to the apical portion of the instrument have recently become available. These include the Heliapical, Canal Master and Flexogates.

Heliapical

This instrument (7.172–7.174) resembles a conventional file in the apical 4–5 mm, the remainder being a narrow blank shank. Care is needed in its use; small sizes may fracture if a continuous-rotational motion is used.

Canal Master

The cutting portion of this instrument (7.175–7.177) resembles a reamer with blunted edges and is reduced to 1–2 mm with a 0.75-mm non-cutting pilot tip. The rest of the instrument consists of a parallel-sided shank of round cross-section, narrower than the cutting tip and very flexible. The most efficient means of cutting is using a clockwise rotary motion through 60°. This instrument has not yet been thoroughly evaluated but early work suggests that it has a potential for breakage.

Flexogates

This unique stainless steel instrument (7.178–7.180) resembles the Canal Master. It consists of a smooth, flexible shank which is circular and small in cross-section. The non-cutting tip is followed by approximately one spiral of fluting on an expanded head carried on the shank. As in the Gates Glidden drills, the Flexogate is made deliberately weak at the handle end of the thin shank to ensure access for removal of broken instruments. These instruments need to be evaluated further.

A number of unconventional instruments have been designed for use in automated handpieces. The Helisonic (7.181–7.183), Rispisonic (7.184–7.186) and Shaper (7.187–7.189), each with a safety tip, have been developed for the MicroMega Sonic Air handpiece. Of these, the Shaper has the most aggressive cutting action.

McSpadden Engine file

This unique instrument, designed to be used in a rotary handpiece at slow speeds (300 r.p.m.) is constructed from a superelas-

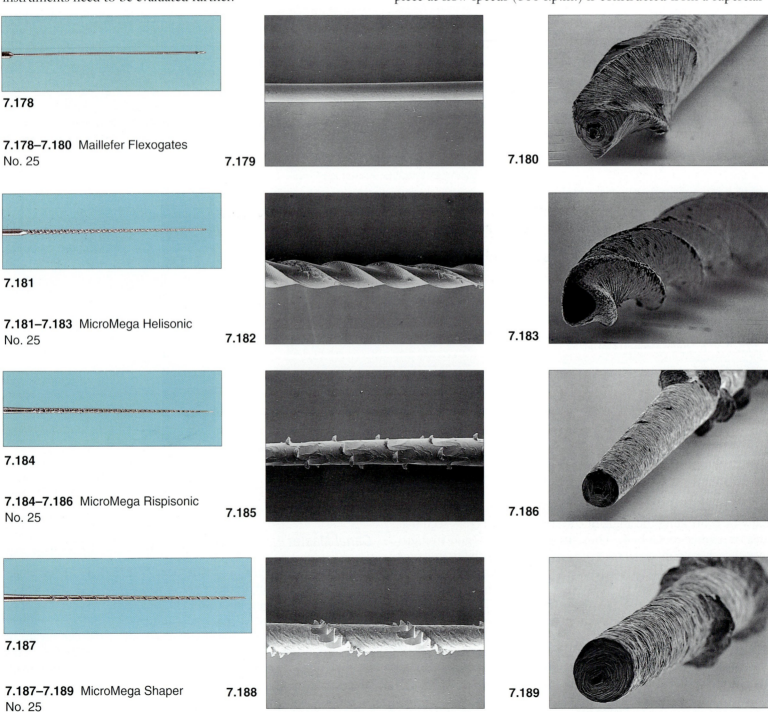

7.178–7.180 Maillefer Flexogates No. 25

7.181–7.183 MicroMega Helisonic No. 25

7.184–7.186 MicroMega Rispisonic No. 25

7.187–7.189 MicroMega Shaper No. 25

tic nickel–titanium alloy (**7.190–7.192**). The instruments are designed to avoid binding into canal walls. This is achieved in one of two ways. In sizes 15–35 flat areas are substituted for blades, and cutting is achieved by a planing action. In sizes 40–60 the same is achieved using two or more spiralled blades (which are not parallel) intersecting along the shaft of the instrument. The most unique feature of this instrument is that it 'pulls' the canal system's contents out rather than forcing them apically.

Irrigants for canal preparation (cleaning)

A variety of chemical agents in fluid form, and sometimes in viscous preparations, has been used to aid canal preparation. Irrigation is one of the most important aspects of canal preparation: irrigants will help to clean those areas of the root canal system that are not directly planed by instruments, providing they are antimicrobial and able to dissolve organic debris. Irrigants perform a number of functions.

Lubrication

Irrigants help to lubricate the action of root canal instruments and aid their passage down narrow curved canals.

Flushing out of gross debris

Irrigants wash out debris, regardless of their chemical action, and help to prevent blockages caused by compaction of accumulated debris. In addition, the chemical action of irrigants is possible only when it wets the substrate sufficiently and none of the available irrigants has a low enough surface tension to allow wetting of the entire root canal system without assistance. The solutions need to be delivered to the appropriate site using a hypodermic needle and syringe (**7.193**). Deep placement of the needle is possible in wide canals before preparation (**7.3**) but in most canals some early coronal preparation is necessary to facilitate access (**7.194, 7.195**). Even then, apical delivery of irrigant is limited, sometimes even once preparation (**7.196, 7.197**) is complete. A

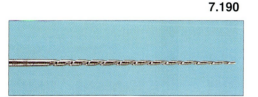

7.190–7.192 McSpadden engine driven nickel–titanium file No. 25

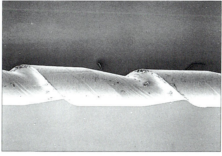

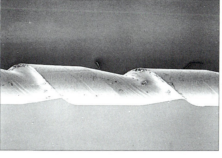

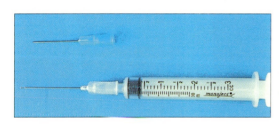

7.193 Hypodermic needle and syringe

7.194, 7.195 Preparation to facilitate needle placement

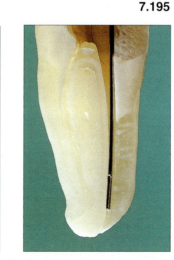

7.196, 7.197 Apical delivery of irrigant may be limited

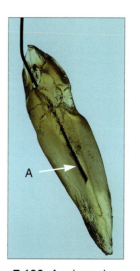

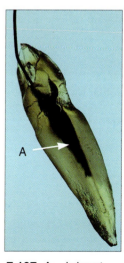

7.196 A = hypodermic needle in cleared canine tooth

7.197 A = irrigant

narrow-gauge needle (27) is recommended for deeper irrigant placement (**7.198**). Use of a smaller needle may render injection slow and difficult because the pressure required is quite high and space should be allowed next to the needle to prevent irrigant extrusion (**7.199**). Several needle designs are available to resolve this problem, most including a perforation in the side of the needle shank (**7.200**). Despite these aids, replacing irrigant in the apical portion of a narrow canal may be difficult. Figure **7.201** shows a canal with irrigant which is saturated with debris. Irrigation replaces the coronal part of the fluid (**7.202**), the depth of replacement being related to that of needle penetration (**7.203**). The apical unreplaced irrigant may be diluted using a file to mix the debris-saturated irrigant in the apical portion with the fresh coronal solution (**7.204**). This procedure (called *recapitulation*) is an important means of avoiding blockage of the apical canal. Frequent replacement of irrigant allows better cleaning.

Dissolution of organic and inorganic material

One of the most important functions of the irrigant is to dissolve pulpal organic debris, but the importance of dissolution of the inorganic component has not yet been satisfactorily determined. Instrumentation of the root canal surface produces a smear layer composed of both organic and inorganic material (**7.205**). Some clinicians believe it is important to remove this layer (**7.206**) because it may harbour bacteria which may later recolonize the

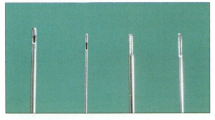

7.198 Different gauges of needle are available in all types

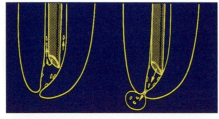

7.199 Needle binding encourages extrusion of irrigant

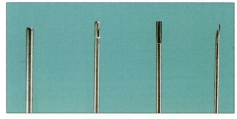

7.200 Needle designs

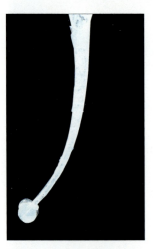

7.201 Canal containing dentine-saturated irrigant

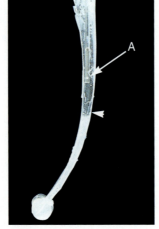

7.202 Fresh irrigant replaces coronal saturated irrigant (arrowed): A = needle tip

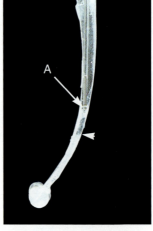

7.203 Deeper needle placement allows deeper replacement of irrigant (arrowed): A = needle tip

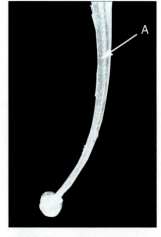

7.204 Recapitulation to remove apical dentine-saturated irrigant: A = small file

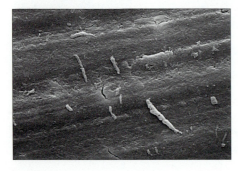

7.205 Smear layer formed by instrumentation

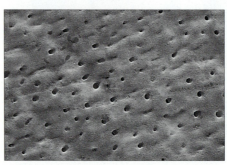

7.206 Smear layer removed

7.207–7.210 Dissolution of extirpated pulp in sodium hypochlorite

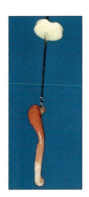

7.207 Immediately after extirpation

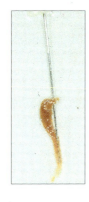

7.208 Immediately after placement in sodium hypochlorite

7.211 Corrosion of Endosonic handpiece by sodium hypochlorite

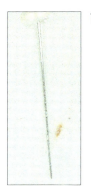

7.209 After 5 min

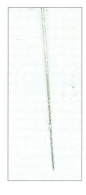

7.212 Rubber dam should be sealed well when using Endosonics

7.213

7.214

7.210 After 10 min

7.213, 7.214 Effervescence in root canals is of dubious value

root canal; however, there is no firm evidence to support this. The opened dentinal tubules may be even more difficult to decontaminate if infected. A range of chelating agents or weak acids may be used to remove the inorganic material.

Antimicrobial effect

The most important function of the root canal irrigant is to destroy all micro-organisms in the root canal. Since the beginning of the century a range of substances has been used to irrigate the root canal, including chemically non-active solutions (water, saline, local anaesthetic), chemically active materials such as enzymes (streptokinase, streptodornase, papain, enzymol, trypsin), acids (30% hydrochloric acid, 50% sulphuric acid, citric acid), alkalis (sodium hydroxide, potassium hydroxide, urea, sodium hypochlorite), chelating agents (various ethylenediaminetetra-acetic acid (EDTA) preparations), oxidizing agents (hydrogen peroxide, carbamide peroxide), antibacterial agents (chlorhexidine, bisdequalinium acetate) and detergents (sodium lauryl sulphate). The few that remain in use are reviewed below.

Chemically inactive irrigants

Water, saline and local anaesthetic are commonly used because of their availability and low cost. However, their only merit is that they are non-toxic to periradicular tissues. They are all equally capable of washing out debris from the canal and lubricating instruments, but none is able to dissolve organic or inorganic debris or exhibits significant antimicrobial effect.

Chemically active irrigants and lubricants

Sodium hypochlorite

This readily available solution is the irrigant of choice. It has been used in concentrations from 0.5 to 5.25 %. It is able to lubricate, wash out debris, dissolve organic tissue (**7.207–7.210**) (and when ultrasonically activated, inorganic debris) and destroys almost all micro-organisms found in the root canal system. Figures **7.208–7.210** show extirpated pulp tissue immediately (**7.208**), 5 min (**7.209**) and 10 min (**7.210**) after placement in sodium hypochlorite. This 'ideal' irrigant does have its drawbacks: it is very caustic, can corrode equipment (**7.211**), bleach clothes and cause a severe reaction if extruded through the periapex in high concentration or volume. A good rubber dam seal is necessary to avoid leakage into the mouth (**7.212**). The bactericidal and solvent properties decrease as the solution is diluted; the latter affected more than the former. These properties may be enhanced by heating the solution. A safer (lower) concentration may be compensated for to an extent by using a larger volume if periradicular damage is of concern.

Oxidizing agents

Hydrogen peroxide (usually 3%) is often recommended as an adjunct in root canal irrigation and several studies report favourable results of alternating its use with sodium hypochlorite. Benefits of using hydrogen peroxide include production of nascent oxygen, which may help to eliminate anaerobic bacteria. The effervescence (7.213, 7.214) may help to displace debris by bulk flow, but this is of dubious value: a counter argument is that the bubbles prevent adequate contact between irrigant and organic debris and thus reduce efficiency. *Carbamide peroxide* is another oxidizing agent found in a commercially available viscous lubricating paste called Glyoxide. The rest of the base is made up of anhydrous glycerol. This material does not possess significant antibacterial or solvent effect.

Chelating agents

Most of these have become popular with the trend for removing the smear layer. A number of commercially available preparations have been used for irrigation in addition to EDTA. These agents are also good lubricants and useful for instrumentation of fine calcified canals. EDTA acts by chelating and binding calcium ions from dentine, softening it. This can speed up preparation of fine calcified canals. Some practitioners have expressed concern about misuse of this material, which may lead to oversoftening and perforations but this is unlikely because the material is self-limiting as it becomes spent; its duration of action is dependent upon its concentration and volume.

As EDTA has no antimicrobial properties and cannot dissolve organic tissue it is of value purely for removing smear layer and speeding enlargement of calcified canals.

Techniques for preparing root canals

There are many ways in which different files and irrigation regimens may be used to achieve specific preparation aims. Some procedures have been well documented, researched and are established models for teaching controlled root canal preparation. The available techniques can be divided into two groups: (1) apical–coronal techniques (7.215), in which working length is established and the full length of canal then prepared, sequentially increasing it in size until the final shape is established. The preparation often ends with refinement of the coronal part; (2) coronal–apical techniques (7.216), in which the coronal portion of the canal is prepared before determining working length. The canal is prepared sequentially from the coronal end to the full working length, which is determined at some point after coronal preflaring.

The second approach is thought to offer the following advantages which make it the preferred approach:

1. It allows early debridement of the coronal part of canal which may contain the bulk of organic and microbial debris, reducing the risk of carrying this material to the apical end and through the foramen.
2. Early coronal widening enables better and deeper penetration of irrigant early in the preparation, which reduces the risk of apical blockage with dentine chips and pulp tissue.
3. Preparation of the coronal portion tends to shorten the effective length of canal, and determining the working length after such enlargement will reduce the problem of its alteration during preparation.
4. It allows better control over apical instrumentation.

There is, however, some resistance to teaching these techniques to the novice because they carry risks of ledging, blocking and perforation, especially if the canal is very narrow. In these cases a compromise is to widen the entire length of the canal to size 10 or 15 before proceeding, which would reduce these risks.

In the following descriptions of the individual techniques it is assumed that adequate access has been gained and that irrigation compatible with the technique is used.

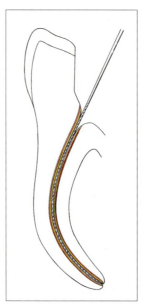

7.215 Apical–coronal preparation techniques
Colour code for file sizes:
Purple = 10
White = 15
Yellow = 20
Red = 25
Blue = 30
Green = 35
Black = 40
White = 45
Yellow = 50
Red = 55

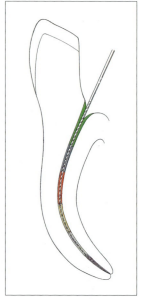

7.216 Coronal–apical preparation techniques

7.217–7.221 Standardized preparation technique using reamers. Coloured areas indicate dentine removed by respective instruments

Apical–coronal techniques

Standardized preparation

The premise of this technique (7.217–7.221) is that most root canals are circular in cross-section in the apical third. The aim is to prepare the root canal by enlarging it sequentially to a selected size as follows.

1. Determine the working length.
2. Introduce the smallest reamer into the canal and rotate it clockwise to engage dentine and then withdraw. Wipe clean and reinsert; repeat until the working length is reached.
3. Repeat with successively larger reamers until the required size is reached apically (size 25 in the illustrated example).
4. A canal shape should be produced which matches the last reamer used and which may then be obturated with a matching solid cone, e.g. silver point.

This technique occasionally works, particularly if the canals are narrow, of circular cross-section and not enlarged to a large size. Use of large reamers may cause canal deviation apically. The technique is unlikely to debride canals with more complicated shapes well and obturation would rely almost entirely on the sealer carried by the silver point.

In order to overcome some of these deficiencies a hybrid technique consisting of reaming the apical third and filing the coronal two-thirds has been recommended. The coronal preparation is obturated by gutta percha. The risk of extrusion of debris in this technique is significant because of the lack of early coronal cleaning and the close fit of the reamer to the canal wall as it is negotiated to the working length (7.222).

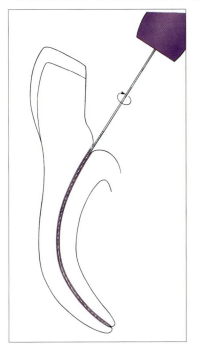

7.217 Dentine removed by size 10 reamer

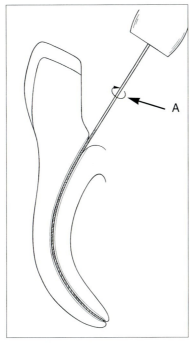

7.218 Dentine removed by size 15 reamer: A = reaming

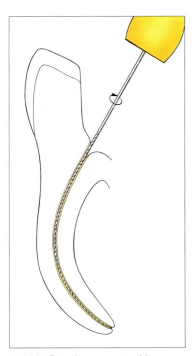

7.219 Dentine removed by size 20 reamer

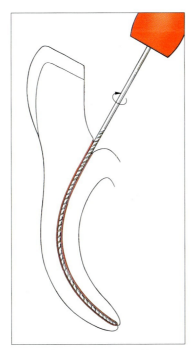

7.220 Dentine removed by size 25 reamer

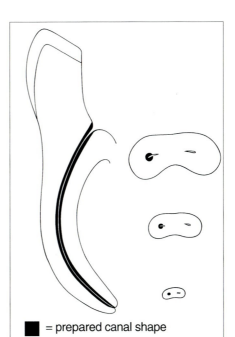

= prepared canal shape

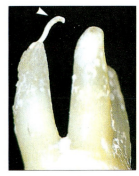

7.222 Apical extrusion of debris

7.221 Longitudinal and transverse sections showing the canal before and after preparation

Step-back canal preparation

This well established technique is currently the one that is most widely used and taught (7.223–7.235), and a number of modifications have been described. In essence, the technique consists of preparing the canal using files with a push-pull motion, to a wider taper than that produced in the standardized technique. The preparation may be modified to obturate the canal in several different ways, but is most commonly filled using the lateral condensation technique. It is interesting to note that there has been a change in emphasis in the reason for canal shaping: whereas canal shaping was previously mainly dictated by the obturation technique, it is now considered to be dictated mainly by the need to clean the canal. A more conservative taper can therefore be produced. The obturation technique is then selected on the basis of final canal shape among other factors. The following steps are taken.

1. Determine working length.
2. Insert the largest file that will fit to the full length without force and file circumferentially until the next size up will reach the full working length. Irrigate copiously.
3. Repeat until a size 25 file, or one or two sizes larger than the first file that binds at the apex will reach the working length in small curved canals. It is important that filing with each size is carried out only until the next size can be accommodated or the terminal file at the working length is just loose to ensure control over the tapered shape.
4. The preparation is flared using each larger file 1 mm shorter than the previous file until it is just loose. If the file reaches its correct length without binding, no more filing should be carried out. After each file it is of paramount importance to recapitulate using a small file to the full working length together with copious irrigation, to ensure and maintain canal patency.
5. Refine the coronal preparation using Gates Glidden drills. It is usually not necessary to go larger than size 3 in the coronal 1–2 mm.

In the absence of sodium hypochlorite this technique is likely to achieve cleaner canals and allows better control over the apical preparation than the standardized technique. However, it is difficult to master and suffers from the disadvantages of apical–coronal preparations: the potential for extrusion of debris, apical blockage and alteration of working length. Another disadvantage is the tendency for canal deviations, particularly when large inflexible instruments are used. Each type of file has its own characteristic problems. The Hedstroem file, for example, tends to pack less apical debris but if used carelessly can produce overflaring and strip perforation.

7.223–7.235 Step-back technique

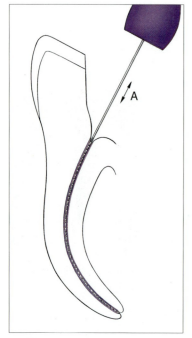

7.223 Filing to full working length (WL) with size 10 file: A = filing

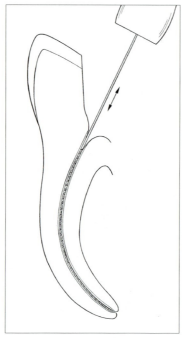

7.224 Filing to full WL with Size 15 file

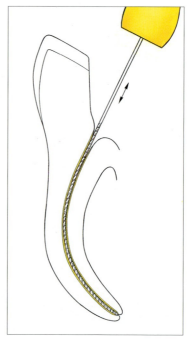

7.225 Filing to full WL with size 20 file

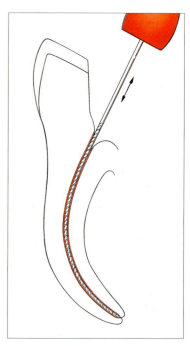

7.226 Filing to full WL with size 25 file

7.223–7.235 Step-back technique–*continued*

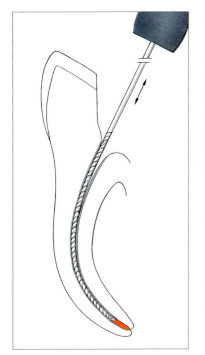

7.227 Stepping back by 1mm from WL at size 30

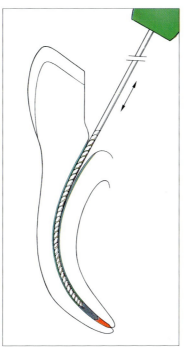

7.228 Stepping back by 2mm from WL at size 35

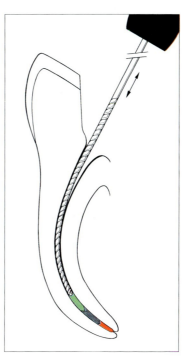

7.229 Stepping back by 3mm from WL at size 40

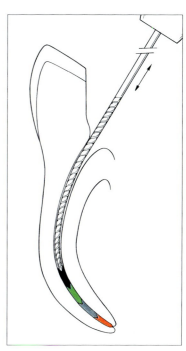

7.230 Stepping back by 4mm from WL at size 45

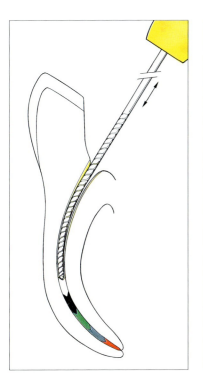

7.231 Stepping back by 5mm from WL at size 50

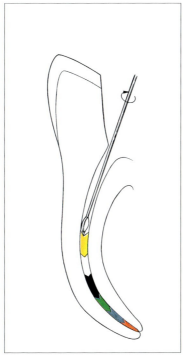

7.232 Refining coronal flare with Gates Glidden size 1

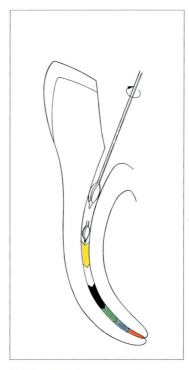

7.233 Refining coronal flare with Gates Glidden size 2

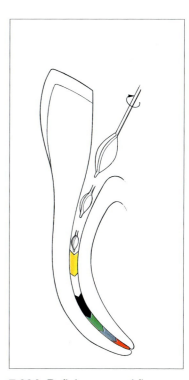

7.234 Refining coronal flare with Gates Glidden size 3

127

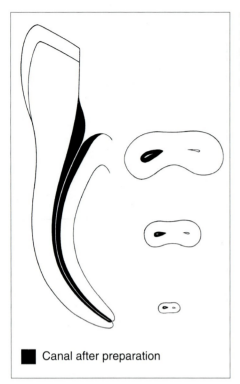

7.235 Step back technique: canal before and after preparation in longitudinal and transverse sections

■ Canal after preparation

The Roane technique (balanced forces)

This relatively new technique (7.236–7.246) uses Flex-R files in a novel clockwise/anticlockwise rotational motion to remove dentine. The technique uses different concepts and terminology. It is a difficult technigue to classify. Three of its main features are as follows. Canals are prepared to predesigned dimensions, of which three are recognised and are designated 45, 60 and 80 according to the size of apical preparation. These dimensions refer to the size of the file used at the third step-back, not to the size of the master apical file. Each step-back from the master apical file at the *periodontal ligament* is 0.5 mm shorter than the previous one. This apical preparation is termed the 'apical control zone'. It is not prepared to the apical constriction/foramen, which is considered too variable, but to the radiographic length corresponding to the periodontal ligament. The technique aims to create its own prepared and standardized apical constriction. The Flex-R files used are not precurved and are used in a controlled rotary motion, which is said to balance forces acting on a file in a curved canal and prevent procedural errors. The file is placed into the canal and turned clockwise 90°, advancing it into the canal and engaging dentine. The cutting motion involves turning the file anticlockwise, using light apical pressure to prevent it from working its way back out. It is necessary to learn how much pressure may be applied to turn instruments without fracturing them. Cycling between clockwise and anticlockwise carries the file to its intended depth. Each clockwise turn may carry the file apically by a millimetre or more.

7.236–7.246 Roane technique

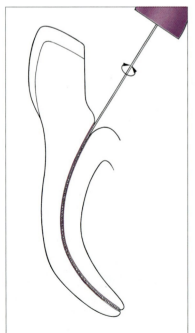

7.236 Size 10 to the full working length (WL)

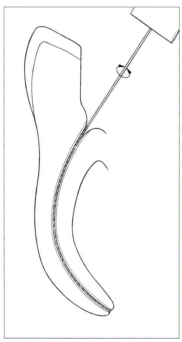

7.237 Size 15 to the full WL

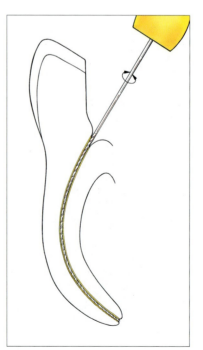

7.238 Size 20 to the full WL

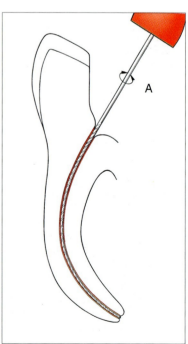

7.239 Size 25 to the full WL: A = clockwise and counter clockwise movement

The stages involved in the technique are described below.
1. Irrigate the coronal part of the canal with 5% sodium hypochlorite.
2. Determine working length to the radiographic apex with the largest file (placed without force). This also helps to determine the size of canal and thickness of root, which will determine selection of predesigned preparation (45, 60 or 80). A guideline to selection of size is presented in **Table 7.2**.
3. Flex-R files are used to the apex to create the 'apical control zone' (**7.247**).
4. Create canal access with Gates Glidden drills by accentuating and smoothing the flare of the coronal two-thirds of the preparation. This stage is carried out just before obturation, so a decision has to be made about single or multiple visit treatment before this stage. The Gates Glidden drills should always remain 3–5 mm short of the radiographic length.

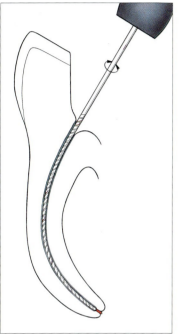

7.240 Size 30, 0.5mm short of WL

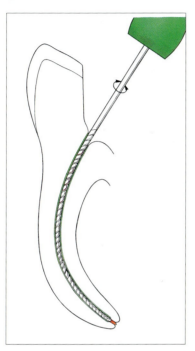

7.241 Size 35, 0.5mm short of WL

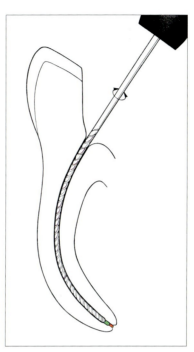

7.242 Size 40, 1mm short of WL

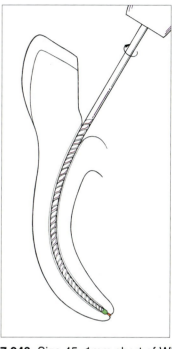

7.243 Size 45, 1mm short of WL

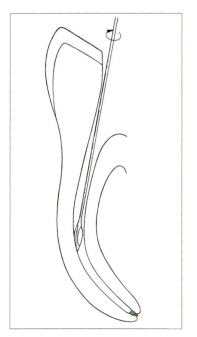

7.244 Gates Glidden size 2 as far as curve allows

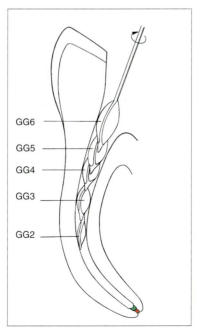

7.245 Gates Glidden size 2–6 to complete flare

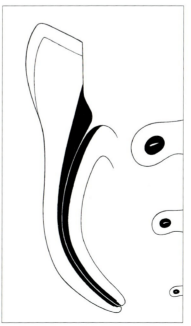

7.246 Longitudinal and transverse sections showing canal before and after preparation

It is possible to maintain quite severe canal curvature with this technique, but the preparations are very wide and the instruments prone to fracture. New tactile sense has to be learned to control the instruments.

Table 7.2 Guide to selection of predesigned preparations

Tooth	Roots	Canals	Preparation size
Maxillary teeth			
Central incisor	1	1	80
Lateral incisor	1	1	80
Canine	1	1	80
First premolar	2	2	45
First premolar	1	2	60
First premolar	1	1	80
Second premolar	1	1	80
Second premolar	1	2	60
Second premolar	2	2 (large)	60
Second premolar	2	2 (small)	45
Molar	3	Buccal	45
Molar	3	Palatal	60
Mandibular teeth			
Incisor	1	1/2	60
Canine	1	1	80
Canine	2	2	60
Premolar	1	1	80
Premolar	2	2 (equal size)	60
Premolar	2	large/small	60/45
Molar	2	Mesials	45
Molar	2	Distals	60
Molar	3	Mesials	45
Molar	3	Distobuccal	60
Molar	3	Distolingual	45/60
Molar	1	1	80

Adapted from reference 15, with permission

Coronal–apical techniques

Step-down technique

This is essentially a modification of the step-back technique and advises the following steps (**7.248–7.261**).

1. Prepare the coronal portion of the canal to a depth of 16–18 mm or to the beginning of the curve using Hedstroem files 15, 20 and 25 in a circumferential filing motion, with anticurvature filing. In narrow, calcified canals sizes 08 and 10 should first be used to enable placement of the Hedstroem files and establish patency. They are also used intermittently between the Hedstroem files to maintain canal patency.

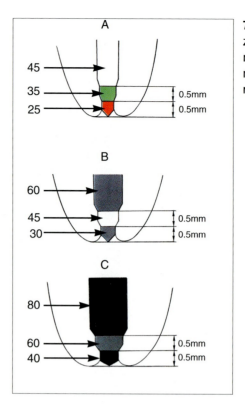

7.247 Apical control zone: A = size 45 preparation; B = size 60 preparation; C = size 80 preparation

7.248–7.261 Step-down technique

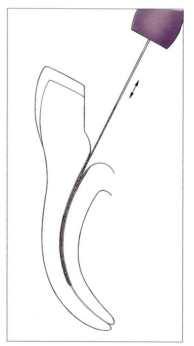

7.248 File with size 10 to 16–18mm or beginning of the curve

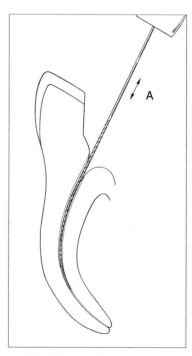

7.249 File slightly shorter than size 10 using Hedstroem size 15: A = filing

2. Gates Glidden drills 1, 2 and 3 are then used to refine the coronal preparation, the No. 3 drill extending 1–2 mm into the canal orifice.
3. Determine working length.
4. Use the step-back technique described above to complete apical preparation.

This technique overcomes many of the disadvantages of the 'pure' step-back technique, and is becoming the technique of choice. Possible disadvantages include formation of ledges, apical blockage and perforation, especially in narrow canals but these may be overcome by careful manipulation of files and frequent recapitulation.

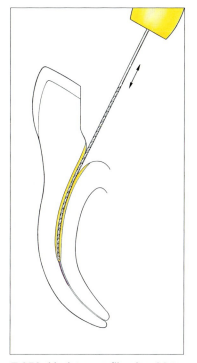

7.250 Hedstroem file size 20 to 16–18mm

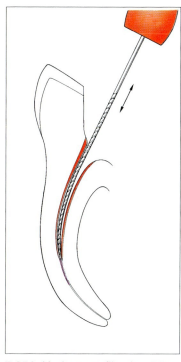

7.251 Hedstroem file size 25 to 16–18mm

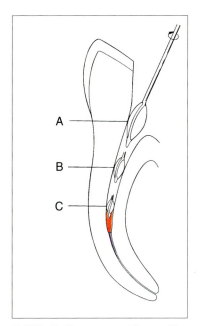

7.252 Refine coronal flare with Gates Glidden drill sizes 1–3: A = Gates Glidden 3; B = Gates Glidden 2; C = Gates Glidden 1

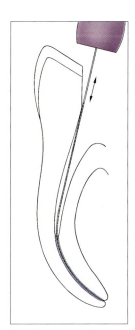

7.253 Size 10 file to full working length (WL)

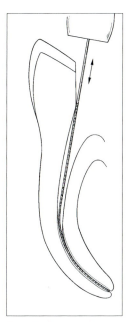

7.254 Size 15 file to full WL

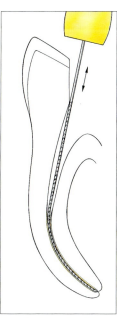

7.255 Size 20 file to full WL

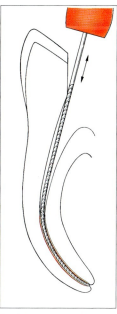

7.256 Size 25 file to full WL

7.248–7.261 Step-down technique–*continued*

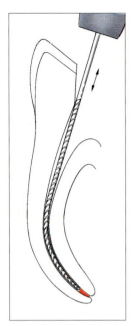

7.257 Size 30 file 1mm short of full WL

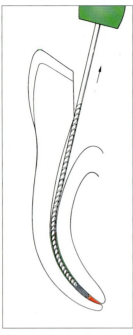

7.258 Size 35 file 2mm short of full WL

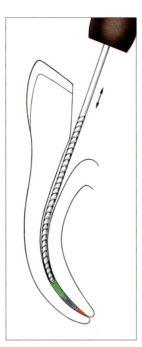

7.259 Size 40 file 3mm short of full WL

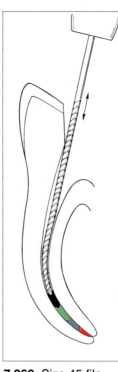

7.260 Size 45 file 4mm short of full WL

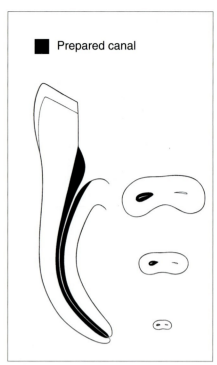

7.261 Longitudinal and transverse sections to show canal before and after preparation

Double-flared technique

This technique was devised with the fundamental principles of the coronal–apical approach in mind. The following steps should be followed (**7.262–7.276**).

1. Irrigate the pulp chamber and introduce a small file into the canal using only gentle push-pull movements to a working length estimated from radiographs. The aim of this is to introduce irrigant into the canal.
2. Take a further radiograph to check the working length.
3. Re-irrigate and introduce a larger instrument into the canal to a depth of about 14 mm (or in any case coronal to the curve). This should be loose in the canal, but is used to file the canal walls.
4. Re-irrigate and introduce the next size down 1 mm deeper into the canal, maintaining instrumentation coronal to the curve, and file the walls gently. The instrument should not bind in the canal.
5. Repeat stage (4) with the next size down.
6. Continue until the working length is reached, taking another radiograph if necessary to establish definitive working length. Once the working length is reached the full length of the canal is prepared to the appropriate size.
7. The canal is now prepared using the step-back technique as described above, except that much less filing is necessary to establish the final taper. Once again, the use of recapitulation is stressed.

This technique was originally recommended for straight canals and in the straight portions of curved canals. It is contraindicated in calcified canals, young permanent teeth and in those with open apices. The principles of the approach (to neutralise canal contents and minimize their extrusion) may be applied to most teeth.

7.262–7.276 Double-flared technique

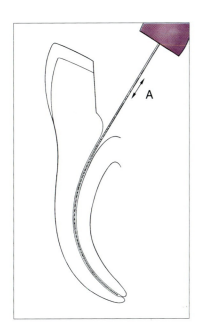

7.262 Introduce small file (No. 10) to full WL: A = without filing

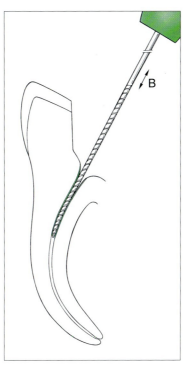

7.263 File to size 35 at about 14mm: B = filing

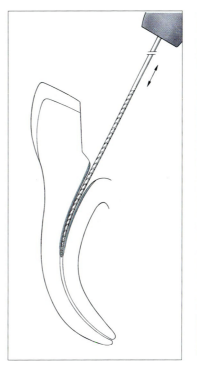

7.264 File with size 30 to 1mm deeper than size 35

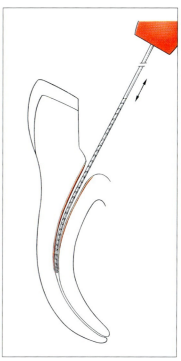

7.265 File with size 25 to 1mm deeper than size 30

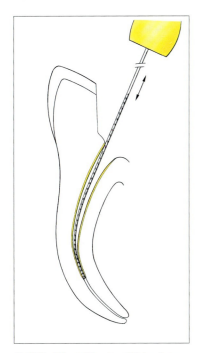

7.266 File with size 20 to 1mm deeper than size 25

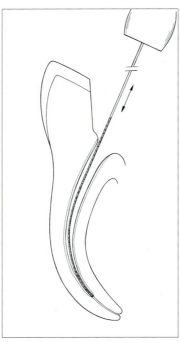

7.267 File with size 15 to 1mm deeper than size 20

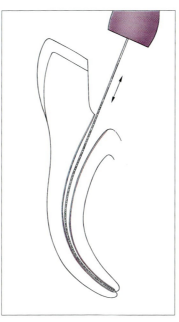

7.268 File with size 10 to 1mm deeper than size 15 (now at WL)

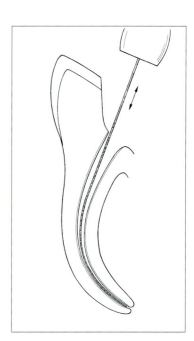

7.269 File with size 15 at WL

133

7.262–7.276 Double-flared technique–*continued*

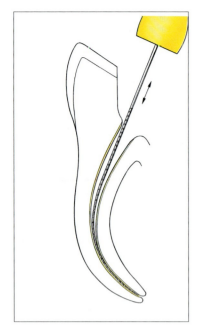

7.270 File with size 20 at WL

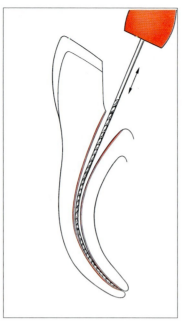

7.271 File with size 25 at WL

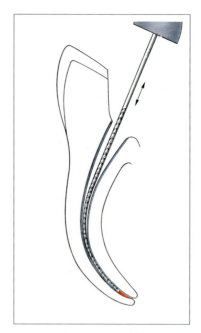

7.272 File with size 30 1mm shorter than WL

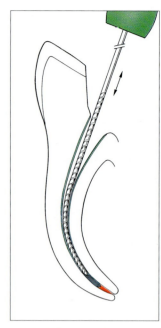

7.273 File with size 35 2mm shorter than WL

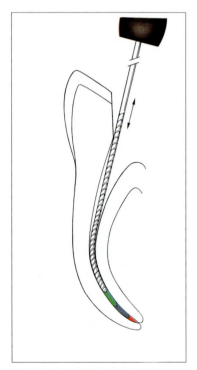

7.274 File with size 40 3mm shorter than WL

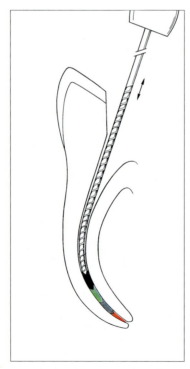

7.275 File with size 45 4mm shorter than WL

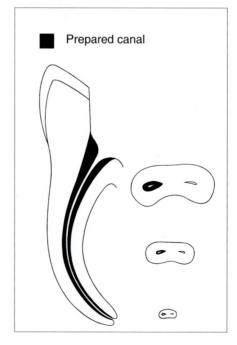

7.276 Longitudinal and transverse sections to show canal before and after preparation

Crown-down pressureless technique

The aim of this coronal–apical technique is to facilitate preparation of curved canals without causing deviation. Rotary action is used to cut dentine with the apical part of files. The following sequence (7.277–7.302) is recommended.

1. Determine radicular access length (the depth to which a No. 35 file penetrates to its point of first resistance). If this is more than 16 mm, the coronal portion of the canal should be prepared to this length. If the file penetrates less than 16 mm, a radiograph should be used to determine whether it is because of canal curvature or calcification. If it is due to beginning of a curve, the canal is prepared to the point of first resistance; if not, the canal is widened with smaller files until the No. 35 file penetrates to 16 mm.
2. Establish a provisional working length at 3 mm short of the radiographic apex.
3. Place a No. 35 file into the canal until it encounters resistance. At this point turn the file two full revolutions without apical pressure. Repeat, using the next file down until the provisional length is reached.
4. Establish the definitive working length with a check radiograph.
5. Repeat the sequence of placing a file and rotating twice without apical pressure until the working length is reached, starting with a No. 40 file.
6. Repeat the sequence, using the next instrument up in size, until the apical portion of the canal has been prepared to the desired diameter.

This technique is effective in maintaining canal shape but the rotary motion inevitably means a preparation of circular diameter. Without the use of appropriate irrigants the canals may not be as clean as in those prepared by techniques using circumferential filing.

7.277–7.302 Crown-down pressureless technique

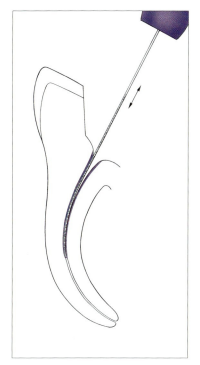

7.277 Widen canal with small files to allow No. 35 to penetrate to 16mm or curve

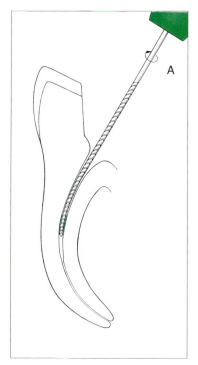

7.278 Rotational cutting with file size 35 to 16mm or curve: A = rotary motion

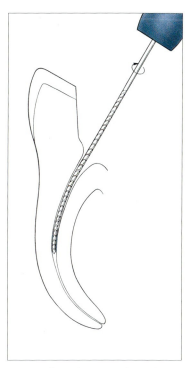

7.279 Rotational cutting with file size 30 as far as it will penetrate without apical force

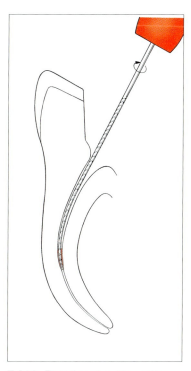

7.280 Rotational cutting with file size 25 as far as it will penetrate without apical force

7.277–7.302 Crown-down pressureless technique–*continued*

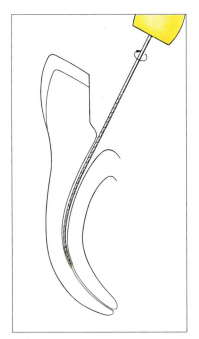

7.281 Rotational cutting with size 20 as far as it will penetrate without apical force

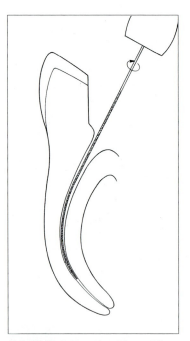

7.282 Rotational cutting with size 15 as far as it will penetrate without apical force

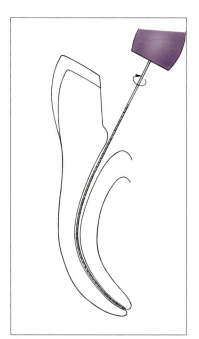

7.283 Rotational cutting with size 10 as far as it will penetrate without apical force

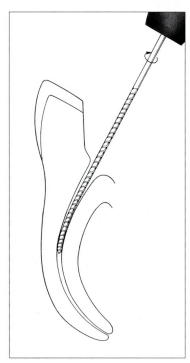

7.284 Repeat sequence– starting with size 40

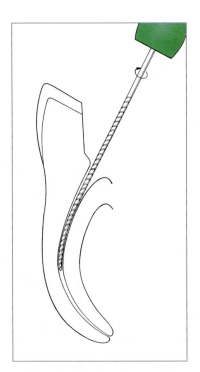

7.285 Rotational cutting with size 35

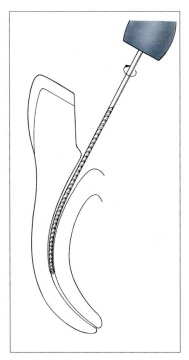

7.286 Size 30 penetrating deeper

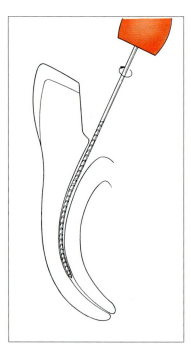

7.287 Size 25 penetrating deeper

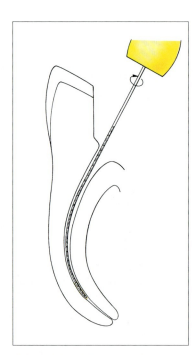

7.288 Size 20 penetrating deeper

7.277–7.302 Crown-down pressureless technique–*continued*

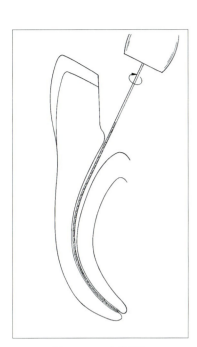

7.289 Size 15 at full WL

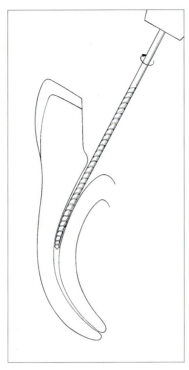

7.290 Repeat sequence starting with size 45

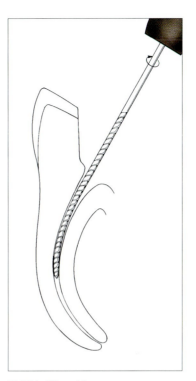

7.291 Size 40

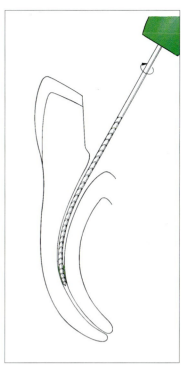

7.292 Size 35

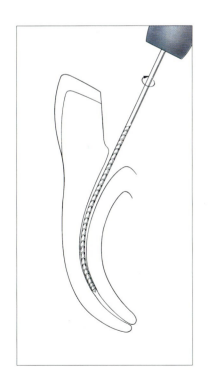

7.293 Size 30

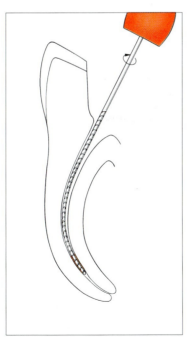

7.294 Size 25

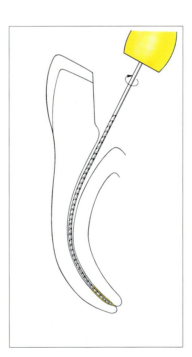

7.295 Size 20 at full WL

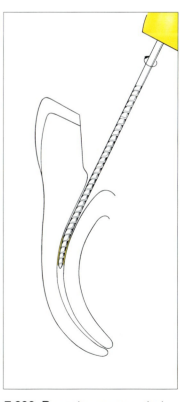

7.296 Repeat sequence starting with size 50

7.277–7.302 Crown-down pressureless technique–*continued*

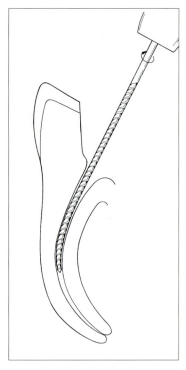
7.297 Size 45

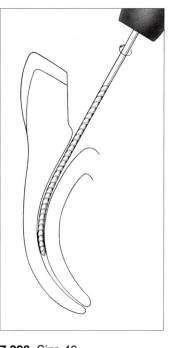
7.298 Size 40

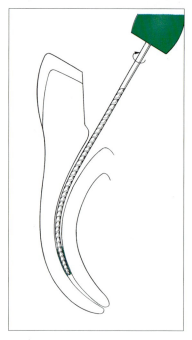
7.299 Size 35

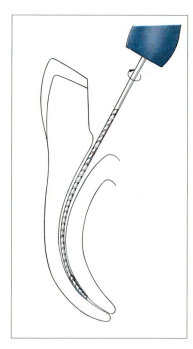
7.300 Size 30:

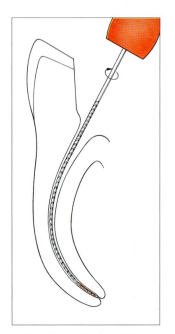
7.301 Size 25 at full WL

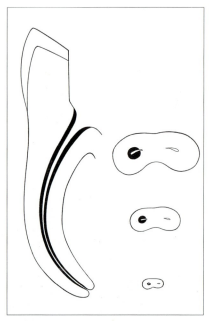
7.302 Longitudinal and transverse sections showing canal before and after preparation

Canal Master technique

This technique uses a revolutionary brand of root canal instrument in a coronal–apical approach. Its aim is to aid the maintenance of curves using a rotary instrument designed so that only the apical 1–2 mm is engaged in dentine removal. The instruments are both hand-held and mechanized. The apical 0.75 mm of the hand instruments is safe-ended to facilitate maintenance of canal curvature and it is claimed that this technique avoids the need for recapitulation. The following sequence (**7.303**–**7.319**) is used.

1. Determine working length.
2. Prepare to the beginning of the curve using the mechanized rotary instruments.
3. Use the Canal Master instruments in step-back fashion to prepare the curve.

Thorough evaluation of this relatively new technique is needed, but early results seem promising in terms of the shape produced. Intermediate file sizes are available, enabling easier negotiation of curves and a progressive development of flare at 0.5 mm intervals. The instruments may have a tendency to fracture. The disadvantages are those of any technique using purely rotary motion.

7.303–7.319 Canal Master technique
N.B. The size of the tip of these instruments is smaller than conventional hand instruments

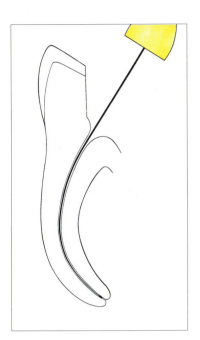

7.303 Size 20 to full WL

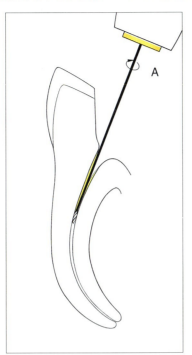

7.304 Size 50 in automated instrument to beginning of curve: A = rotary motion

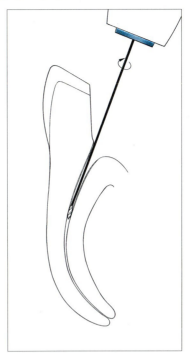

7.305 Size 60 in automated instrument to beginning of curve

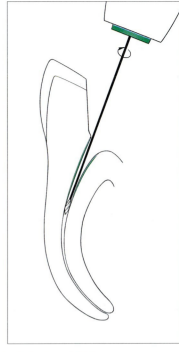

7.306 Size 70 in automated instrument to beginning of curve

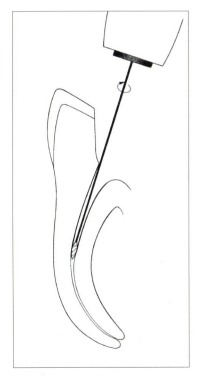

7.307 Size 80 in automated instrument to beginning of curve

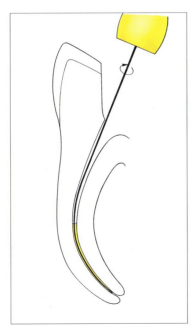

7.308 Size 20 to full WL

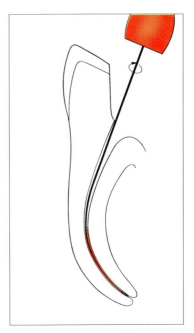

7.309 Size 25 to full WL

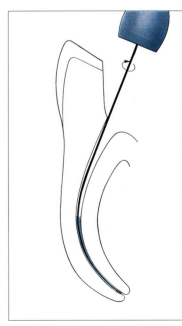

7.310 Size 30 to full WL

7.303–7.319 Canal Master technique—*continued*

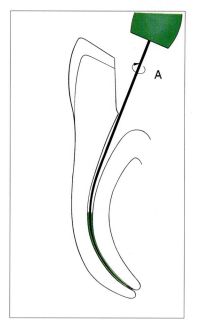

7.311 Size 35 to full WL: A = rotary motion

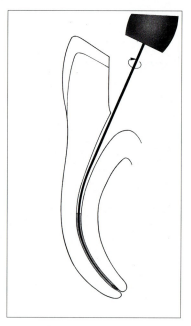

7.312 Size 40 to full WL

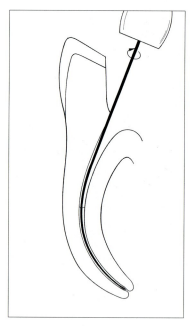

7.313 Size 45 to full WL

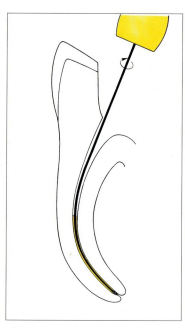

7.314 Size 50 to full WL

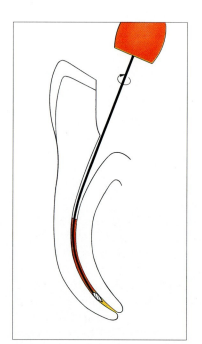

7.315 Size 55 1mm shorter than WL

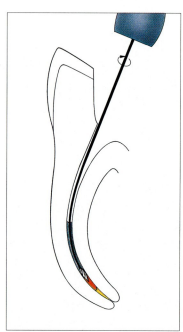

7.316 Size 60 2mm shorter than WL

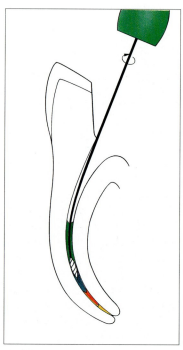

7.317 Size 70 3mm shorter than WL

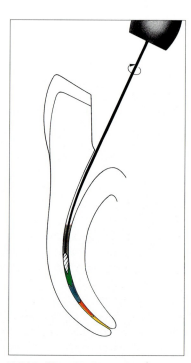

7.318 Size 80 4mm shorter than WL

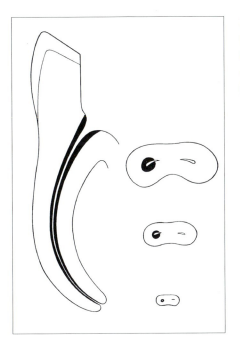

7.319 Canal Master technique: Longitudinal and transverse sections of canal before and after preparation

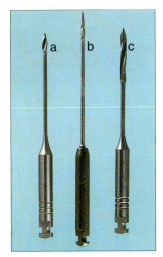

7.320 (a) Gates Glidden; (b) Canal Master 'U'; (c) Peeso reamer

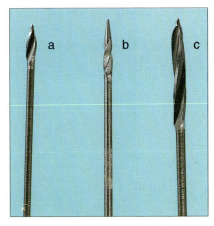

7.321 (a) Gates Glidden; (b) Canal Master 'U'; (c) Peeso reamer

Hybrid techniques

The instructions given above describe general principles only and should not be followed 'cook-book' style, except in the early stages of learning. Most experienced operators mix the desirable aspects of different techniques to suit individual needs.

Preparation using automated devices

Preparation of root canals with hand instruments is both hard work and time consuming. Most operators are attracted by the idea of using an automated instrument that will make root canal preparation easier and quicker. Many automated devices are available, all of which have advantages and disadvantages but none of which provides better control or produces a more predictable shape than hand-operated instruments. The main disadvantage of automated instruments is the loss of tactile sense, and therefore lack of control of where and how much dentine is removed from the root canal wall. Further considerations of automated devices are the ergonomics, the facility of changing files, the time taken to sterilize the handpiece and general maintenance, which must all be added to the preparation time. Which automated device is 'best' is a matter of personal preference.

Classification of devices

A simple classification is given below according to the type of movement imparted to the cutting instrument.

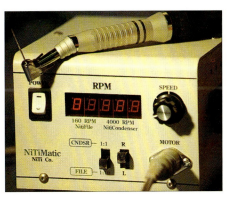

7.322 16:1 gear reduction unit (NiTiMatic)

Rotary

Used in a slow running standard handpiece such as Gates Glidden, Peeso and Canal Master (**7.320**, **7.321**). All these instruments should be used only in the straight part of the root canal.

A new 16:1 gear reduction handpiece has been introduced (The NiTiMatic, available from NT company, Shallowfield Road, Chattanooga, TN 37421, USA), which is run at 300 r.p.m. (**7.322**). Two different types of nickel–titanium file have been designed specifically for the handpiece. The flexibility and resistance to fracture of these files allow preparation of severely curved root canals. The files are manufactured with an off-centre tip that facilitates negotiating around curvatures and ledges. No comparative studies are available to date.

Reciprocal quarter turn

This uses a special handpiece (**7.323**) which contrarotates the instrument through 90°. The Giromatic (**7.324**) was introduced in 1964 and still has a following. A second handpiece, with a similar movement, is the Endo-Cursor, which has a press button chuck and will take hand instruments. The Kerr's Endolift has a vertical component in addition to the rotation but is little used. A variety of canal instruments is available for use with the Giromatic:

- Giro-pointer: 16 mm long orifice opener;
- Giro-broach or cleanser;
- Giro-file, a Hedstroem configuration;
- Giro-reamer;
- Heli-girofile, with three cutting blades in cross-section.

Vertical

The Canal Finder system (available from Societé Endotechnic (SET), 6 Traverse des Hussards, 13005 Marseilles, France) is a specialized handpiece with a vertical movement of 0.3–1.0 mm and a free rotational movement (**7.325**). Increasing vertical pressure will stop the vertical movement. The free rotational movement allows the tip of the instrument to move away from an obstruction in the wall of the root canal. The instrument designed for the handpiece, the Canal Master, is a Hedstroem file with a safe-ended tip.

A modified, speed reducing handpiece with a 4:1 step down, the Canal Leader (produced by SET, Haupstrasse 3, Olching, Germany) (**7.326**), is available. It has a vertical movement of 0.4–0.8 mm and a contrarotational movement which is restricted to 30° (**7.327**). Both of these movements depend on the speed of the micromotor and the resistance within the root canal: the greater the resistance the more the movement is restricted. Three cutting instruments are available: a K-File with a safe ended tip for narrow canals; a more aggressive Hedstroem file; and a universal file, which is a flexible Hedstroem file with a safe-ended tip.

Random

The W & H handpiece, called an Excalibur (**7.328**), produces a random lateral vibrational movement. The instruments are modified K-files and the handpiece is run at 20 000–25 000 r.p.m. The authors have found the handpiece somewhat bulky in the posterior part of the mouth.

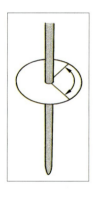

7.323 Reciprocal quarter turn

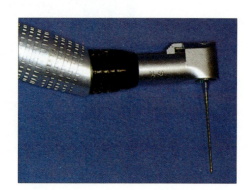

7.324 Giromatic

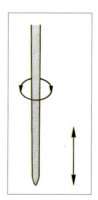

7.325 Vertical movement with free rotation

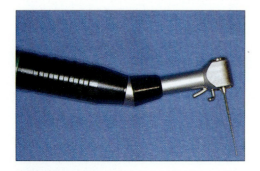

7.326 Canal Leader

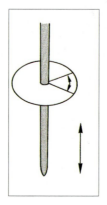

7.327 Vertical and rotational movement

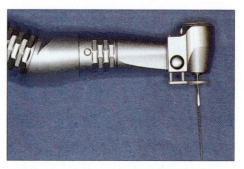

7.328 Random movement (Excalibur)

Sonic oscillation

These include the Sonic air 1500 and the Megasonic 1400 (**7.329**), produced by MicroMega, and a similar handpiece produced by Endostar. A vibrational wave form is imparted to the file shank. The handpiece will accept Rispi files, Heli-sonic files and Shapers. Rispi files are used in the coronal two-thirds of the root canal and the Shaper in the apical one-third. The displacement of the tip of the file is adjusted to 1.0 mm for maximum efficiency. It has been reported that when lateral movement is stopped in the canal a vertical movement of approximately 100 µm is evident (**7.330**). The movement of the file shank creates a form of acoustic microstreaming (**7.331**) with two areas of turbulence, one around the mid shank and the other at the tip.

Ultrasonic oscillation

There are two methods of generating ultrasonic oscillations in the file shank: magnetostrictive (**7.332**) and piezoelectric (**7.333**). The piezoelectric is the most common type on the market; it is more powerful than the magnetostrictive method and does not require water cooling. The magnetostrictive stack requires water cooling, which means that if sodium hypochlorite is used as the irrigant, the water must be led away from the stack via additional tubing, making the handpiece both clumsy and expensive. In both types the greatest amount of movement in the file is at the tip. Two types of file are used: a modified K-file and a diamond-impregnated file for the straight part of the canal. The magnetostrictive type can, with care, produce a tapered canal

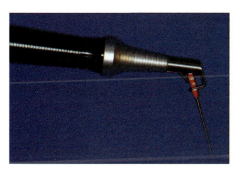

7.329 Sonic air

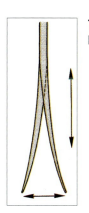

7.330 Sonic oscillation

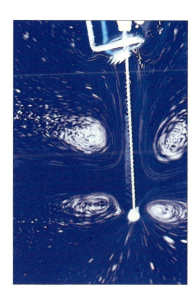

7.331 Microstreaming effect with sonic oscillation

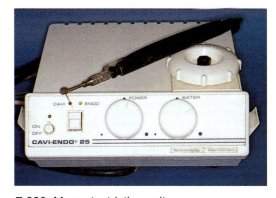

7.332 Magnetostrictive unit

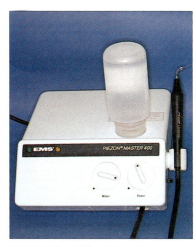

7.333 Piezoelectric unit

shape because the tip is constrained by pressing against the wall of the canal. The piezoelectric units are more powerful and so less easy to constrain at the tip of the file, which may produce apical widening and ledges in curved canals (7.334).

Current feeling is against using ultrasonic units for shaping curved root canals. The main advantage of using ultrasound in root canals is the cleaning effect; 7.335 shows the irrigant passing down the shank of the file. The main cleaning effect is thought to be due to acoustic microstreaming; 7.336 illustrates the turbulence along the shank of the file when immersed in a fluid. The size of file recommended by the authors is 10 or 15 because these are the most flexible and therefore less likely to produce ledges; also, a small file allows more space between the shank and the canal wall for the irrigant. Continuous irrigation is recommended, and it is interesting to note that the temperature of the irrigant within the canal does not increase. There is evidence to show that, provided sodium hypochlorite is used, cleaner root canal walls may be obtained than with hand instruments and an irrigation syringe.

Ultrasonic units are useful for the removal of posts, fractured instruments (see Chapter 13) and coating the canal walls with sealer before filling.

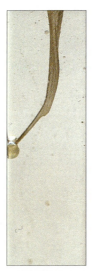

7.334 Ledge formation and apical widening

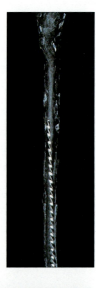

7.335 Irrigant passing down shank

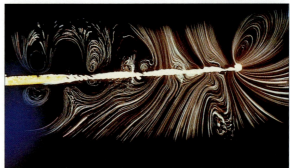

7.336 Acoustic microstreaming

8 Intracanal medication and temporary seal

Rationale for intracanal medication

The rationale behind intracanal medication is to destroy residual micro-organisms and their toxins and to remove organic tissue. This objective is mostly fulfilled during canal preparation but the complexity of root canal systems is such that not all microorganisms or remnants of pulp tissue are removed. Furthermore, the dentinal tubules of canals with necrotic pulps may be invaded by anaerobic bacteria. The medicament should inhibit microbial recolonization of the cleaned parts of the root canal system by preventing residual microorganisms from growing and new organisms invading through lateral communications and coronal access.

Ideally the medicament should

1. Destroy all root canal microorganisms.
2. Have a lasting antimicrobial effect.
3. Be unaffected by organic material.
4. Help to remove residual organic tissue.
5. Penetrate the root canal system and dentinal tubules.
6. Not irritate periradicular tissues or have systemic toxicity.
7. Have anodyne properties.
8. Induce a calcific barrier at the junction with periradicular tissues.
9. Have no effect on the physical properties of the temporary filling material.
10. Not diffuse through the temporary filling material.
11. Be easily placed and removed.
12. Be radio-opaque.
13. Not stain the tooth.

No single root canal medicament meets all these requirements and it is therefore not surprising that a great range of different materials has been tested, many empirically or on the basis of research *in vitro*. Little clinical research appears to have been undertaken on the efficacy of these materials, and usage tends to be based on personal preference. The vast array of materials may be divided for analysis into groups of like chemical structures and mode of function.

Phenol-based agents

These include phenol, parachlorophenol, camphorated monoparachlorophenol, metacresyl acetate, cresol, creosote, eugenol and thymol, and once were the most commonly used agents. The antimicrobial effect of these agents has only been proven *in vitro*. Unfortunately, the essential good contact between microorganisms and the agent, which is possible *in vitro*, is difficult to achieve within the root canal system. A pledget of cotton wool soaked in the solution and placed in the pulp chamber is not sufficient: the characteristic strong-smelling vapours are not concentrated enough to destroy micro-organisms. The solutions exhibit antimicrobial properties only when used in sufficient volume and concentration, (i.e. the canals must be flooded). Furthermore, their antimicrobial effect is not long-lasting. These solutions are able to diffuse through the temporary filling material and cause an unpleasant taste in the mouth; some even soften the filling material.

Phenol

Phenol is no longer used because of its toxicity – it was replaced by monochlorophenol, which has lower toxicity and improved antimicrobial effect.

Camphorated monochlorophenol (CMCP)

A solution of CMCP may be made by dissolving monochlorophenol crystals in camphor. Work *in vitro* suggested that weaker solutions were more effective as antimicrobial agents and more dilute solutions have been used clinically.

Metacresyl acetate

Metacresyl acetate, or cresatin, has been favoured by some clinicians because it was thought to have low irritation potential and anodyne action but the latter is unproven. Most products containing this compound are therefore now largely out of favour because of their limited antimicrobial effect (in both range and duration), toxicity and lack of other positive features.

Aldehydes

These materials (formaldehyde-containing preparations, formocresol, glutaraldehyde) have mainly been used in paedodontics, and their efficacy in this respect is covered in Chapter 16. They have no role in the treatment of permanent teeth. Formaldehyde-containing materials have been used for their antimicrobial and fixative properties but they are very toxic to periradicular tissues and furthermore fixed pulp tissue is potentially antigenic.

Glutaraldehyde also has the potential to cause hypersensitivity.

Halides

These include sodium hypochlorite and iodine–potassium iodide. Sodium hypochlorite fulfils the most important criteria of antimicrobial effect and tissue dissolution, but its efficacy is limited because chemical reaction depletes its effect. In addition, because the canal would need to be flooded, sodium hypochlorite may interact with the temporary filling material.

Iodine–potassium iodide appears to be of low toxicity and highly antimicrobial *in vitro*. It is easily made by mixing 4 g potassium iodide and 2 g iodine in 94 ml water. The root canal needs to be flooded but its long-term clinical effectiveness is not known. This material has probably not gained favour because of its potential for allergic responses and tooth staining.

Antibiotics

Topical application of antibiotics (such as bacitracin, neomycin, polymyxin, chloramphenicol, tyrothricin and nystatin) in the root canal has been popular with some clinicians because of a few uniquely favourable properties: they are not toxic to periradicular tissues, do not stain teeth and are active in the presence of organic material. No single antibiotic is active against all microorganisms found in the root canal, so a combination of antibiotics with different ranges of activity is used, usually in paste form. Objections that have been raised to the use of antibiotic pastes include the possibility of resistant strains, possible sensitization of the patient and development of an allergic response. Although a few cases of allergic response have been recorded, there is no overwhelming evidence against the use of topical antibiotics. However, the efficacy of most of these preparations has not been thoroughly tested.

Steroids

Steroids (prednisolone, triamcinolone, hydrocortisone) have been used in root canals mainly for pain relief but there is no positive clinical evidence of the anodyne properties of steroids. These materials have no other beneficial quality and therefore may be mixed with other antimicrobial agents such as calcium hydroxide. The commercially available paste popularly used in this manner is Ledermix, which also contains the antibiotic tetracycline. However, mixing these materials may reduce the effect of individual components rather than providing synergism.

A disadvantage of using steroids is that they depress defence mechanisms, including inflammation. Their use may also bring the risk of inducing a bacteraemia, a particular hazard in patients susceptible to infection of damaged tissue or prosthetic replacements, e.g. those with infective endocarditis and prosthetic heart valves.

Calcium hydroxide

This material is very popular as an intracanal medicament, as it is effective against most root canal pathogens. It is also able to denature bacterial endotoxin and organic tissue, making it more susceptible to dissolution by sodium hypochlorite. The duration of antimicrobial effect depends on the concentration and volume of the paste but is considered to be long-lasting. The material is irritating if extruded and may cause localized necrosis, which is self-limiting. Extrusion may be accompanied by severe pain lasting 12–24 hours. For this reason some clinicians prefer to mix calcium hydroxide with a steroid paste.

The material's ability to cause localized necrosis may help to form a hard calcific barrier at the junction with the periradicular tissues. Necrotic tissue forms the matrix for calcification, and calcium hydroxide is therefore useful for closing wide apices (**8.1, 8.2**) and intracanal repair of perforations (**8.3–8.5**) and horizon-

8.1, 8.2 Closure of wide apices

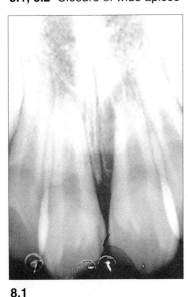

8.1

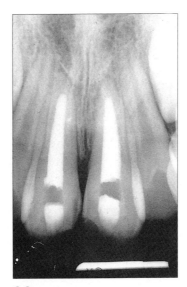

8.2

8.3

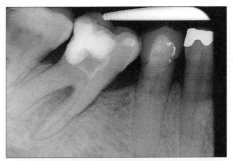

8.3–8.5 Intracanal repair of perforation in the furcal aspect of the mesial root of 6̅|

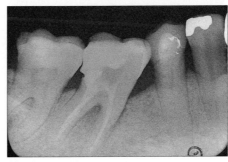

8.4

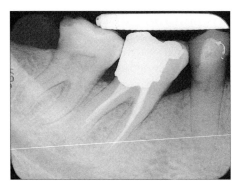

8.5 **8.6–8.8** Treatment of horizontal fractures where apical fragment has vital pulp tissue

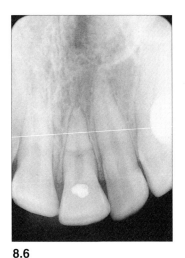

8.6

8.7

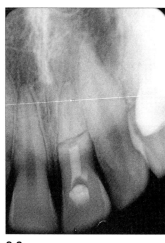

8.8

8.11–8.13 Non-resolution of replacement resorption, despite root canal treatment

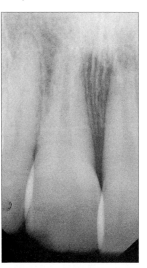

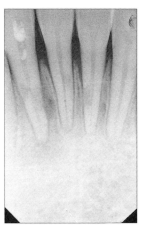

8.9 External inflammatory resorption in mandibular right lateral incisor and replacement resorption in left central incisor

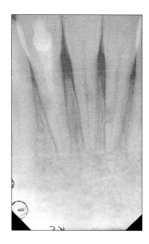

8.10 Resolution of inflammatory resorption following canal debridement and calcium hydroxide dressing in right lateral incisor

8.11

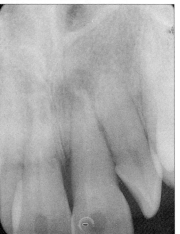

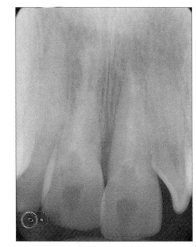

8.12

8.13

tal fractures (**8.6–8.8**) before obturation.

Calcium hydroxide is also readily available, inexpensive, simple to place and simple to remove from the root canal system. It does not stain the teeth, or affect temporary dressings. Another benefit attributed to calcium hydroxide is the ability to dry weeping canals. The reason for this effect is unclear but it is probably related to elimination of residual infection and possibly inactivation of toxins. Calcium hydroxide has been recommended for treatment of external inflammatory resorption. Its mode of action is probably related to its antimicrobial properties. Figures **8.9** and **8.10** show both external inflammatory resorption (right lateral incisor) and external replacement resorption (left central incisor); the latter does not respond to calcium hydroxide treatment as demonstrated by the case shown in **8.11–8.13**.

Calcium hydroxide preparations

Many commercially available products (e.g. Multical, Pulpdent, Hypocal, Rootcal, Reogan) contain calcium hydroxide with other ingredients. The constituents of these commercial products vary widely: the calcium hydroxide content is about 34–50%, barium sulphate 5–15%. The remainder is water and methyl or hydroxymethyl cellulose. Other antiseptic materials such as chlorothymonol may be added.

The disadvantages of commercially available materials are that the most important ingredient (calcium hydroxide) is diluted and the pastes may be difficult to place with any degree of control. Many clinicians prefer to use the pure-grade calcium hydroxide powder, which can be mixed in a ratio of 7:1 with barium sulphate powder for radio-opacity. The resultant mixture, which should be stored in an airtight bottle, may be mixed with water, saline or local anaesthetic (without vasoconstrictor) to a paste of the required consistency (**8.14**). The powder may also be added as a thickener to commercial products, but it may adversely affect its rheological properties.

Placement of calcium hydroxide

The method of placing calcium hydroxide is usually a matter of personal preference. A range of manual and automated techniques may be used depending upon the consistency of the preparation. The more fluid, commercially available, pastes may be applied with files or paper points but these methods are unlikely to reach all aspects of the root canal system. Some recommend the use of spiral fillers or an ultrasonically activated file.

The stiffer pastes may be loaded using conventional amalgam carriers or intracanal carriers such as the Messing Gun (**8.15**). The paste can be packed down to the position required using pluggers or files (**8.16–8.19**). Packing large pellets of a hard mix may cause periapical discomfort if air is trapped apical to the calcium hydroxide; it is better to break up the dressing into smaller portions within the canal before packing these apically.

Removal and replacement of calcium hydroxide

Calcium hydroxide is relatively easily removed by washing and irrigating with water or sodium hypochlorite solution (the latter is preferable because it will allow further dissolution of residual organic debris). Sometimes the calcium hydroxide may become very well compacted in a narrow canal, giving the impression of a blockage. It is important to use sufficient water and a small file to negotiate past the blockage. An ultrasonically activated file is very

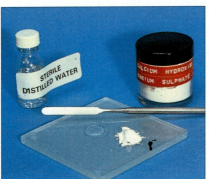

8.14 Preparation of calcium hydroxide paste with powder and water

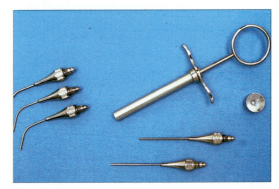

8.15 Messing gun

8.16–8.19 Placement of calcium hydroxide

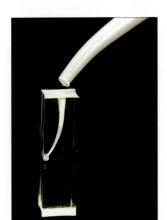

8.16 Placement of calcium hydroxide with amalgam carrier

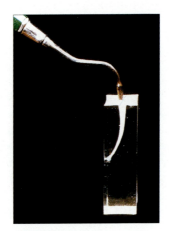

8.17 Coronal compaction into the canal with a narrow amalgam plugger

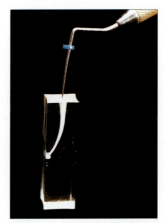

8.18 Breakage of calcium hydroxide mass in canal into small pellets with plugger

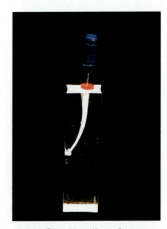

8.19 Small pellets from **8.18** carried apically with a file or plugger

effective at removing calcium hydroxide dressings.

The period for which a calcium hydroxide dressing is retained depends on the objective of the dressing. If a routine intracanal dressing is required, a few days is likely to be sufficient; to arrest a weeping canal it may be necessary to dress with a stiff paste for 1–2 weeks. If a substantial amount of paste has been resorbed (**8.20, 8.21**), more frequent dressings with stiffer pastes may be required. Dressing and irrigation are continued until weeping is resolved.

The use of calcium hydroxide to induce a calcific barrier at the periodontal ligament (at the apex in immature teeth, at fractures and perforations) requires longer periods of dressing. In the first instance, dressing should be changed at 2 weeks to evaluate the degree of loss or contamination (it also allows further opportunity to irrigate the canal system with sodium hypochlorite and reduce the microbial and organic contamination). The dressing may then be left in place and healing reassessed at intervals of 3–4 months. Criteria for assessment of healing include absence of intracanal bleeding or exudate, absence of symptoms, tactile evidence of a barrier and radiographic evidence of bone resolution adjacent to the site of calcific repair (**8.22, 8.23**). Incompletely formed apices can take up to 24 months before a complete barrier forms but are mostly complete by 9 months.

The duration of dressing in cases of dental trauma and root resorption is discussed in Chapters 12 and 13.

Calcium hydroxide may also be used as a long-term dressing, or as a short-term root filling if treatment cannot be completed for logistical reasons or if the tooth needs to be reviewed to assess outcome of treatment (for example, perio-endo cases: see **8.24, 8.25**). There is positive advantage to the routine dressing of root canals with calcium hydroxide.

Temporary seal

Following canal preparation and dressing a temporary seal is placed in the access cavity to prevent microleakage of microorganisms and saliva, which may inactivate the medicament and allow bacterial regrowth.

The integrity of seal depends on strength and durability of the material and the marginal seal. The access cavity is designed to provide retention and resistance form in the apical and coronal

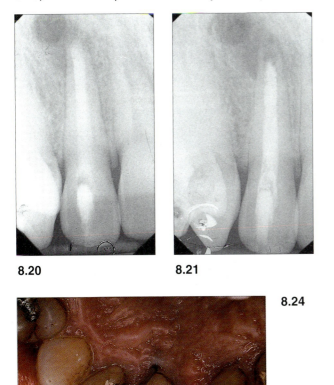

8.20, 8.21 Resorption of calcium hydroxide paste with time

8.24, 8.25 Canal debridement and dressing with calcium hydroxide may aid diagnosis of a perio-endo lesion

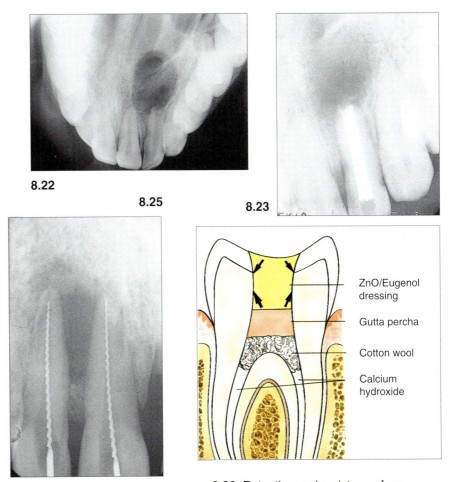

8.22, 8.23 Periapical resolution following canal debridement and calcium hydroxide dressing

8.26 Retention and resistance form of an access cavity

directions (**8.26**).

It is customary for the access cavity seal to be placed as a double layer. Warmed stick gutta percha is placed over cotton wool in the access cavity before applying the definitive sealing material (**8.26, 8.27**). The gutta percha and cotton wool help to separate the intracanal medicament from the temporary seal and prevents particles of the material falling into the canal during its removal.

Materials

Materials available for temporary seal include zinc oxide/eugenol (preferably reinforced), Cavit, glass ionomer, polycarboxylate, zinc phosphate and resins.

Zinc oxide/eugenol cement

The material of choice is zinc oxide/eugenol because it has proven ability to seal against microorganisms. It is not very strong or durable and therefore IRM and Kalzinol should be used. These materials are best used to restore a conventional access cavity rather than a larger defect.

To effect a good seal, proper manipulation of this sticky material is essential. It should be adapted with apical pressure from the centre of the cavity outwards or it may pull away from the margin (**8.28**). When mixed to a high powder/liquid ratio the material is very durable (**8.29**). In the case shown the patient did not attend for 2 years after placement but the IRM dressings were still intact when seen. In the second case (**8.30**), a low powder/liquid ratio resulted in surface loss of material over a period of 3 months.

The only disadvantage of using zinc oxide/eugenol is its incompatibility with composite restorations. If this is likely to be a problem a non-eugenol dressing should be used.

Glass ionomer cements

Glass ionomer cements have been recommended because of their adhesive properties. However, the need to use the material in bulk means that setting contraction may be significant and can cause the integrity of at least part of its margin to be compromised.

Other materials

Other cements, such as zinc phosphate and zinc polycarboxylate, provide durable seals and reasonable marginal integrity at high powder/liquid ratios, but do not possess the same antimicrobial activity as zinc oxide/eugenol.

Cavit is popular because it is available in a ready-to-use form. It is essentially 'plaster', and can give a reasonable seal over periods of about a week, but is not very durable. It does possess some antimicrobial effect but is not as strong as zinc oxide/eugenol. Its so-called 'self-repairing' capacity is related to its ability to absorb moisture and expand. Because of its lack of physical strength it needs to be used in adequate depth, considered to be about 3.5 mm. Restoration of large cavities with Cavit results in cracks within it and leakage.

The latest access restorative materials are made of resins. An example is *Term*, which is also a hygroscopic material and which may be useful for larger cavities.

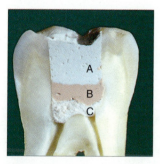

8.27 Double-layered dressing of access cavity: A = zinc oxide/eugenol dressing; B = gutta percha; C = cotton wool

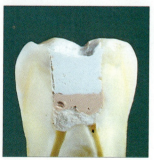

8.28 The IRM dressing tends to pull away from the cavity wall opposite to that being adapted unless adapted with apical pressure

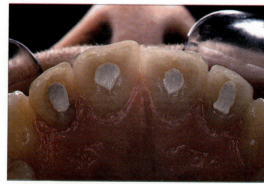

8.29 IRM dressing with a high powder: liquid ratio after 2 years

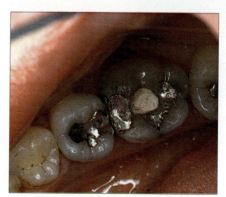

8.30 IRM dressing with a low powder:liquid ratio after 3 months

9 Obturation of the root canal system

Rationale for obturation

The aim of filling the root canal system is to prevent recontamination by micro-organisms, either from those microbes left in the canal after preparation or from new invaders from the coronal access or lateral communications. The root filling should therefore be able to destroy residual micro-organisms and adapt adequately to root canal walls to prevent their passage or growth. It should also prevent leakage of molecules capable of supporting microbial growth or initiating a periapical defence response. The degree of seal required is dictated by the smallest molecule capable of initiating and sustaining periapical inflammation. Unfortunately, our knowledge of the pathogenesis of periapical lesions does not extend to such detail and in the absence of such information it would seem wise to seal the canal system as well as the materials available allow.

When to root fill

Root canal treatment has traditionally been performed over multiple visits, partly because root canal systems are complex and unpredictably variable. Two or more visits therefore allow an opportunity to gauge the efficacy of canal cleaning as judged by commonly accepted clinical criteria. These are:

1. Absence of pain and swelling.
2. No tenderness to percussion.
3. Absence of tenderness to palpation of the associated oral mucosa.
4. No demonstrable patent sinus.
5. Absence of persistent exudate in the canal (dry canal).
6. An odour-free canal.

Persistence of symptoms is taken to indicate residual infection, prompting re-evaluation of the tooth's canal anatomy, its state of contamination and the need for further cleaning or preparation.

Recently there has been a trend, especially among specially trained endodontists, towards completing the treatment in a single visit. The rationale behind this is that obturation at a second visit may allow recontamination of the canal system in the intervening period and therefore jeopardize the outcome. Single-visit treatment also offers the advantages of only one application of local anaesthetic and rubber dam, reduced overall treatment time and therefore reduced cost (it may therefore be more acceptable to patients). The advantage to the operator is better familiarity with the canal system at the time of filling. However, the operator and patient risk severe fatigue with this technique and the root canal is not easily accessed for drainage in the event of an acute flare-up after treatment. Specific indications for such an approach include root canal treatment of teeth with vital pulps (where multiple visits may expose the canal system to the risk of microbial contamination and reduce chances of success) and the need for an immediate post crown. If a probationary period is essential, an alternative is to restore aesthetics and function with an immediate temporary overdenture, which allows an undisturbed temporary access seal.

The only absolute contraindication of a single visit approach is persistent weeping from the root canal. Indeed, this contraindicates obturation at any time and may need a surgical 'through and through' approach to stop it. Complex anatomy with long, narrow, curved canals may render single visit treatment more difficult or prevent it altogether.

Properties of root filling materials

The ideal root filling material exhibits the following properties.

1. It is antimicrobial.
2. It does not irritate periapical tissues but promotes periapical healing.
3. It possesses no systemic toxicity.
4. It has good flow characteristics.
5. It adapts well to canal walls, to the extent of being adhesive.
6. No dimensional changes occur after placement.
7. It is not susceptible to disintegration by moisture and tissue fluid.
8. It is radio-opaque.
9. It has good manipulative characteristics and is easy and quick to place.
10. It is easily removed for post-space preparation and retreatment if necessary.
11. It does not stain dentine.
12. It is cheap.

Many obturation materials and techniques are available but none satisfies all of these criteria. Effective use requires an appreciation of the properties of the materials and their manipulation characteristics. As well as compatibility between the material, instruments and technique it is important that the shape of the prepared root canal will facilitate their use.

Gutta percha

The most widely used and accepted material for obturation of flared root canals is gutta percha (*trans*-polyisoprene). Gutta percha may exist in one of three forms: two crystalline stereo forms (α and β) and an amorphous or molten form (**9.1**). All three play a part in obturation of root canals. For practical reasons it is important to understand the relationship between the three forms. Gutta percha harvested from trees is mainly α phase and is used in the latest thermoplasticized techniques (or so the manufacturers claim). Conventional gutta percha points are made from the β phase, which transforms to α phase when heated to 42–49

°C. On continued heating the crystalline form is lost to give the amorphous melt at 53–59°C (the exact temperatures depend on the brand used). These phase transformations are associated with volumetric changes (**9.2**), which have obvious relevance to the obturation of root canals. Gutta percha heated to a higher temperature shrinks more on cooling. If cooling is also associated with a phase change, as seems likely, then the shrinkage is even greater. The practical implication is that heated gutta percha requires pressure to compact it as it cools to prevent contraction gaps from developing (**9.3, 9.4**).

Commercially available gutta percha is compounded with a number of substances to modify its properties (**Table 9.1**). The exact composition varies between manufacturers and batches: this accounts for the variation in properties.

The different formulations of gutta percha are used in a number of techniques:

1. Cold lateral condensation.
2. Warm lateral condensation.
3. Warm vertical condensation.
4. Thermocompaction and hybrid technique.
5. Injection technique using thermoplasticized gutta percha.
6. Thermoplasticized gutta percha carried on a solid core.
7. Diffusion technique.

In all except the last of these techniques, a sealer is needed as an adjunct to filling root canals.

Use of sealers

The purpose of a sealer is to fill the irregular spaces between the canal wall and gutta percha points. It is applied to root canal walls, and thinly to individual gutta percha points where appropriate. Sealers should have adequate mixing properties and working time in addition to the desirable properties of root filling materials.

Sealers are usually a cement formulation mixed to a paste which sets by chemical reaction. Many contain zinc oxide/eugenol (e.g. Roth's, Grossman's, Kerr's, Procosol, Wach's, Tubliseal and CRCS sealers). Most sealers have a powder/liquid formulation and relatively long setting times, but some (e.g. Tubliseal) have a paste/paste formulation, with a shorter setting time, particularly in the presence of moisture and heat. A new Tubliseal formulation has been developed with an extended working time.

Sealers may also contain radio-opacifiers, such as barium sulphate, precipitated silver or bismuth salts in addition to zinc oxide and eugenol, and resins such as stabylite, hydrogenated rosin ester, hydrogenated resin, oleoresins and polymerized resin. Some sealers also contain antibacterial substances (e.g. Tubliseal contains thymol iodide). CRCS sealer also contains calcium hydroxide – but this is unlikely to be of much therapeutic benefit because most of it is chelated by the eugenol. Sealapex, a paste/paste formulation, is another material containing calcium hydroxide. It does not contain eugenol, but is based on a polymeric reaction. It releases calcium hydroxide and is thought to be

Table 9.1 Percentage composition of conventional gutta percha points

Gutta percha	20
Zinc oxide	60–75
Metal sulphates	1.5–17
Waxes/resins	1–4

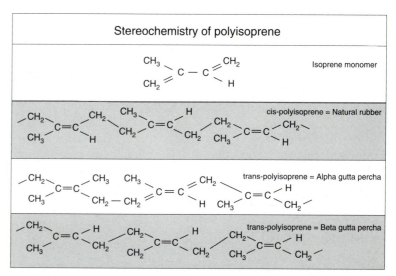

9.1 Structural formulae for isoprene, rubber, gutta percha (α and β phases)

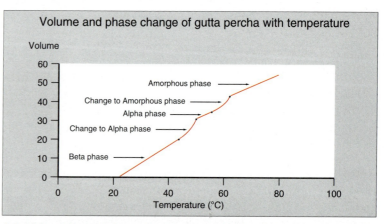

9.2 Volumetric and phase changes associated with heating gutta percha

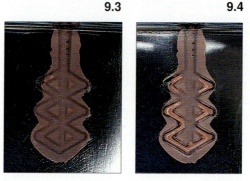

9.3, 9.4 Shrinkage of thermoplasticized gutta percha after placement

relatively soluble but is associated with very favourable healing with cementum formation around the foramen (**9.5, 9.6**).[1] Despite the presence of calcium hydroxide it is not regarded as very antibacterial and so may be appropriate for use with vital pulpectomies.

Non-eugenol sealers include AH26 and Diaket, both of which set by polymerization. AH26, an epoxy resin, was modified from an industrial adhesive. Its main advantage is its long setting time. Although the manufacturers claim that one of its constituents, hexamethylene tetramine, helps to make it biologically inert, AH26 has been found to provoke severe reactions, possibly because it releases formaldehyde during the early setting phase. Diaket is a polyvinyl resin formed from the reaction of keto complexes with metal salts. It is insoluble in water but does dissolve in organic solvents. Its adhesiveness to dentine is offset by difficulty in manipulation.

Preparation and application of sealers

Good sealer consistency aids manipulation, so proper mixing is important. Paste/paste formulations give a standard consistency and the powder/liquid formulations allow greater variability. The desirable consistency for most of the zinc oxide/eugenol sealers is shown in **9.7**: it should be sufficiently viscous that a string of the smoothly mixed material may be lifted. It may then be carried and applied to the root canal walls in several ways, the choice of which is a matter of personal preference.

The walls may be coated with sealer carried on paper points, files or the master gutta percha point or spreader (**9.8, 9.9**). Use of an ultrasonically activated file without irrigant is a very effective way of coating canal walls. Problems with this method include staining of the sealer (**9.10**), presumably by metal from the file, and accelerated setting caused by heat from the activated file.

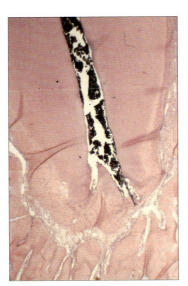

9.5 Low-power view of healing by cementum formation when Sealapex is used. (Black particles are residual Sealapex and root filling material) (courtesy of Professor M. Tagger)

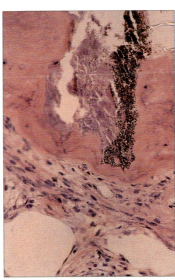

9.6 High-power view of **9.5** (courtesy of Professor M. Tagger)

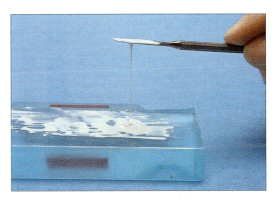

9.7 Desirable consistency of sealer

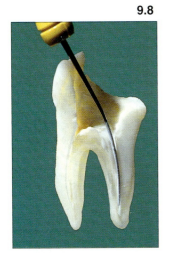
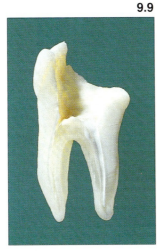

9.8, 9.9 Application of sealer to canal wall

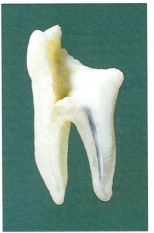

9.10 Sealer may stain if endosonically placed

Cold lateral condensation technique

This is the most widely used obturation technique. Tapered cones of gutta percha are placed in the canal and condensed with a metal spreader. A standardized gutta percha point, matching the master file size (**9.11**), is used as the master point to plug the apical foramen. Non-standardized gutta percha points, which have a range of different tapers (**9.12**), are used as accessory points to fill the rest of the canal. Spreaders are available in a range of sizes: those which match the non-standardized gutta percha points are preferable (**9.13**). Spreaders may be long handled (**9.14**) or similar to files (i.e. finger spreaders (**9.13**): these are less likely to split roots). Prerequisites for effective obturation include a regularly tapered canal and accessory gutta percha points and spreaders with a compatible taper (**9.15**). If the canal taper varies along its length different tapers of gutta percha points and spreaders may be used in the different portions (**9.16**). Spreader size is selected by placing it in the canal to the full length (**9.17**). If the optimal spreader does not fit to the full working length (**9.18**) then either a narrower spreader is chosen or the canal taper is modified.

A standardized gutta percha point is selected to ensure that the apical foramen is occluded to prevent subsequently placed gutta percha and sealer extruding (**9.19, 9.20**). The point is selected by matching it with the file that just snags in the apical portion of the canal at the full working length. Inaccuracy in standardization of instruments and gutta percha points may cause mismatch between their sizes, in which case an appropriate size is selected to achieve close apical fit. If the point proves to be small the tip may be cut by the necessary amount. Unfortunately, the apical portion of the canal is not always circular in cross-section (**9.21–9.24**), which makes it difficult to plug the apical foramen with a conventional master point (**9.25**). Furthermore, when the apical foramina are circular, multiple exits may be present (**9.26–9.28**).

The master point may be customized to fit variations in form by dipping the apical 1 mm of the master point into chloroform for one second (**9.29**) and placing it into the wet canal to the full length, effectively taking an impression of the apical portion of the canal (**9.30**) (if the canal is not wet the gutta percha may adhere to the canal walls). The gutta percha point is then allowed to dry out before final placement. This customized gutta percha

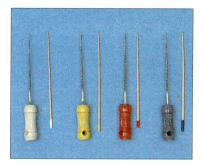

9.11 Standardized gutta percha points match files

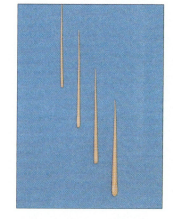

9.12 Non-standardized gutta percha points have different tapers

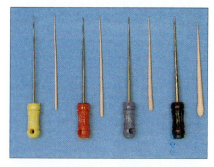

9.13 Non-standardized gutta percha points should be used with matching spreaders

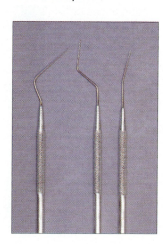

9.14 Long-handled spreaders

9.15, 9.16 The taper of the canal should be matched with spreader and accessory points

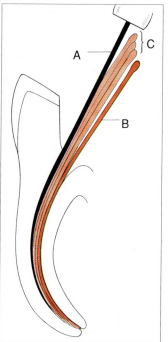

9.15 A = spreader; B = master point; C = accessory points

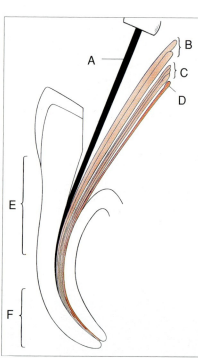

9.16 A = spreader; B = wide accessory points; C = narrow accessory points; D = master point; E = wide taper; F = narrow taper

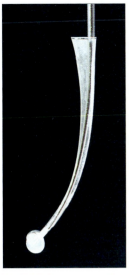

9.17 Select spreader size by trying fit in canal

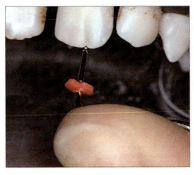

9.18 Spreader unable to reach full length

9.19, 9.20 Selection of master gutta percha point to occlude apical foramen

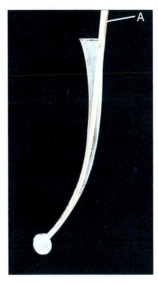

9.19 A = gutta percha point

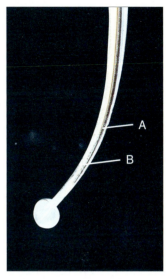

9.20 A = spreader; B = gutta percha

9.21–9.24 Irregular nature of apical foramina

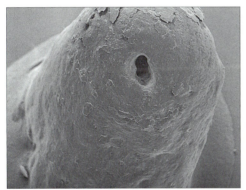

9.21

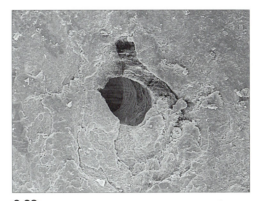

9.22

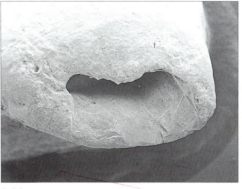

9.23

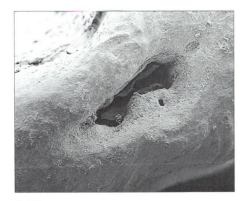

9.24

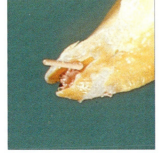

9.25 Irregular foramina may allow extrusion of gutta percha

point will not reseat if it is not replaced in the correct orientation. If this technique is effectively performed, adequate obturation of apical anatomical irregularities in the canal system is possible (**9.31, 9.32**).

Some canals may be wider than the largest available gutta percha point. In such cases a customized master point may be rolled using several large gutta percha points (**9.33–9.35**). These are softened by heating in a flame and rolling into a cone between two glass slabs. When ready the point is chilled in water and tried in the canal. If it is too large it may be resoftened and rerolled; if too small, the tip may be clipped with a pair of scissors until it fits at the apex.

Accessory points are chosen to match the selected spreader(s), measured for length and marked by notching to help prevent extrusion (**9.36**). The canal walls are coated with sealer and the master point placed to the full length. The spreader is inserted as far as possible and is used to compact the point against the canal

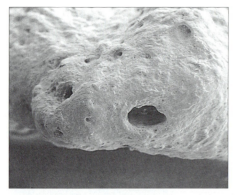 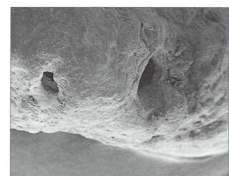 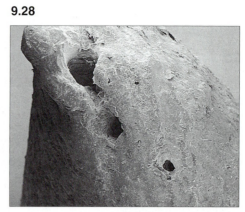

9.26–9.28 Multiple apical foramina

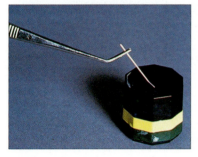

9.29 Chloroform dip technique

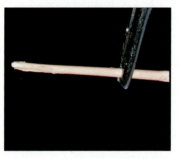

9.30 Impression of apical foramen

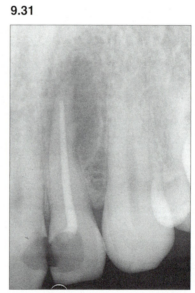 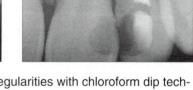

9.31, 9.32 Filling apical canal irregularities with chloroform dip technique

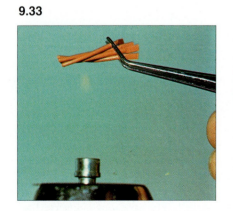 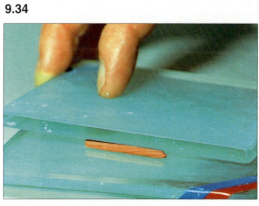 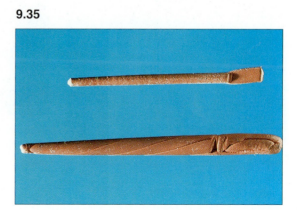

9.33–9.35 Customizing master point

wall. In a curved canal it may be helpful to compact the gutta percha against the inner curve so that the more rigid spreader can follow the gentler outer curve (**9.37, 9.38**). In this way the spreader is less likely to impale the master gutta percha point and pull it out (**9.39**). The spreader is left in place for a few seconds to allow the gutta percha time to deform and flow under pressure to adapt to the wall. The spreader is then freed by slight clockwise and anticlockwise rotary movements and removed. The first accessory point is then placed into the space created by the spreader and the condensation repeated (**9.40, 9.41**). The process is repeated until the canal is filled (**9.42–9.47**). Once the canal is filled beyond the curve, the spreader is inserted into the middle of the gutta percha mass and used to compact circumferentially (**9.48, 9.49**). The number of accessory points used depends on the relative size of the points and the canal. In the wider coronal part of the canal it may be possible to use widely tapered points, reducing the number required.

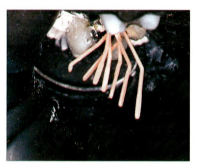

9.36 Marking accessory points for length

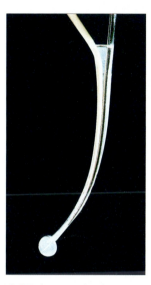

9.37 Long axis view

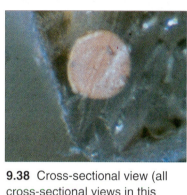

9.38 Cross-sectional view (all cross-sectional views in this series courtesy of Dr F. Weine)

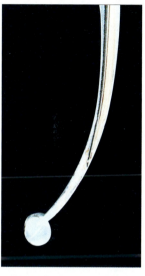

9.39 Spreader impaling gutta percha point

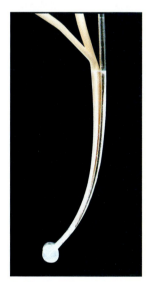

9.40 Longitudinal view—one accessory point

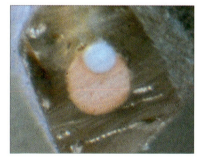

9.41 Cross-sectional view—one accessory point

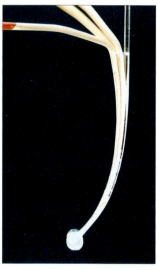

9.42 Longitudinal view—two accessory points

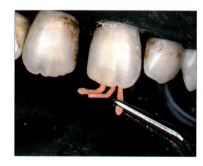

9.43

9.37–9.49 Stages of cold lateral condensation technique

In well tapered canals good results may be obtained (**9.50**, **9.51**), but in irregularly shaped canals it may not be possible to achieve close compaction (**9.52**). Cold compacted gutta percha points deform and adapt to canal walls very well (**9.53**), even spreading into lateral canals (**9.54**).

Two common criticisms of cold lateral condensation are the potential for root fracture (**9.55**) and the waste of gutta percha, which remains outside the canal (**9.56**).

Canal morphology has an important influence on the procedure for obturation. When two canals join in the apical part, it is

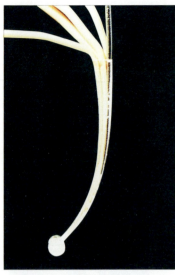

9.44 Longitudinal view–three accessory points

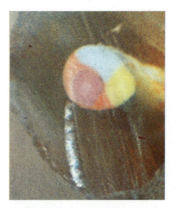

9.45 Cross-sectional view–three accessory points

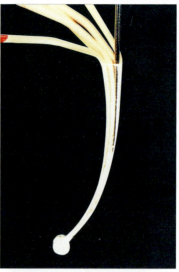

9.46 Longitudinal view

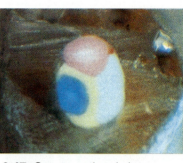

9.47 Cross-sectional view

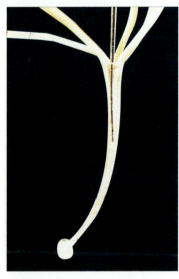

9.48 Longitudinal view

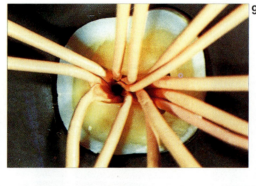

9.48, 9.49 Spreader inserted in the middle of gutta percha in straight part of canal

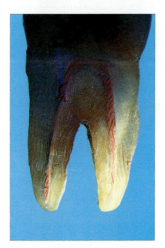

9.51 Quality of obturation of well tapered canals with cold lateral condensation

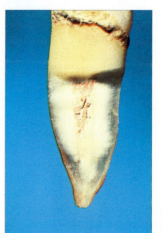

9.52 Poor compaction in irregularly tapered canal

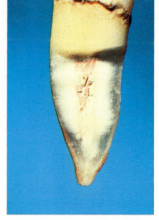

9.50 Quality of compaction of gutta percha removed from well tapered canal

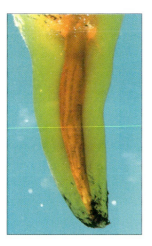

9.53 Adaptation of gutta percha in well tapered canal–cleared tooth

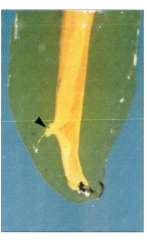

9.54 Gutta percha point deformed into lateral canal during cold condensation (arrowed)

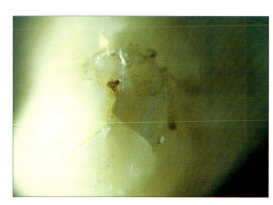

9.55 Root end fracture caused by cold lateral compaction of gutta percha

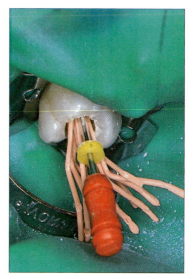

9.56 Wastage of gutta percha in cold lateral condensation technique

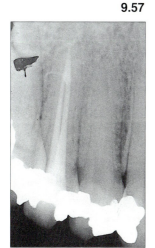

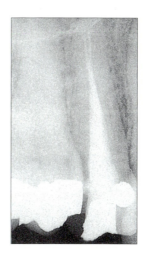

9.59 Obturation of canal that divides apically

9.57, 9.58 Obturation of canals that join apically

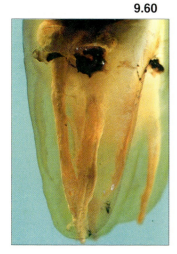

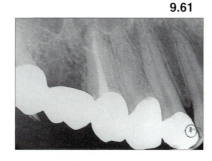

9.60, 9.61 Better adaptation of warmed gutta percha to irregular canals

best to place master points in each simultaneously to prevent occlusion of the unfilled canal with sealer (**9.57, 9.58**). Accessory points are then placed alternately in each canal. If a single canal divides into two, one canal should be obturated first up to the division and then the second (**9.59**).

Warm lateral condensation

The force necessary to compact and adapt cold gutta percha to irregular canal walls encourages the use of heat: softened gutta percha is more easily adapted with less force (**9.60, 9.61**), facilitating filling of irregularly tapered root canals.

This technique is identical to cold lateral condensation in principle and in the early stages. After the master point and some accessory points are compacted, heat may be applied in a number of ways. Heat carriers (**9.62**) may be heated in the flame (**9.63**) and inserted in the mass of gutta percha in the canal (**9.64**), if possible to within about 2 mm of the working length. After the initial plunge, the carrier is rotated through about 45° as it cools to prevent it from sticking to the gutta percha. The carrier is then removed and the gutta percha cold condensed with a conventional spreader to compensate for any contraction on cooling. Further gutta percha points are then added and the procedure repeated until the canal is filled. Commercially available instruments such as Caulk/Dentsply's Endotec (**9.65**), Analytic Technology's Touch n' Heat device (**9.66**), Degussa's Thermopact and Almore International's Endo-Temp may be used for carrying the heat.

Figure **9.67** compares the sizes of the Endotec and Touch n' Heat carriers. The Endotec is operated by a rechargeable battery and is capable of achieving temperatures up to 350°C (there is no evidence that this transient temperature affects the periodontium but it may affect the properties of gutta percha). The Endotec has two spreader tips, the small one equivalent to a size 30 file and the large to size 45 (**9.68**). The larger size is inflexible and not very suitable for curved canals. The Touch n' Heat is a battery powered, rechargeable heat carrier, but the batteries are carried in a separate box with a cable link rather than in the handle as in the Endotec. It is capable of providing a range of high temperatures instantly.

An ultrasonically activated spreader may also be used for warm lateral condensation (**9.69, 9.70**). Ultrasonic vibration generates considerable heat and is able to produce well compacted root fillings, but this technique needs to be researched further.

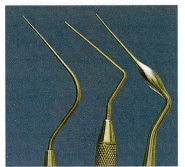

9.62, 9.63 Heat carriers

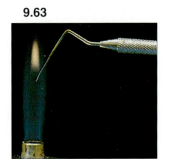

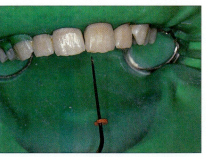

9.64 Insertion of heated carrier into canal

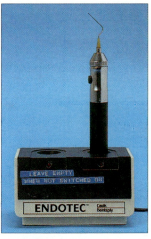

9.65 Endotec (Caulk/Dentsply)

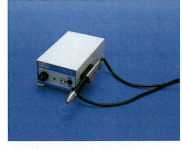

9.66 Touch n' Heat (Analytic Technology)

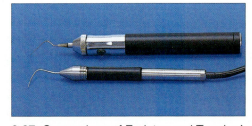

9.67 Comparison of Endotec and Touch n' Heat spreaders

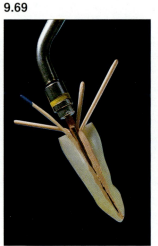

9.69, 9.70 Ultrasonic lateral compaction of gutta percha

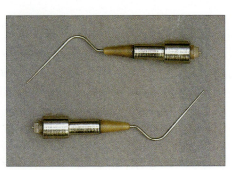

9.68 Spreader tips (small, large) for Endotec

Warm vertical condensation

In this technique pluggers with flat-ended tips (**9.71, 9.72**) are used to compact warmed gutta percha apically in a series of steps, beginning with the apical portion and gradually backfilling the canal (**9.73**). The technique relies on capturing the maximum cross-sectional area of gutta percha with the tip of the plugger and pushing it apically without the plugger binding against the canal walls (**9.74**). This means that the series of pluggers of different sizes, graduated at 5-mm intervals, are prefitted into the canal and premeasured (**9.75**). Too small a plugger would simply plunge through the gutta percha (**9.76**); one too wide would bind against the canal walls and could split the root (**9.77**). The smallest plugger should reach within 5 mm of the working length to achieve good apical compaction without extrusion. The width and rigidity of the pluggers necessitate a more widely tapered canal preparation than that for lateral condensation. The technique is not easy to use in very curved canals, where the rigid pluggers may not negotiate the curvature and could result in apical voids (**9.78**).

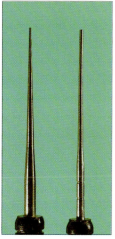

9.71 Finger pluggers

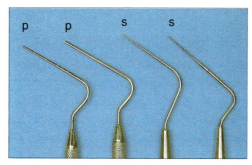

9.72 Long-handled pluggers (p) compared with spreaders (s)

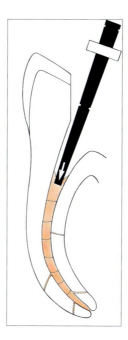

9.73 Warm vertical condensation

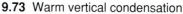

9.74 Plugger should capture maximum cross-sectional area of gutta percha without apical binding

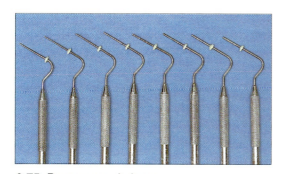

9.75 Premeasured pluggers

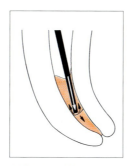

9.76 Small plugger is ineffective

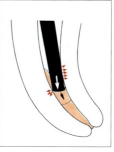

9.77 Plugger binding apically may split root

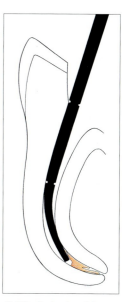

9.78 Apical voids may result in very curved canals

Procedure

The prepared canal walls are first coated with sealer. The selected master point is a non-standardized gutta percha point with the apical tip cut off. It is fitted to achieve apical tug-back at about 1 mm from the working length (**9.79**). If the canal diameter is wider than the first point, a second point is fitted. Gutta percha protruding from the canal orifice is removed with a hot instrument (**9.80**). The widest plugger is now used to compact the gutta percha into the canal using 2–3 mm vertical strokes (**9.81**). A series of overlapping strokes is used if the canal is wider than the plugger (**9.93**). The heat transfer instrument, heated to cherry red, is again plunged into the mass of gutta percha to a depth of 3–4 mm and quickly withdrawn (**9.82**) (a high temperature ensures that a mass of gutta percha is not removed with the carrier). The appropriate plugger is then used as already described (**9.83**).

Each time this sequence is repeated some gutta percha is removed with the heat carrier and a smaller plugger is placed closer to the working length (**9.84, 9.85**). It is rarely necessary to compact closer than 5 mm from the working length.

The coronal part of the canal is then backfilled by introducing 3–4 mm sections of gutta percha and repeating the sequence of heating and vertical compacting (**9.86–9.93**).

This technique is able to fill accessory anatomy very well and if performed carefully will provide a homogenous root filling (**9.94**). Inadequate control over the depth of insertion of pluggers may result in voids (**9.95**).

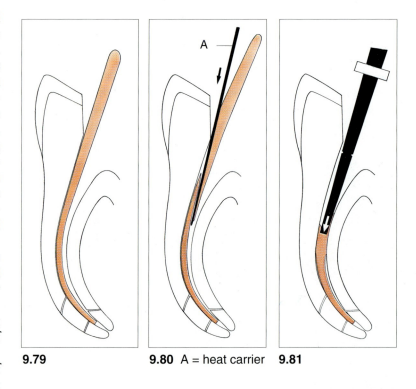

9.79–9.93 Procedure for warm vertical condensation

9.79   **9.80** A = heat carrier   **9.81**

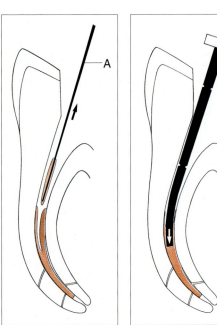
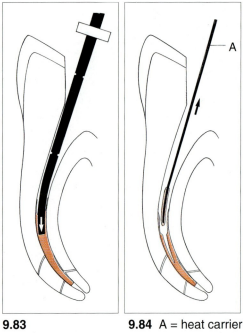
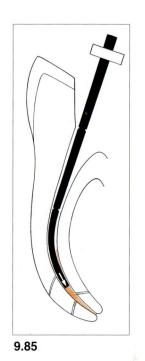
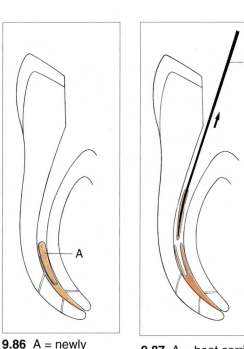

9.82 A = heat carrier   **9.83**   **9.84** A = heat carrier   **9.85**   **9.86** A = newly added 3–4 mm section of gutta percha   **9.87** A = heat carrier

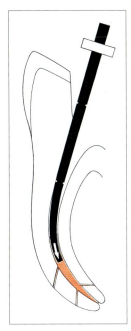 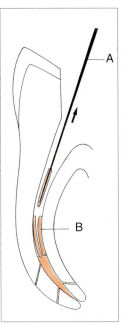 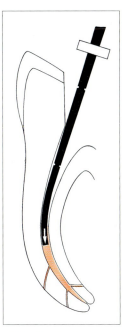 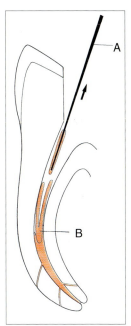 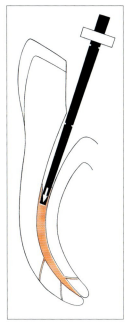 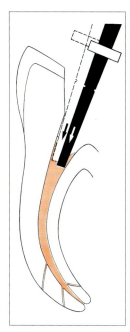

9.88 Vertical compaction

9.89 A = heat carrier; B = newly added gutta percha

9.90 Vertical compaction

9.91 A = heat carrier; B = newly added segment of gutta percha

9.92 Vertical compaction

9.93 Final vertical compaction with overlapping strokes

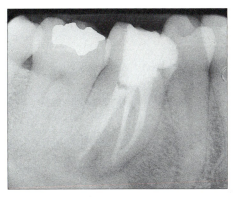

9.94 Filling of accessory anatomy using warm vertical condensation

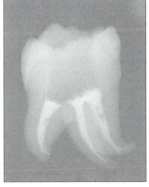

9.95 Voids produced during warm vertical condensation

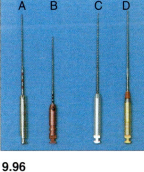

9.96

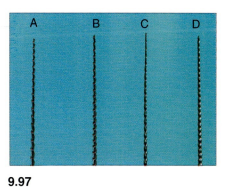

9.97

9.96, 9.97 Variety of thermocompactors: A = Maillefer Gutta condensor; B = McSpadden nickel–titanium thermocompactor; C = Quickfill compactor; D = Zipperer thermocompactor

9.98   9.99

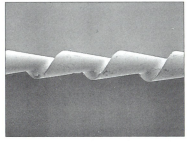

9.98, 9.99 Maillefer Gutta-condensor (SEM views)

Thermocompaction

In this technique friction between gutta percha and a rotating 'reverse file' generates heat to soften the gutta percha and feed it apically. Thermocompactors available have different designs which determine their properties (**9.96, 9.97**). Those available include the Maillefer Gutta-condensor (**9.98, 9.99**), McSpadden nickel–titanium thermocompactor (**9.100, 9.101**), Zipperer thermocompactor (**9.102, 9.103**) and Quickfill compactor (**9.104, 9.105**).

The attractions of the technique include speed and conservative use of gutta percha. The idea, first introduced by McSpadden, consisted of using a reverse Hedstroem file in a high-torque conventional handpiece rotated at speeds of 8000–10 000 r.p.m. As the activated thermocompactor is advanced into the canal containing a single gutta percha point, it becomes tangled with it and plasticizes and feeds it to the apex. As it does so the thermocompactor is pushed coronally out of the canal. The operator can feel this backpressure and allows the instrument to withdraw under its own pressure.

Use of speeds higher than recommended may result in a poorer seal. Another potential disadvantage is damage to periodontal supporting tissues by overheating (**9.106–9.109**), including resorption and ankylosis, but if heat transfer to the supporting tissues is great enough, the demonstrated damage to the supporting tissues may occur with any technique employing heated gutta percha. Other criticisms of the technique include extrusion of filling material (**9.110**), gouging of canal walls (**9.111**) and fracture of the thermocompactor.

9.106–9.109 Histological sections to show effect of thermocompaction on the periodontium (courtesy of Dr E. Saunders)[2]

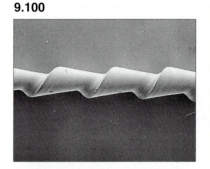
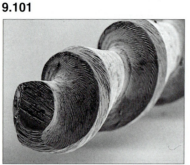

9.100, 9.101 McSpadden nickel–titanium thermocompactor

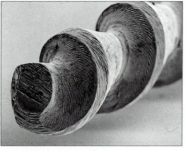

9.102, 9.103 Zipperer thermocompactor

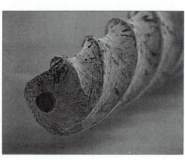
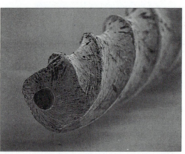

9.104, 9.105 Quickfill compactor

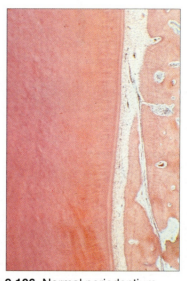

9.106 Normal periodontium

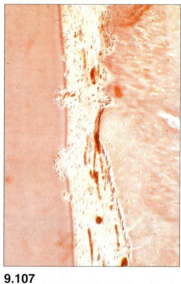

9.107

9.107, 9.108 Various degrees of resorption seen on the root surface following thermocompaction

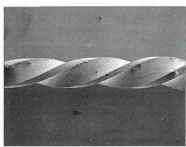
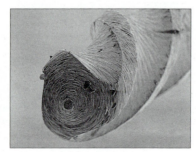

9.108

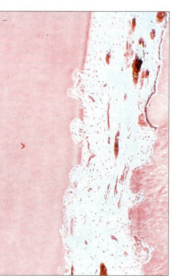

9.109 Ankylosis following thermocompaction

The old design of thermocompactor has now been superseded by one made of more flexible nickel–titanium (**9.100, 9.101**). Another more robust thermocompactor is the Gutta-condensor (**9.98, 9.99**), which is less likely to fracture.

Tagger recommended a hybrid technique, in which the apical part of the canal is filled using cold lateral condensation and the remainder backfilled with the thermocompactor. This technique overcomes the lack of apical control inherent in pure thermocompaction, speeds obturation and reduces wastage of gutta percha. An effective homogenous filling may be obtained (**9.112**) but the results are variable, reflecting the lack of control inherent in the technique. The variability of different brands and batches of gutta percha may also contribute to unpredictability.

Injection of thermoplasticized gutta percha

This technique involves injecting molten gutta percha into the root canal system. Easy in principle, the technique requires considerable practice to master and has its shortcomings.

To prevent underextension the delivery needle should be placed within 3–5 mm of the working length (**9.113**). Inadequate control of temperature can cause poor results (**9.114**). As the gutta percha cools in the canal, it shrinks and therefore requires pressure to compensate for the shrinkage. An incremental technique with vertical condensation gives a better result and is useful for filling accessory anatomy (**9.115**). Overextension is also a potential problem and may be overcome by using a hybrid technique in which the apical portion of the canal is filled using lateral condensation, excess gutta percha removed with a hot instrument and the remainder vertically condensed before the canal is backfilled with thermoplasticized gutta percha.

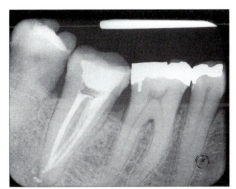

9.110 Extrusion of root filling material following thermocompaction

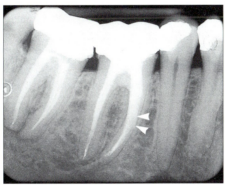

9.111 Gouging of canal walls in mandibular first molar during thermocompaction (arrowed)

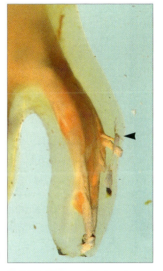

9.112 Filling of lateral canal using thermocompaction

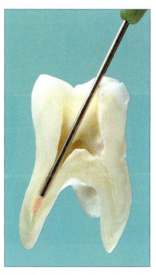

9.113 Underextension of gutta percha because of short delivery needle

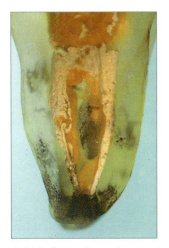

9.114 Poor obturation due to lack of temperature control

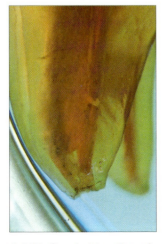

9.115 Good obturation of accessory anatomy

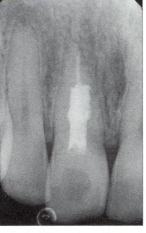

9.116 Obturation of internal resorption defect

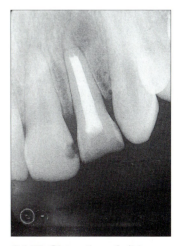

9.117 Obturation of wide, straight canal

The injection technique should always be used with a coating of sealer on the canal walls and is particularly useful in filling irregularly shaped wide canals: internal resorption defects (**9.116**), backfilling wide, straight canals (**9.117**), incompletely formed roots with induced apical barriers are particular indications (**9.118**). If healing has not occurred at the apex and a complete barrier has not formed, thermoplasticized gutta percha can be used in a 'through and through' surgical technique (**9.119–9.122**). The injection technique is also useful in retrograde filling of some canals during surgery (**9.123–9.127**). In the case shown, after the extruded silver point was removed and the canal cleaned with a file (**9.124**), the Ultrafil system was used to fill the canal (**9.125, 9.126**). Figure **9.127** shows healing 3 months postoperatively.

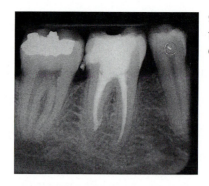

9.118 Obturation of incompletely formed roots or blunderbuss canals

9.119–9.122 'Through and through' obturation using injection techniques

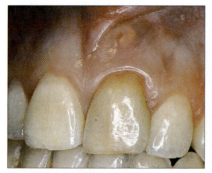

9.119 Persistent sinus over |1

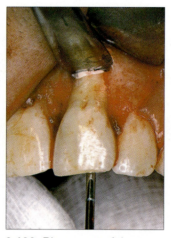

9.120 Placement of thermoplasticised gutta percha by injection

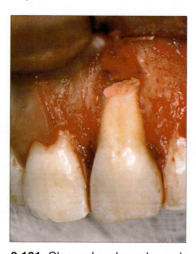

9.121 Cleaned and condensed apical seal

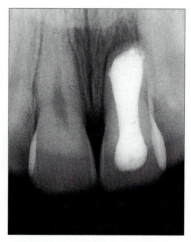

9.122 Post obturation radiograph

9.123–9.127 Use of injection technique in retrograde procedure

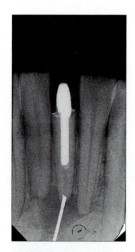

9.123 Large, wide post and extruded silver point

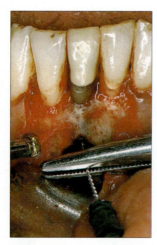

9.124 Retrograde canal filing

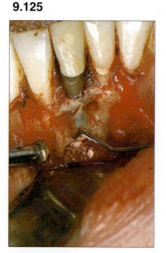

9.125

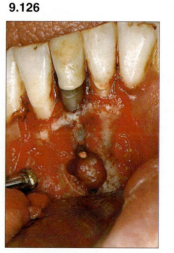

9.126

9.125, 9.126 Retrograde obturation with injection of thermoplasticised gutta percha

9.127 Healing 3 months postoperatively

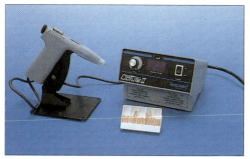

9.128 Obtura system

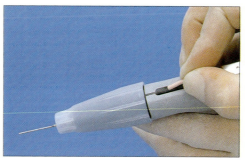

9.129 Loading Obtura gun with gutta percha

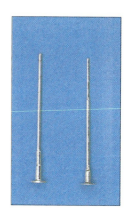

9.130 Disposable silver needles for Obtura

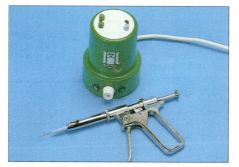

9.131 Ultrafil system

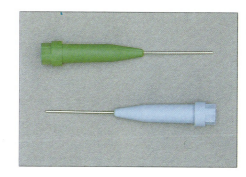

9.132 Prefilled gutta percha cannules for Ultrafil

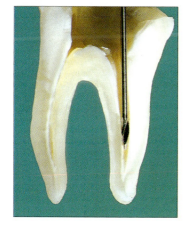

9.133

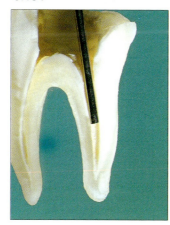

9.134

9.133, 9.134 A wide canal is necessary for adequate needle placement

Two delivery systems are available, which are suitable for the specific indications described but not for routine filling of all root canal systems.

Obtura system

This system (**9.128**) consists of a control unit and a pistol-grip syringe designed to accept gutta percha pellets available with the system. The exact composition of the gutta percha is not known. The pellets are placed in the barrel of the syringe (**9.129**), where they are heated to a temperature of 160°C. When molten, the gutta percha is extruded through disposable silver needles (available in a range of sizes: 18, 20, 22, and 25 gauge) (**9.130**). The extruded gutta percha has a temperature of 62–65°C and may remain soft for 3 minutes.

Ultrafil system

This system (**9.131**) heats gutta percha to 70°C. It consists of a heater and a separate pistol-grip injection syringe. In contrast to the Obtura system, the gun contains no heating element. The gutta percha is provided in prefilled cannules (**9.132**): regular set (white), endoset (green) and firm set (blue), each with different rates of hardening and total shrinkage. The firm set hardens much faster than the other two. The regular set exhibits the least shrinkage on cooling. The cannules have a standard needle which is equivalent in size to a No. 70 file or No. 2 Gates Glidden drill.

The need to place the tip of the needle to within 3–5 mm of the working length means that wide canal preparation is essential (**9.133, 9.134**). The needle may be curved if necessary, taking care not to obstruct the flow. Cannules are placed in the heater for at least 15 minutes to allow sufficient softening of the gutta percha. If unused at one sitting the cannules may be reheated but should be discarded if they are left in the heater for more than 4 hours. Once removed from the heater, a cannule loses heat rapidly and has a working time of less than 1 minute. The gun with the cannule should therefore be returned to the heater for further softening.

The injection procedure is technique sensitive. The trigger should be squeezed slowly and steadily: undue haste causes excessive pressure which can fracture the cannule (**9.135**) or extrude gutta percha through the back of the cannule (**9.136**). As gutta percha is injected, the developing back-pressure is used to work the needle slowly out of the canal.

Thermoplasticized gutta percha carried on a solid core

A number of α phase gutta percha techniques have recently been marketed. Their unique feature is that the gutta percha is heat-softened and carried to the canal on a carrier or core resembling a file, the apical part of which may or may not be left behind in the canal as part of the root filling. The original product of this type (marketed after Dr Johnson) was the Thermafil endodontic obturator.

Technique using Thermafil endodontic obturators

The manufacturers claim that α phase gutta percha is essential to the technique because it has better flow characteristics when thermoplasticized. The gutta percha is moulded into a non-standardized thick parallel-sided point with a central carrier of stainless steel, titanium or plastic (**9.137**). More recently, the gutta percha has been shaped into a tapering cone to avoid wastage.

The coronal portion of the carrier (and in the case of the plastic carrier the handle as well) has markings and a rubber stop to facilitate length control. The gutta percha normally covers the first two or three graduation marks at 18, 19, 20 mm and must be cut away if required. The carriers have ISO standard dimensions with matching colour coding, with the exception of the small plastic carriers (Nos 25, 30, 35), which have an incrementally greater taper. Plastic carriers are relatively flexible. Sizes below 40 are made of a liquid plastic crystal and are not soluble; sizes 45 and above are made from a polysulphone polymer and may be dissolved in organic solvents. Metal carriers, particularly titanium, are relatively rigid, so flutes or spiralling are used to make them more flexible.

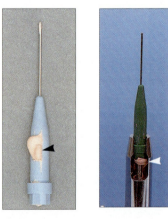

9.135 Fracture of cannule due to haste or inadequate heating

9.136 Extrusion of gutta percha through the back of cannule

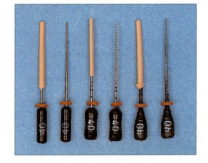

9.137 Thermafil obturators with different carriers. Left–right: titanium, stainless steel, plastic obturators shown with and without the gutta percha

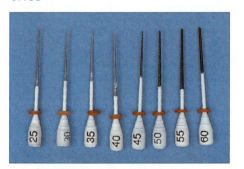
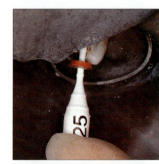

9.138, 9.139 Blank plastic carriers used to verify selection of size

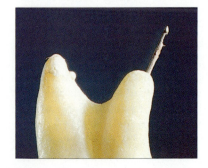

9.140 If carrier is too small it may be extruded

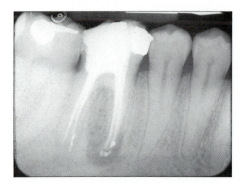

9.141 Inadequate length control with Thermafil

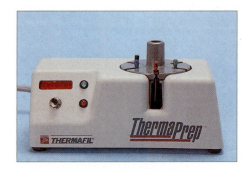

9.142 ThermaPrep oven

Blank plastic carriers are available to gauge the appropriate size for a canal (**9.138, 9.139**). If the selected obturator is too small the carrier with gutta percha may be extruded (**9.140**) and if it is too large the root filling may end short (**9.141**). In the case shown in **9.141** the distal root canal had three canals. The central one has been filled short; another is overextended. In addition sealer has extruded in the mesial root.

As in any obturation technique, the canal must be correctly shaped and cleaned. The generally accepted flared preparation is suitable. Overflaring may cause poor coronal seal. The walls of the canal are coated with a sealer.

The gutta percha is softened in a flame or a custom provided ThermaPrep oven at 115°C (**9.142**) and then placed in the canal. Plastic carriers cannot be heated in a flame but metal carriers can. When heating in the flame, obturators should be passed through the relatively cooler blue zone of the flame a few times (**9.143**): if passed through the hotter part of the flame the gutta percha will ignite (**9.144**). The obturator is considered ready for insertion in the canal when the gutta percha takes on a sheen and begins to expand. Maximum and minimum times should be observed for heating in the oven and if left in the oven longer than the designated time the obturators must be discarded.

When the obturator is ready, it is seated in the canal to the full working length without twisting or forcing. As it is seated excess gutta percha collects at the canal orifice (**9.145**) but does not appear to be completely stripped from the carrier. If the canal has a wide taper, some vertical compaction may be possible (**9.146**). Metal carriers are prenotched for separation but plastic carriers may be cut with a heated instrument or a sharp stainless steel inverted cone bur in a conventional handpiece.

In teeth with multiple canals it is important to ensure that excess gutta percha does not block other canals. This may be achieved either by placing damp cotton wool pledgets into the orifices of the other canals or by trimming away some of the coronal gutta percha off the obturator to minimize overflow of excess material. In roots with two or more canals which may be joined by anastomoses (**9.147**) it is best to place obturators sequentially without delay, or flow of sealer and gutta percha from one canal into another may partially block adjacent canals and prevent adequate obturation without further instrumentation.

This technique has many advantages: it is quick and relatively easy (although some initial learning is required); it provides a seal equivalent to that gained using lateral condensation; it is extremely effective in filling the canal system by virtue of its

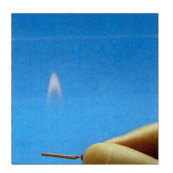

9.143 Heat the metal carrier obturator in the blue zone of a flame

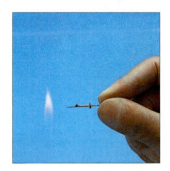

9.144 Heating in the red zone of a flame causes ignition of gutta percha

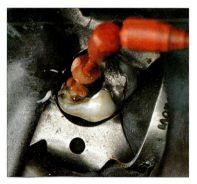

9.145 Seating of obturator

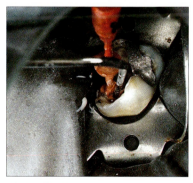

9.146 Vertical compaction alongside carrier

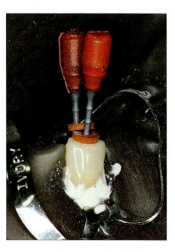

9.147 Rapid placement of obturators in roots with possible canal ramifications

excellent flow characteristics (**9.148–9.150**). Figure **9.151** shows two molars filled with Thermafil, an apical delta having been filled in the mesiobuccal root of the first molar. However, as it is still a new technique there is no long-term clinical follow-up.

Potential problems include extrusion, post-space creation and retreatment. When plastic carriers are used post space is created by first drilling away the plastic carrier with a round bur until it is flush with the canal orifice, then removing the coronal portion with Peeso drills and specially designed non-end cutting Prepi burs to prevent lateral perforation (**9.152–9.154**).

The procedure for metal carriers is more difficult and technique sensitive. The need for post space must be considered at the time of insertion. The technique requires prenotching of the carrier but is not recommended for titanium carriers. Gutta percha is first removed at the required level using a bur and the carrier notched using a diamond bur as the obturator is slowly rotated. The cross-sectional diameter of the carrier is reduced to approximately 0.06 mm (**9.155**). The notch is considered sufficient when the apical portion may be bent by applying light lateral pressure against a fingertip. There should be no rebound and there should be sufficient strength in the residual metal to allow apical pressure for seating along its long axis (this is tested by its ability to indent a fingertip without collapsing). Considerable practice is required to achieve a satisfactory notch. The heated obturator is inserted to the working

9.148–9.150 Roots rendered transparent by clearing show good filling of accessory anatomy using Thermafil obturators

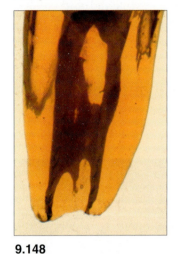
9.148

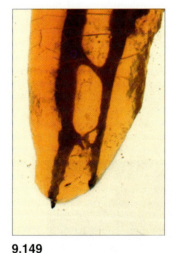
9.149

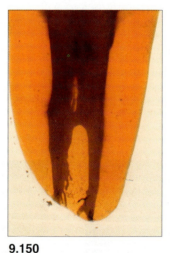
9.150

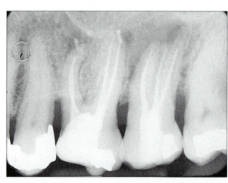
9.151 Molars filled with Thermafil obturators

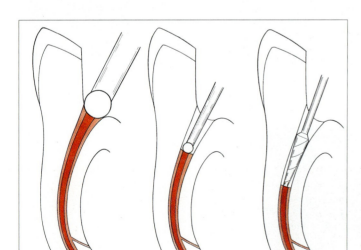
9.152 Post-space preparation when using Thermafil plastic carrier obturators

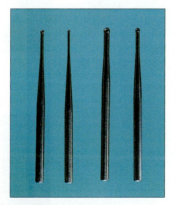
9.153 Prepi burs: low-power view

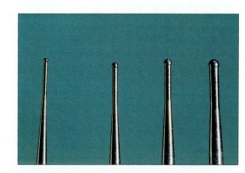
9.154 Prepi burs: high-power view

length without rotation, which may cause the tip to separate prematurely: if this does happen a radiograph should be taken to determine the position of the separated tip. If the tip is at or beyond the middle one-third of the canal the handle is used to push the tip to the apex (provided the gutta percha is still sufficiently plastic). If the tip is in the coronal third of the canal, the tip is removed using Hedstroem files after the gutta percha has hardened. Once fully seated, the coronal part of the carrier is separated by applying apical pressure and turning the handle anticlockwise. Twisting the carrier clockwise in direction may cause an improperly notched carrier to screw through the apex. If post space is required immediately the handle is removed together with the gutta percha (**9.156**); if post space is not required immediately the rubber stop is slid down to the canal orifice and the carrier withdrawn, leaving the gutta percha behind (**9.157**). The gutta percha is then compacted vertically after placing damp cotton wool over the canal orifice. Effective post-space preparation is therefore possible but is a technique-sensitive procedure.

Retreatment of canals with Thermafil obturators may prove difficult. The degree of difficulty is dictated by the ability to remove the carriers. Gutta percha may be removed using a solvent and Hedstroem files, but carriers jammed in the canal may be difficult to remove, especially if prenotched. In such circumstances periapical surgery may be required; root resection has not so far been a problem.

The Thermafil technique requires some refinement but appears on the short-term basis to be a promising one.

Alphaseal and Successfil

Other materials based on a similar concept are Alphaseal and Successfil. Both these techniques provide the gutta percha in a syringe which is heated in custom-made ovens: **9.158** shows the Alphaseal oven. The softened gutta percha is extruded onto a conventional file or thermocompactor, which is used to carry the material into the canal (**9.159, 9.160**).

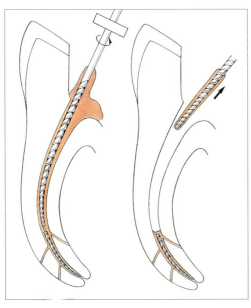

9.155 Prenotching of metal carrier for post-space preparation

9.156 Post space creation when using metal carrier obturators

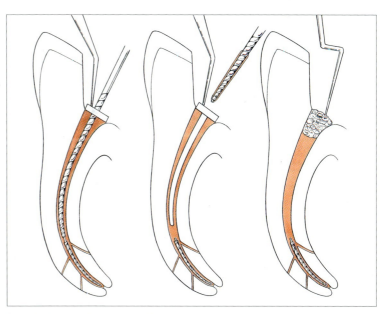

9.157 Removal of coronal part of carrier when post space is not required immediately

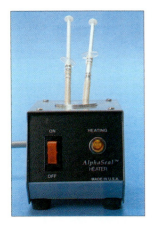

9.158 Alphaseal oven

9.159

9.160

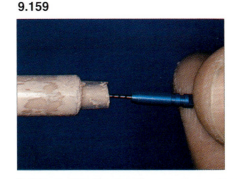
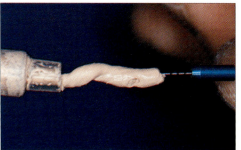

9.159, 9.160 Coating thermocompactor with Alphaseal gutta percha

In a recent modification of the technique (the Multiphase gutta percha obturation technique) two different phases of gutta percha are used. The McSpadden thermocompactor (**9.100, 9.101**) is coated with heated Phase 1, a β phase gutta percha. This is a relatively viscous material with poor adhesive and flow characteristics. The Phase 1 is then coated with an outer layer of Phase 2, an α phase gutta percha with a tacky consistency and good flow characteristics. The gutta percha is then placed in a sealer-coated canal to the working length without rotation. The condensor is then withdrawn 0.5–1 mm from the working length and activated. A Nitimatic motor (**9.161**) may be used to control the speed, which should be between 1000 and 5000 r.p.m. As the thermocompactor is activated it will attempt to 'back-out'. This should be resisted without apical advancement of the condensor. This position is maintained for no longer than 2 seconds and the condensor slowly withdrawn under its own pressure along one side of the canal without stopping rotation. The overall condensation time is approximately 6 seconds.

Extracted teeth, filled and rendered transparent, show a remarkable ability of the Alphaseal gutta percha to fill accessory anatomy (**9.162–9.164**), ramifications (**9.165, 9.166**) and apical deltas (**9.167–9.169**) with a good apical seal: clinical cases obturated with this technique show a similarly impressive result (**9.170–9.174**). In conjunction with nickel–titanium engine file preparation, the technique will maintain and fill severely curved canals (**9.175–9.177**). A further claimed advantage of this method

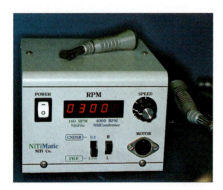

9.161 Nitimatic speed/torque control motor

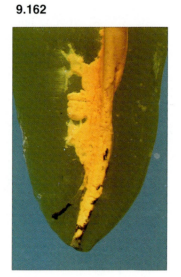
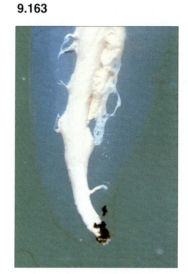
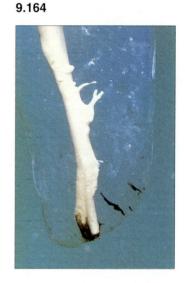

9.162–9.164 Ability of Alphaseal to fill accessory canal anatomy

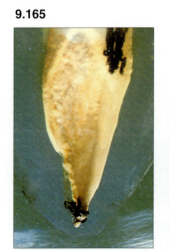
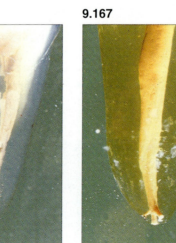
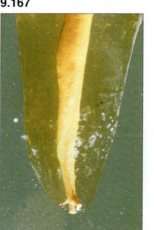
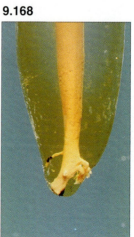
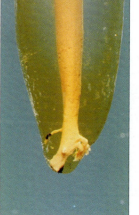

9.165, 9.166 Filling of ramifications between canals with Alphaseal

9.167–9.169 Filling of apical deltas with Alphaseal

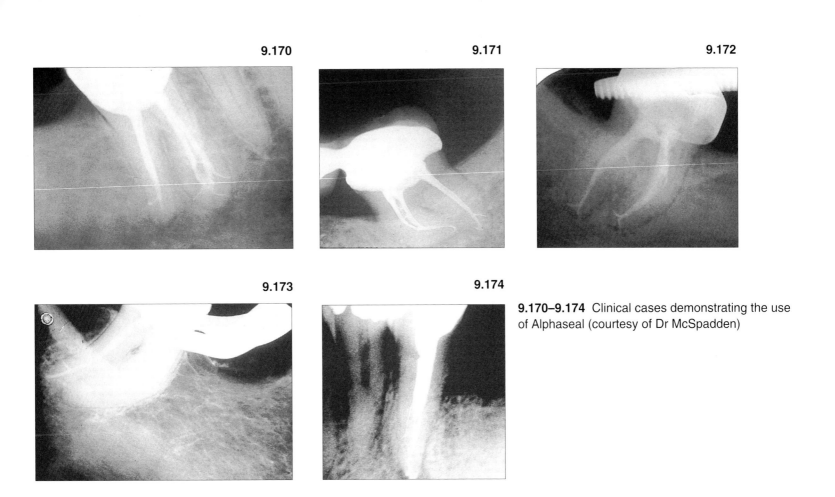

9.170–9.174 Clinical cases demonstrating the use of Alphaseal (courtesy of Dr McSpadden)

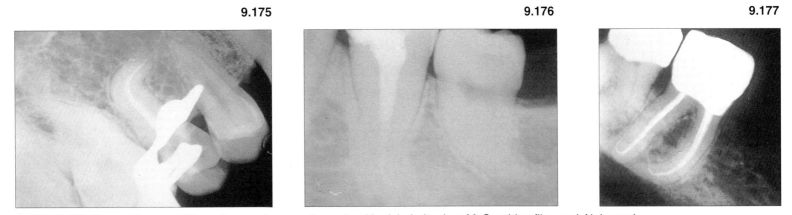

9.175–9.177 Preparation and filling of severely curved canals with nickel–titanium McSpadden files and Alphaseal

is that apexification of 'blunderbuss' roots is not necessary because control over apical placement is good (**9.178**).

This technique is very promising but needs broader clinical testing.

The Successfil technique may be combined with the Ultrafil gutta percha to backfill in the so-called *'Trifecta'* system. However, none of these new techniques has been satisfactorily tested yet.

Quickfill

The latest variation on this technique, Quickfill, provides α gutta percha coated on a thermocompactor (**9.179**). This does not need to be heated in a flame but is plasticized by frictional heat generated by running in a conventional handpiece (**9.180–9.182**). The technique is neat and easy to use. Some of the results on extracted teeth rendered transparent have been impressive (**9.183**), but there is a tendency for voids (**9.184, 9.185**) and the apical seal is not as good as the other α phase techniques. There is little clinical or scientific information on this new technique yet.

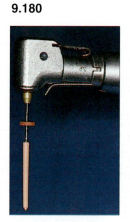
9.180

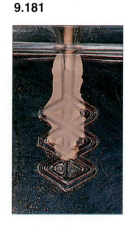
9.181

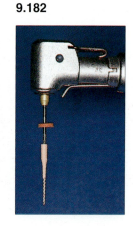
9.182

9.180–9.182 Obturation with Quickfil

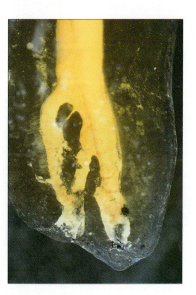

9.178 Good apical control in wide canals

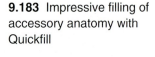

9.179 Quickfil

9.183 Impressive filling of accessory anatomy with Quickfill

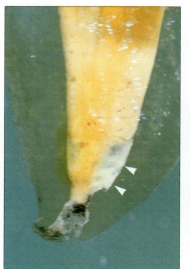
9.184

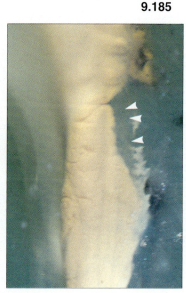
9.185

9.184, 9.185 Voids are sometimes seen with Quickfill obturation (arrowed)

Diffusion techniques

The principle of these techniques is to use gutta percha to fill canal systems without conventional sealers. Instead, gutta percha is partially dissolved in a solvent such as chloroform so that the plasticized gutta percha acts as a sealer (**9.186**). Radiographic results are sometimes reasonable (**9.187**) and sometimes not (**9.188**). The technique has been widely used in Scandinavia but is being discouraged because of the carcinogenic potential of chloroform. In addition, the softened gutta percha shrinks for prolonged periods afterwards so a relatively poor seal is obtained.

Single point technique

This technique, once widely used, relies on preparation of the root canal to a round cross-sectional diameter in the apical portion using reamers. A silver point matching the size of the last reamer is then cemented into the canal. Many good operators have achieved successful results with this technique but complex root canal anatomy may be left undebrided and unfilled (**9.189**), which may cause late failures (**9.190, 9.191**). Corrosion of silver points may cause the seal to deteriorate (**9.192, 9.193**). If sectional points are used to provide post space then late problems

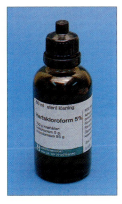

9.186 Chlororesin

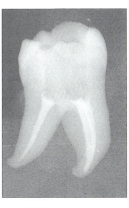

9.187 Reasonable radiographic result with chloropercha technique

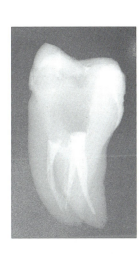

9.188 Less good result obtained using the same technique as in **9.187**

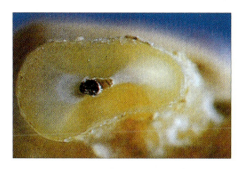

9.189 Undebrided and unfilled canal following use of silver point

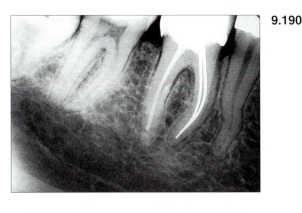

9.190

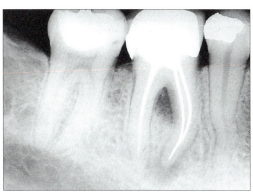

9.191

9.190, 9.191 Late failure associated with silver points

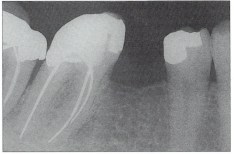

9.192

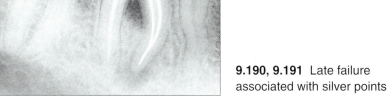

9.193

9.192, 9.193 Apical corrosion of silver points removed during retreatment is not uncommon

may occur as in the case shown in **9.194–9.197**: after 6 years the point became uncemented and dislodged. If the sectional silver point breaks at an incorrect level in the canal, further treatment may be difficult (**9.198**). Problems may be posed both with conventional retreatment and surgical apical treatment.

Use of formaldehyde-containing materials

Formaldehyde-containing materials (such as Endomethasone, N2, R2CB, Reiblers paste and Spad) have been popular. It has been claimed that these materials allow speedy completion of root canal treatment because cleaning and shaping can be compromised, as the formaldehyde can help to eliminate residual infection and mummify residual tissue, but this claim has never been satisfactorily proven. Used with adequate cleaning and shaping and confined within the root canal system, the materials may give successful results. Medicated root filling materials, which can cause irreversible damage to bone, soft tissues and nerves, are to be avoided: many cases of extrusion of material into the inferior dental canal causing permanent paraesthesia or anaesthesia of the lower lip and chin, accompanied by bouts of severe pain, have been documented (**9.199, 9.200**).

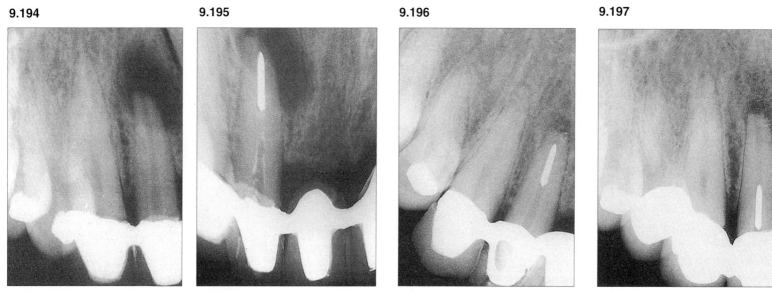

9.194–9.197 Late problems due to sectional silver point technique. A maxillary incisor with a radiolucent area (**9.194**) was root-filled using a sectional silver point (**9.195**). Follow-up radiographs were taken four years later (**9.196**) when it could be seen that healing was taking place, but a small area still persisted. In the final radiograph (**9.197**), two years afterwards, it is clear that the silver point had become disloged because it did not fit.

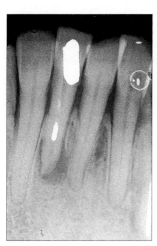

9.198 Problems due to premature separation of apical sectional silver point

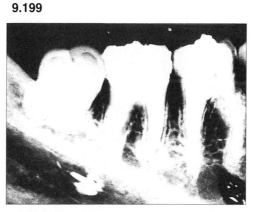

9.199, 9.200 Extrusion of formaldehyde-containing materials into the inferior dental canal

10 Perio-endo lesions

In a perio-endo lesion either pulpal disease mimics periodontal disease or periodontal disease mimics an endodontic problem. Diagnosis may be difficult because it is not possible to determine the histological state of the pulp from clinical signs and symptoms and in many situations it is not clear whether the pulp has been affected. Many lesions are referred to as perio-endo cases because both entities are apparently involved.

It is well known that micro-organisms and their toxins from a necrotic pulp may leach out of the root canal system through the apical foramina and/or lateral canals and damage the attachment apparatus and surrounding bone. It should also be noted that a vital and inflamed pulp may affect the surrounding bone. The extent to which disease within the periodontium can affect the pulp via the apical foramina and lateral canals is not clear. In most cases the apical foramina, containing the main blood vessels to the pulp, must be involved before the pulp disintegrates. When a lateral canal alone is involved only mild degenerative changes occur in most cases. The incidence of lateral canals overall is 40–50%, although in the furcations of molar teeth (particularly in the mandible) it rises to 63%. Root planing, by removing cementum, may expose dentinal tubules and lateral canals but evidence as to whether this jeopardizes the vitality of the pulp is conflicting.

Potential anatomical communication

The close relationship between the pulp and the periodontium is illustrated by considering the number of potential pathways of communication.

Apical foramina

In anterior teeth a single canal tends to lead into one apical foramen although multiple foramina do occur (**10.1**). In posterior teeth the incidence of multiple foramina is high. The position of the major apical foramen varies and may be found up to 2 mm from the apex of the root.

Lateral canals

The incidence of lateral canals, which may occur anywhere along the surface of the root, is high (see Chapter 6). A radiolucency occurring on the lateral surface of the root may be due to a lateral canal, a fractured root or a periodontal lesion. In **10.2** three mandibular incisors have been root treated: the isolated radiolucency near the gingival margin of the right central incisor is due to a lateral canal on the distal root surface. **10.3** shows a blade implant forming part of a fixed three unit bridge. The mesial abutment, the mandibular first premolar, has a radiolucent area around the apex and the distal root surface. The tooth has been inadequately root treated. The cause of the bone loss is not obvious. Retreatment of the premolar root shows a lateral canal on the distal aspect of the tooth (**10.4**).

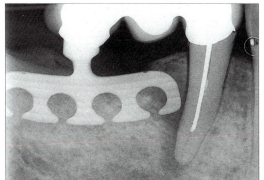

10.3 Blade implant and periradicular radiolucency

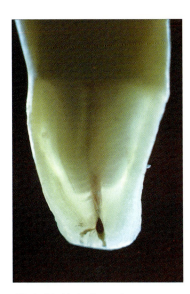

10.1 Multiple foramina

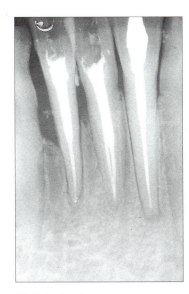

10.2 Lateral canal

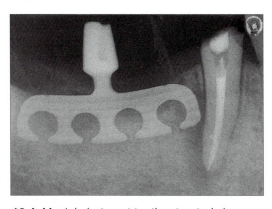

10.4 Mesial abutment tooth retreated shows lateral canal

Dentinal tubules

There is some discussion concerning the effect of toxins passing through dentinal tubules in the furcation of molars. Recent work suggests that the permeability of dentine is lower than was originally thought and it is unlikely that periodontal disease would affect the pulp even after the loss of cementum and some peripheral dentine in the furcation: it is also unlikely that a diseased pulp would affect the periodontal tissues unless a furcation canal is present. The bone loss in the furcation of the mandibular second molar in **10.5** was explained by the presence of the lateral canal seen on completion of the root treatment (**10.6**).

Root fracture, horizontal or vertical

Fractures of the root that involve the pulp form a potential perio-endo lesion, which will form when micro-organisms invade the fracture line. Vertical fractures, which involve the crown as well as the root, have a poorer prognosis because the communication with the oral cavity continuously re-infects the crack. Horizontal root fractures, provided they do not communicate with the oral cavity and the pulp remains vital, will not produce a perio-endo lesion. **10.7** shows a right incisor which was fractured some years previously: the canal has sclerosed but there is no evidence of infection. In **10.8** the mandibular first molar is fractured vertically and has become infected.

Congenital groove

A congenital groove is usually found in the palatal aspect of lateral or central incisors, more rarely in the palatal root of maxillary molars. These grooves may be difficult to detect clinically. In **10.9** a palatal groove is visible in the right central incisor. The groove may be so deep that the pulp and periodontal ligament communicate (the central incisor in **10.10** and **10.11** appears to have two canals, such is the depth of the groove: when root treatment was completed some sealer had been extruded into the groove in the mid-root area). If grooves become infected the prognosis is generally poor, particularly if the groove is deep. However, it may be treatable, as in the case illustrated in **10.12–10.15**. A flap was reflected and the relatively shallow groove ground away. Three months later it was not possible to probe into the defect.

Root resorption

In its advanced stages internal resorption may perforate through the wall of the root; external cervical resorption may also expose the pulp. Extensive internal resorption, which has perforated the root wall, is shown in **10.16** and **10.17**.

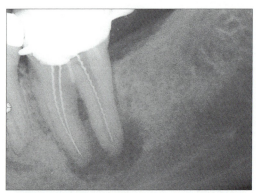

10.5 Furcation bone loss

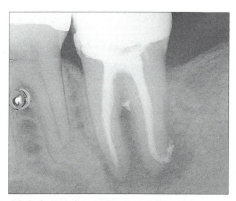

10.6 Lateral canal

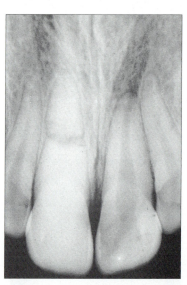

10.7 Old horizontal root fracture

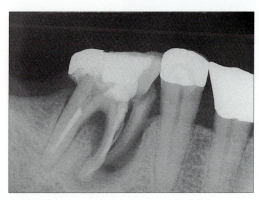

10.8 Infected vertical root fracture

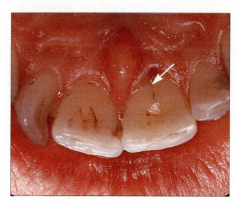

10.9 Congenital groove

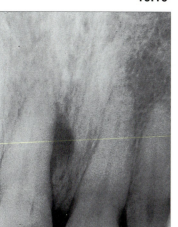
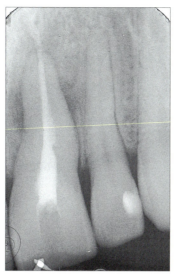
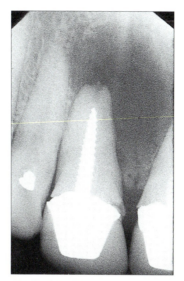
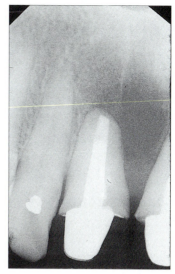

10.10, 10.11 An apparent second canal is a congenital groove. The arrow shows sealer which has extruded into the groove

10.12 Maxillary central incisor with a palatal groove and a Dentatus screw acting as a root filling. A large peri-radicular area is visible

10.13 Periapical area has reduced, but remaining healing has been prevented by a groove

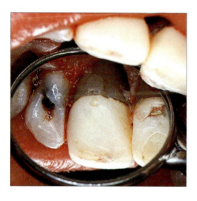

10.14 Palatal flap raised, revealing groove. This was removed with a bur

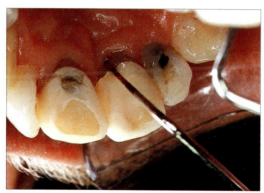

10.15 Three months later the pocket was not probeable

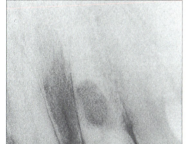
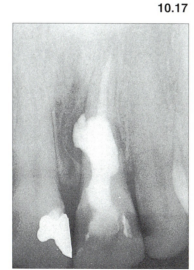

10.16, 10.17 Internal resorption, which has perforated

Iatrogenic perforation

Procedural accidents do occur; for example, the floor of the pulp chamber may be perforated with a bur while attempting to locate a canal entrance (**10.18**), or the wall of a root may be perforated while a post hole is being prepared (**10.19**) (see Chapter 13).

Classifying perio-endo lesions

These lesions are classified to help assess the prognosis and plan the treatment. Several classifications have been made in the literature but some of these are misleading. The lesions are difficult to categorize for two reasons.

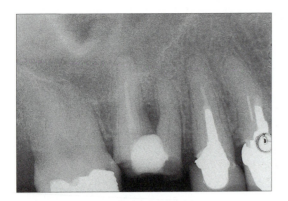

10.18 Iatrogenic perforation

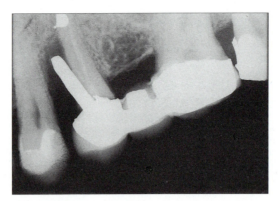

10.19 Misplaced post

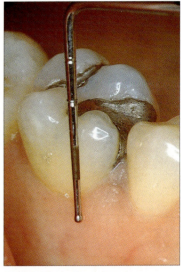

10.20 Periodontal probe

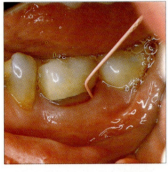

10.21 Gutta percha point in pocket

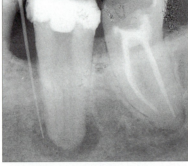

10.22 Demonstrating a periodontal pocket using gutta percha

1. It is not possible clinically to establish either the histological state of the pulp, or in a pulpless tooth whether pulpal death was caused by periodontal disease.
2. Periodontal disease is caused by the interaction of specific micro-organisms and host susceptibility.

The classification adopted in this book is simple:

1. Lesions of endodontic origin;
2. Lesions of periodontal origin;
   a when the pulp responds positively to vitality testing;
   b when the pulp is diseased or necrotic.

Diagnosis and treatment

The three main diagnostic methods used are measuring periodontal pocket depth and noting the width; pulp vitality testing; and taking parallel radiographs.

Figure **10.20** shows probing with a periodontal pocket probe, **10.21** and **10.22** probing with a gutta percha point. The probe should be fine to allow easy access but should have a blunt tip to prevent damaging the pocket floor. A flow chart summarizing the approach to treatment is given in **10.23**.

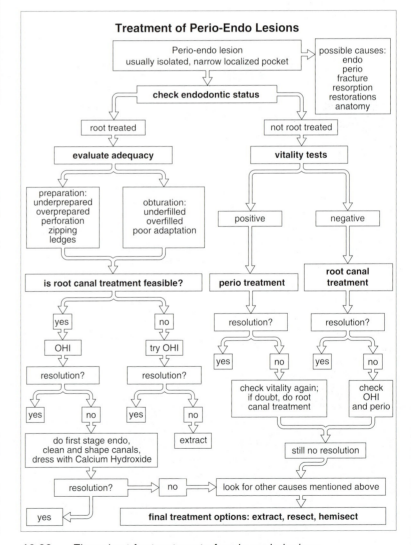

10.23 Flow chart for treatment of perio-endo lesions

Lesions of endodontic origin

The teeth have diseased or necrotic pulps and periodontal probing shows normal pocket depth except in one area. The reason for the non-vitality of the pulp is usually evident (**10.24**).

Root canal treatment is carried out on the tooth and the prognosis is good (**10.25**). Periodontal treatment is rarely required.

Lesions of periodontal origin

Clinical and radiographic examination will show whether the periodontal lesion is limited to one tooth or is generalized throughout the mouth. It is important to check pulp vitality. The teeth are examined for mobility, and re-examination at a later date will demonstrate the success of the treatment.

Pulp responding to vitality testing

When the pulp responds to a vitality test it is probably due to generalized periodontal disease and the patient is treated accordingly. If the lesion affects a single tooth a local cause should be sought – for example, a foreign body (such as a fish bone) that has been forced into the gingival crevice or a congenital groove in the maxillary lateral or central incisor. Restorations with ledges (**10.26, 10.27**) or enamel pearls overlying the furcation may produce local periodontal lesions. The effects of a misplaced pin may be seen in **10.28**.

Appropriate periodontal treatment is carried out. Any overhanging restorations are replaced to allow the patient to clean the area. If they become infected, congenital grooves have a poor prognosis.

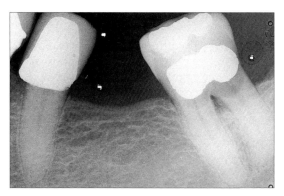

10.24 Obvious reason for non-vitality of the pulp

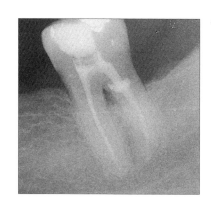

10.25 Root treated tooth

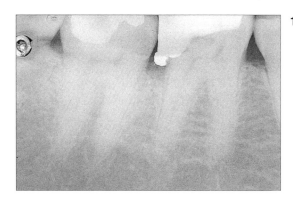

10.26   **10.27**

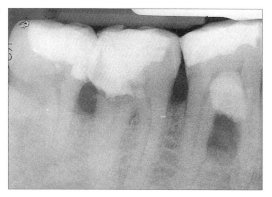

10.26, 10.27 Restorations with ledges

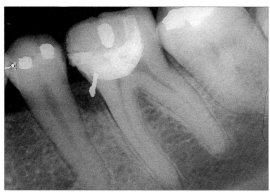

10.28 Misplaced pin

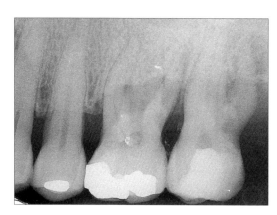

10.29 Generalized periodontal disease

Diseased or necrotic pulp

If a tooth is pulpless it should be established whether this is due to advanced periodontal disease generalized throughout the mouth (**10.29**). In cases of generalized periodontal disease several teeth may be mobile. If the lesion is local the cause should be found. The pulp in the distal abutment to the bridge of **10.30** is non-vital and there is periodontal involvement. Root canal treatment was carried out and a radiograph taken 7 months later (**10.31**) shows good healing. Vertical root fractures, or internal or external resorption which has perforated through the wall of the root, may cause pulpal necrosis.

The prognosis for this group of lesions is generally poor, particularly if the death of the pulp has been caused by periodontal involvement of the main apical vessels.

Root canal treatment and root resection

Periodontal treatment around multirooted teeth may necessitate the removal of one or more roots. This treatment requires careful planning as both periodontal surgery and root canal therapy are needed. Before treatment is undertaken the alternatives should be examined, particularly whether extraction and some form of fixed prosthesis would be the best course of action.

Before root resection is carried out several factors should be considered.

Functional tooth

The tooth should be a functional member of the arch.

Root morphology

The roots should be separate with some inter-radicular bone so that the attachment apparatus is not damaged when a root is removed. Generally, the root separation in the first mandibular molar is better than in the second molar. Figure **10.32** shows a mandibular first molar with good root separation; for periodontal reasons it was decided to remove the mesial root. The mesial root was treated and the distal root resected (**10.33**). The mandibular first molar in **10.34** has roots that are fused; root resection is contraindicated in this case. Surgical access must be sufficient to allow correct angulation of the handpiece for root removal, and a small mouth may contraindicate the procedure.

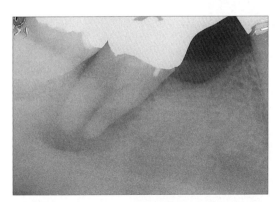

10.30 Periradicular bone loss due to non-vital pulp

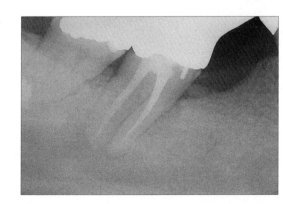

10.31 Good healing 7 months later

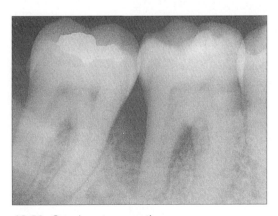

10.32 Good root separation

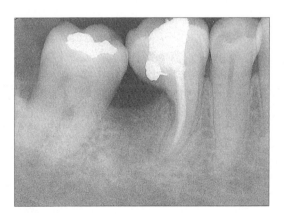

10.33 Resection of distal root

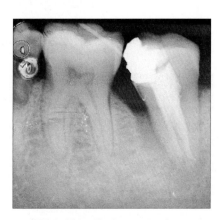

10.34 Mandibular second molar with fused roots

Root filling

It must be possible to provide root canal treatment, which has a good prognosis.

Tooth restorable

Sufficient supracrestal tooth structure must be present to allow the tooth to be restored: **10.35** shows a mandibular molar which can be restored but is a borderline case. In **10.36** tooth destruction is below the crestal level, the tooth is not restorable. The gingival finishing line of the restoration must be cleansable by the patient.

Suitability of patient

The patient must be capable of maintaining a high standard of oral cleanliness around the sectioned teeth and should be a suitable candidate for the lengthy operative procedures.

All teeth that require root resection must be root treated. The surgery, particularly the timing between surgery and root canal treatment, must be planned with care.

Teeth with vital pulps

Ideally, root canal treatment should be performed on the tooth before surgery. The pulps are extirpated and the canals prepared and obturated in the normal way; in the root(s) to be resected the canal does not need to be filled to the full working length although the coronal portion must be well condensed. One method is to widen the coronal straight portion of the canal using Gates Glidden burs and condense amalgam into it (**10.37, 10.38**).

In some cases it becomes apparent during periodontal surgery that a root or roots should be resected and the tooth root filled 10–14 days later. The vital pulp stump may be left exposed or covered with a zinc oxide preparation. Surprisingly the pulp causes little or no discomfort when it is left exposed for the short period before root treatment.

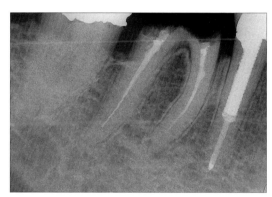

10.35 Tooth may or may not be restorable

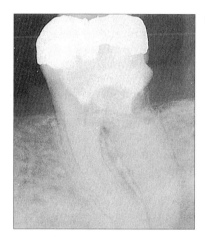

10.36 Non-restorable tooth

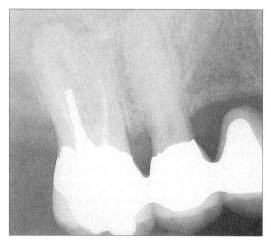

10.38 Amalgam placed in palatal root before resection

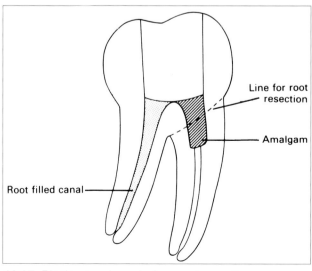

10.37 Placing amalgam before root resection

Pulpless teeth

In many cases it is impossible to estimate the extent of the destruction caused by the necrotic pulp. The necrotic pulp should be removed and the canals cleaned, dressed with calcium hydroxide and the access cavity sealed. The tooth is left for a period of 2–3 months, after which the periodontium is reviewed and a decision made as to whether a root requires resection. If the tooth is to be retained root canal treatment should be completed.

11 Surgical endodontics

Indications for surgery

Modern understanding of the biological basis for performing endodontic treatment has brought into question many of the traditional reasons given for undertaking surgical procedures.

Decisions regarding the need for surgery should be based on the principles that underpin endodontic technique, the degree of practitioner expertise, and the short- and long-term best interests of the patient.

The surgical approach can give rise to complications and the long-term success of surgical procedures is no higher than non-surgical ones. The need for surgery should always be questioned and surgery should not be embarked upon when the only positive indication seems to be operator convenience. Very few true indications exist for performing even the most practised surgical endodontic procedure, apical surgery.

The surgical approach is often prescribed when conventional endodontics is impossible or unlikely to succeed. Common indications quoted are the sclerosed canal or unfavourable canal anatomy. Surgery is not positively indicated when a conventional approach to search for the sclerosed canal or negotiate the anatomical complexity is possible.

The surgical approach is most often prescribed in situations where conventional techniques have not succeeded (**11.1**). Surgery may be indicated if conventional retreatment is impossible or if retreatment is unlikely to achieve a better result; however, non-surgical retreatment should always be considered and where possible undertaken (**11.2**) in preference to surgical retreatment.

Where failed root fillings (**11.3**), fractured instruments (**11.4**), and metal posts (**11.5**) cannot be removed, surgical access to the root canal system may be the only treatment means available (**11.6**–**11.8**).

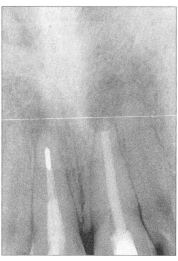

11.1 Failed endodontic treatment

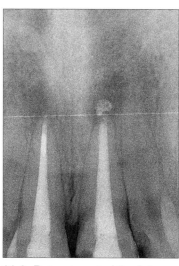

11.2 Retreatment of the failure

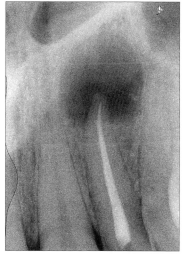

11.3 Failed endodontic treatment

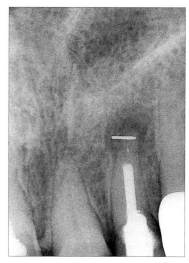

11.4 Fractured instrument in tooth

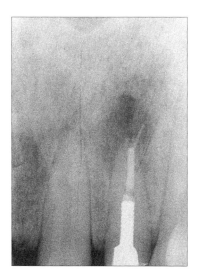

11.5 Metal post in tooth

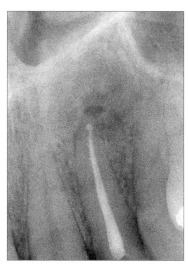

11.6 Surgical retreatment of failed endodontics (**11.3**)

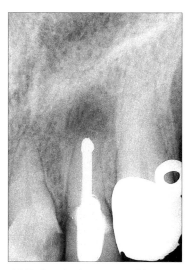

11.7 Surgical removal of fractured instrument (**11.4**)

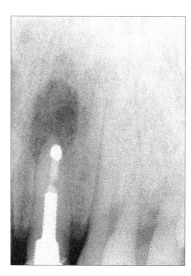

11.8 Surgical retreatment of tooth with a metal post (**11.5**)

The presence of an overextended root filling (**11.9**), although quoted as an indication for surgical treatment, is not a valid reason in itself for surgery. Conventional retreatment followed by a period of observation may be all that is required to effect successful repair (**11.10**).

Conventional root treatment is always the preferred method of dealing with an irreversibly damaged pulp, and is becoming increasingly important in the treatment of failed surgical cases (**11.11**). Retreatment demonstrates a lateral canal.

Surgical endodontics is indicated, and may be considered a useful adjunct to conventional endodontics, in the three areas of incision and drainage, apical surgery and reparative/corrective surgery.

Incision and drainage

Incision to establish drainage (**11.12**) of inflammatory exudate and pus from a fluctuant swelling is normally undertaken when drainage through the root canal is difficult. Releasing the products of acute inflammation helps bring the condition under control. Antibiotics should be required only if there are systemic effects from the infection or if drainage cannot be established. The incision of an intraoral fluctuant swelling is normally achieved with the aid of a surface analgesic. Where an injection is required this should be performed with care, avoiding inflamed tissue. Drainage is accomplished using either a scalpel blade or a wide-bore needle and disposable syringe; a drain is not normally required.

Patients occasionally present in pain with acute symptoms in a tooth which cannot be drained through the root canal and which has no fluctuant swelling. The infection is confined to cancellous bone and drainage is attempted by a process known as *cortical trephination*. An incision is made through the mucoperiosteum and the cortical bone is penetrated using a rotary instrument. Local analgesia is required for this procedure. This is not an easy task to perform and always carries the risk of damaging the underlying root.

Apical surgery

In broad terms the principles that govern this type of surgical procedure demand good presurgical planning, including a preoperative radiograph using a paralleling technique (**11.13**). Pain control measures are required in securing adequate analgesia. Attention must be paid to incisions (**11.14, 11.15**), mucoperiosteal flap reflection design (**11.16**) and bone removal before performing the chosen procedure. An immediate postoperative check radiograph is taken before flap replacement and suturing (**11.17**). The patient is instructed in postoperative instructions and after care and is reviewed periodically (**11.18**) when radiography (**11.19**) should be performed to confirm favourable healing.

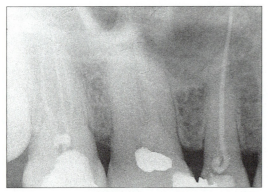
11.9 Overextended failed root filling

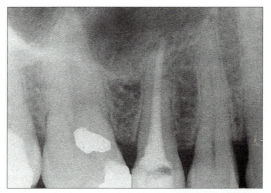
11.10 Conventional retreatment of the failure

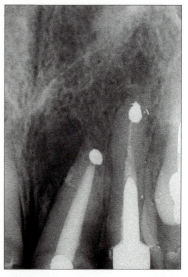
11.11 Conventional retreatment of failed surgical case

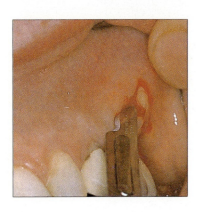
11.12 Drainage by incision

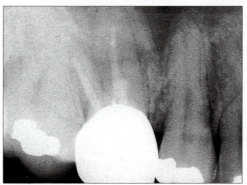
11.13 Preoperative radiograph

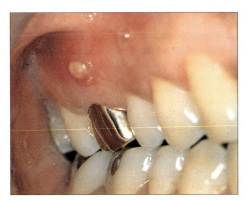
11.14 Pre surgical incision

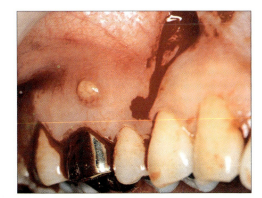
11.15 Surgical incision

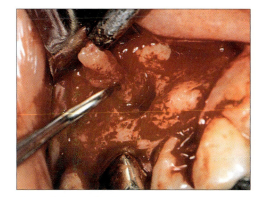
11.16 Flap reflection

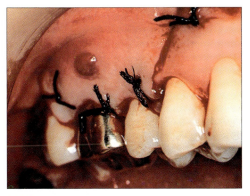
11.17 Suturing

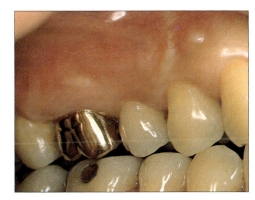
11.18 Clinical review

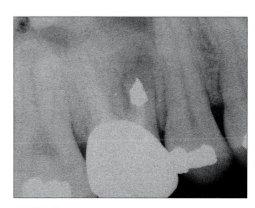
11.19 Postoperative radiograph

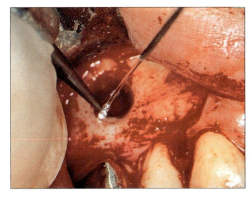
11.20 Apical seal

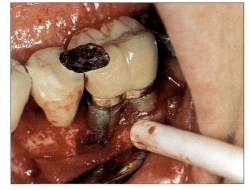
11.21 Vertical root fracture

Periradicular curettage involves removing any soft tissue lesion from around the root apex or lateral surface of a pulpless tooth. Root cementum and excess root filling material may be curetted at the same time. There is a trend towards the use of ultrasonic devices to perform this curettage, which may also help eradicate extraradicular infection. The procedure is rarely performed on its own because, even when there is what appears radiographically to be an adequately condensed root filling, residual infection may be present.

Curettage is generally a part of apicectomy and root end filling. This involves resection of the apical portion of the root and placement of a restoration in a cavity cut into the apical extent of the pulp canal system (**11.20**). The resection of the apical part of the root allows access to the root canal for seal placement.

Apical surgery may also be carried out in a situation where it is necessary to reflect a flap in order to examine the root and surrounding tissues, often when searching for a vertical root fracture (**11.21**). The appropriate treatment is usually carried out at the same time. Biopsy is performed if there is doubt about the cause and nature of a periapical lesion. The lesion is removed completely, placed in a transport medium (such as formol saline or fixative) and sent for histological evaluation. Samples of diseased soft tissue removed during the surgical procedure should routinely be sent for histopathological examination: serious pathology has been identified in this manner.

Reparative/corrective surgery

Surgery may be required to repair defects in a root surface created by iatrogenic and pathological influences.

Perforations result from resorption, caries and mechanically created root defects. The outcome of repair depends to a great extent on the size, location and length of time the perforation has been present. Small iatrogenic perforations may be treated by a non-surgical approach using calcium hydroxide as a long-term medicament when tissue repair and healing needs to be encouraged. The prepared canal space may usually be sealed using a conventional obturation technique.

Persistent clinical symptoms and bone resorption usually indicate a need for surgical sealing of perforations (**11.22, 11.23**). Surgical management depends upon the access and the relationship with the crestal bone level and epithelial attachment.

Root resection

This consists of removing an entire root from a multirooted tooth without removing the corresponding portion of the crown. Indications include periodontal disease, resorption, root fracture, unrestorable roots or roots that are unsuitable for conventional root treatment. Root resections are more commonly performed on maxillary molars (**11.24, 11.25**). Long tapered fissure and diamond burs are particularly useful in removing the root and shaping the furcation area to create a shape which is conducive to good plaque control. Flap reflection and bone removal and remodelling are usually essential in these situations.

Tooth resection

Cutting off a root with its associated coronal tooth structure is termed tooth resection. The separated part of the tooth may be removed or separately restored. Tooth resections are performed using long tapered diamond burs and a vertical cut approach in maxillary (**11.26**) and mandibular (**11.27**) molars. The vertical and lateral extent of the cut may be determined using a periodontal probe and silver points or metal wire to act as guides for the cut.

11.22, 11.23 Surgical repair of a perforation

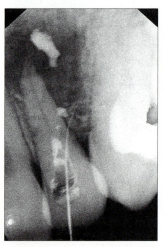
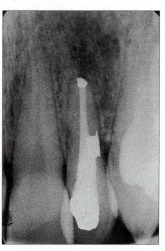

11.22   11.23

11.24, 11.25 Root resection of a maxillary molar

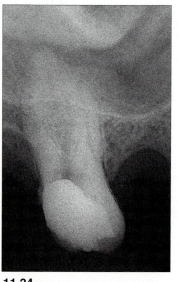
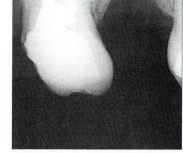

11.24   11.25

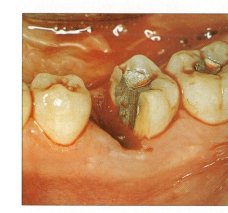

11.26 Tooth resection of a maxillary molar

11.27 Tooth resection of a mandibular molar

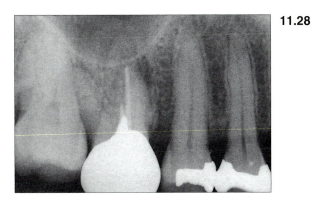

11.28

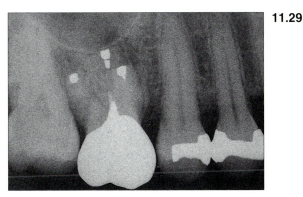

11.29

11.28, 11.29 Intentional replantation of a molar

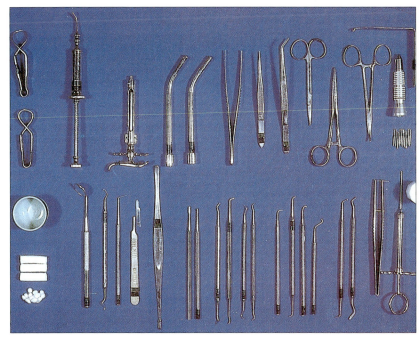

11.30 A basic surgical kit. **Top row (left–right):** Towel clips, Hunt's syringe, syringe for local anaesthetic, aspirator tips, mouse-tooth forceps, college tweezers, scissors, suture needle holder, curved needle holder, handpiece (straight) burs, angled flap retractor. **Bottom row (left–right):** Galley pot, cotton wool rolls, cotton buds, mirror, Briault probe, straight probe, scalpel handle and no. 15 blade, periosteal elevator, tungsten carbide straight chisels (2), excavators (3) and Mitchell trimmer, custom-made amalgam condensers (4), Baldwin amalgam burnisher, double-ended flat plastic KG retro-amalgam carrier, Messing amalgam gun

Intentional replantation

In intentional implantation a tooth is replaced in its socket following deliberate avulsion. This is usually carried out when there is no other option to retain the tooth. While the tooth is out of the mouth, apicectomy and root sealing is normally performed (**11.28, 11.29**). Successful clinical management requires two operators, one looking after the extraction site while the other attends to the treatment of the tooth. The reinserted tooth is splinted for a period of 5 days.

Armamentarium

A complete armamentarium should be available for surgical endodontic procedures. A normal (**11.30**) layout should include

Sterile towels
Gauze swabs and ribbon
Plastic bowl for saline
Irrigating syringe
Scalpels No. 15
Periosteal elevator
Periosteal retractor
Hooked, curved and angled probes
Front surface mirror and small mirrors to view large lesions
College tweezers
Surgical round and tapered burs
Cavity preparation burs
Bone curettes
Periodontal curettes
Angled and straight handpiece
Ultrasonic unit and tips
Miniature handpiece
Carver, condenser and burnisher
Tissue forceps
Needle holder for a 16 mm needle containing 4/0 black silk suture
Surgical scissors
Local anaesthetic equipment
Aspiration equipment
Instruments for canal preparation and obturation

Anaesthesia and pain control

Surgical procedures conducted on conscious patients should be accompanied by a complete absence of pain. In most cases local anaesthesia is used.

The object should be to achieve profound and long lasting anaesthesia and adequate haemostasis: local anaesthetic solutions containing 1:80 000 adrenaline should be used to secure haemostasis.

Great care must be taken to ensure that the nerve block techniques of injection provide the desired level of anaesthesia, and that supplementary infiltration injections provide the right level of vasoconstriction by involving the whole surgical site. To be effective, infiltration injections should be deposited at the level of the root apices just superficial to the periosteum.

Pain during an operation is most distressing and may normally be avoided by inducing a predictably high level of analgesia through good local anaesthetic injection techniques using 2% solution of lignocaine and 1:80 000 adrenaline. This produces a long lasting analgesia and reduces bleeding at the operation site.

Maxillary anaesthesia

In the maxilla, in addition to buccal, labial, and palatal infiltration techniques, greater palatine and long sphenopalatine nerve blocks may be required. The greater palatine nerve is blocked by placing anaesthetic at the junction of the alveolar process and the horizontal palatal bones. Following palatal infiltration in the anterior region to blanche the incisive papilla, the sphenopalatine nerve is blocked by depositing local anaesthetic into the incisive foramen (**11.31**).

Mandibular anaesthesia

In the mandible, inferior dental blocks need to be supplemented with buccal and lingual infiltrations.

The pain experienced following surgery differs quite markedly from patient to patient. Analgesic drug therapy should be selected and prescribed on an individual basis. For mild to moderate discomfort non-narcotic analgesics, which have far fewer side effects than narcotic analgesics, are the pain relief of choice.

Non-narcotic analgesics should be given 1–3 hours before the procedure, in advance of the pain and inflammation associated with prostaglandin production.

The choice of drug will depend upon the health of the patient, existing drug therapy, and possible history of adverse reactions. Aspirin and paracetamol are still the most widely prescribed analgesics for moderate dental pain. Diflunisal and ibuprofen, non-steroidal anti-inflammatory drugs, may be used if preferred.

Up to 50% of patients are susceptible to 'the placebo effect': a well informed patient who is confidently directed to commence a suitable analgesic regime before surgery is less likely to encounter problems postoperatively.

Flap design and reflection

Flaps have been designed to fulfil specific needs in different surgical situations. The general requirements of flaps include having an adequate blood supply, providing an unobstructed view of the operating site and possessing clear, well defined margins. Flap incisions should be made through periodontally healthy soft tissue, over sound bone and should avoid bony protuberances.

Two types of mucoperiosteal flap are used in surgical endodontics: full flaps and limited flaps. The essential difference is that full flaps involve the marginal and papillary soft tissues whereas the limited flaps are submarginal and do not involve the marginal and papillary tissues.

Full flaps

Full flaps (**11.32**) may be described as rectangular, trapezoid, triangular and horizontal. The rectangular and trapezoid flaps have two vertical relieving incisions, the triangular flap has one and the horizontal flap has none. The absence of relieving incisions in the horizontal flap restricts access and its use is limited. The trapezoid flap has a wide base and the relieving incisions produce an obtuse angle at the gingival margin. The angulated incision is thought likely to produce greater disruption of the vasculature in a region where the vessels tend to be vertically oriented. For these reasons, the triangular flap is most applicable to the posterior segments and the rectangular flap lends itself to the anterior region.

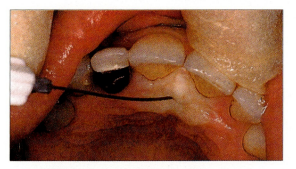

11.31 Blanching the incisive papilla

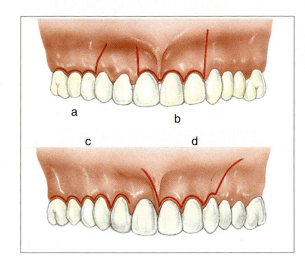

11.32 Full flaps: a triangular; b vertical; c horizontal; d trapezoid

The relieving incisions commence in alveolar mucosa and pass through the attached and marginal gingivae to end in the region of the mesial or distal aspects of the teeth so that the papillae are never bisected by the flap.

The full rectangular and triangular flaps appear to be applicable to most endodontic situations.

Full flap reflection should be initiated in the relieving incision in the region of the attached gingivae, elevating the periosteum from the alveolar bone. The elevator should then be edged coronally to lift the marginal and papillary tissue with a minimum of trauma. Elevation should proceed in an apical direction. If a sinus tract is present it may be necessary to resort to the use of a scalpel blade to assist the reflection of the flap.

Once reflected the flap is held passively away from the operative site with a retractor. The retractor must always rest on the bone and not on the reflected tissues. Retractor-induced tissue damage impairs healing.

Limited flaps

These (**11.33**) include the semilunar and Leubke–Ochsenbein flaps. The aim of both flaps is to maintain the integrity of the gingival margin. The only virtue of the semilunar flap appears to be the ease with which it is replaced and sutured: limited access and inevitable scarring (**11.34**) are its main drawbacks. The Leubke–Ochsenbein flap does not involve crestal bone and may have an application when dealing with crowned anterior teeth; however, at least 2 mm of attached gingivae needs to remain intact to prevent delayed healing and tissue shrinkage. This design is limited to patients with a wide band of attached gingivae and scarring is less of a problem.

Bone removal and root resection

Once the flap is retracted the next priority is to locate the root tip: if a sinus is present or if the lesion perforates the buccal alveolar plate this is a fairly simple matter but where the root apex is not so obvious a sharp straight probe may be used to feel for the tooth in the apical region. When the root tip has been located the overlying bone is removed using a round bur in a 'paring' motion until the root becomes visible. The apical lesion can be curetted at this stage. Complete removal of granulation tissue is a requirement in order to eradicate extraradicular infection, which may be responsible for a lesion's non-resolution. Complete removal of the lesion is also required for the purpose of biopsy, which should be performed routinely.

Root resection is performed using a tapered fissure bur until the apical extent of the main root canal becomes visible. There is also no requirement to remove valuable root substance to access the base of the apical lesion. When the bony cavity has been cleared and the bleeding controlled the canal may be enlarged, cleaned and prepared for the reception of the apical seal. This is normally achieved using latch burs in a miniature handpiece. A number of cavity designs are available; however, the major difficulty encountered in retrograde cavity preparation, because of limited access, is in preparing a cavity along the axis of the root canal. This hinders successful cleaning of the apical portion of the canal system. There is a move to the use of reverse filing techniques in order to overcome this problem, using bent hand files held in artery forceps and ultrasound to prepare and clean the apical portion of the root canal. Less emphasis is being placed on the need for bevelled sectioning of the root.

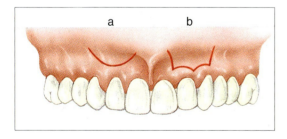

11.33 Limited flaps: a semilunar; b Leubke–Ochsenbein

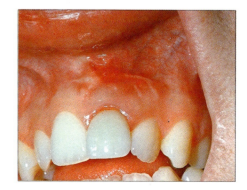

11.34 Semilunar flap scarring

Sutures and suture removal

Wound closure is an essential part of the surgical process for uneventful healing and involves replacing the flap and suturing.

The flap should be returned to its original position. The use of a gauze soaked in normal saline under finger pressure can assist in the process. When the flap is in the correct position it can be stabilized using sutures.

Suturing techniques should be adopted to stabilize the repositioning of the flap. Following suturing it is advisable to recompress the stabilized flap using a saline-enriched gauze. Four styles of suture are generally used alone or in conjunction:

The interrupted suture (**11.35**)
The single sling suture (**11.36**)
The vertical mattress suture (**11.37**)
The anchor suture (**11.38, 11.39**)

The vertical mattress suture has the advantage of not involving the incision site. If black silk sutures are used the patient should use a chlorhexidine mouthwash before and after surgery.

Sutures may be removed in 2–4 days; it is preferable to remove them earlier rather than later.

Decompression

Large periradicular lesions may be treated by the process known as decompression. If a large lesion is lined with epithelium and the cavity becomes filled with high molecular weight proteins fluid is attracted to the cavity by osmotic pressure. Decompression procedures aim to disrupt the integrity of the lesion wall and eliminate the osmotic effect.

The lesion is penetrated through the mucoperiosteum and cortical plate between adjacent teeth. The patency of the opening is maintained by inserting a flanged cannula, and the marsupialized

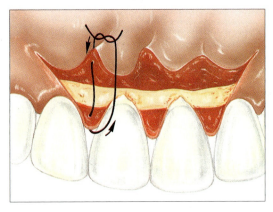

11.35 The interrupted suture

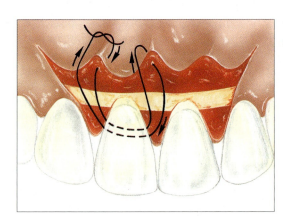

11.36 The single sling suture

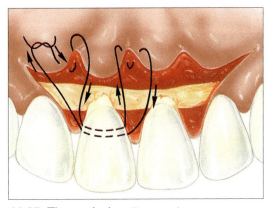

11.37 The vertical mattress suture

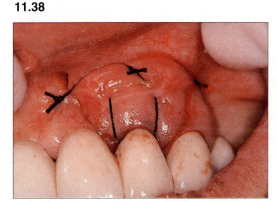

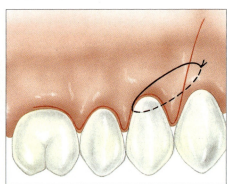

11.38, 11.39 The anchor suture

lesion may be irrigated daily by the patient (**11.40–11.44**). Termination of decompression should be based on radiographic and clinical criteria.

The advantages of this technique include reduction in the risk of damaging either adjacent vital teeth or anatomical structures.

Achieving seals

The main objective of most surgical endodontics is to provide a seal. The material used should be compatible with the oral tissues, non-resorbable, and adaptable to the site to be sealed. Many materials are available which, if used correctly, will satisfy the clinical requirements of a seal.

The most commonly used materials currently in use are amalgam, zinc oxide based materials, and glass ionomers. Preference seems to be moving towards zinc oxide materials and away from amalgam. The outcome of treatment is likely to be influenced more by the way in which a surgical procedure has been conducted than the particular sealing material used.

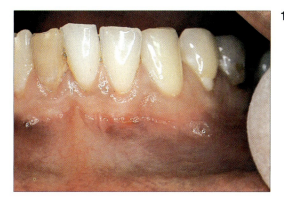

11.40

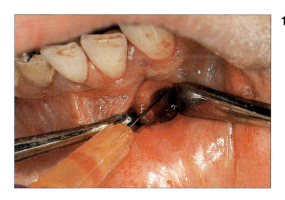

11.41

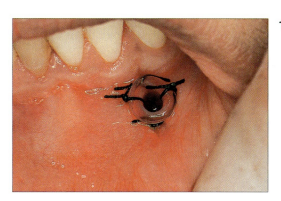

11.42

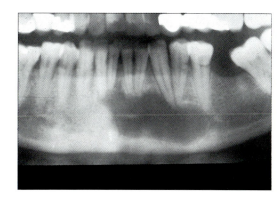

11.43

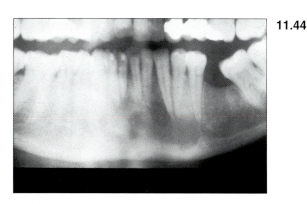

11.44

11.40–11.44 Decompression

12 Emergency endodontics

One of the most satisfying aspects of endodontic treatment is caring for the patient in pain. This can normally be achieved in a short period of time without jeopardizing the overall treatment plan.

It is probably true to say that over 85% of patients attending the dentist in pain are suffering from pulpal or periapical disease. The operator's aim, in providing emergency care, is to remove the pain and control the inflammation or infection that is present.

Emergencies of pulpal origin

Clinical reversible pulpitis is characterized by pain of short duration produced by extremes of temperature and sweet food. The teeth do not tend to be sensitive to palpation or percussion. The pain is usually of dentinal origin in situations where there is exposed sensitive dentine, early dental caries, and leaking restorations. Radiographically there should be no widening of the periodontal ligament space unless the pulpitis is induced by occlusal trauma, creating inflammation within the periodontal ligament and pulp. Treatment involves removing the source of dentinal irritation. In the case of sensitive dentine, fluoride varnish may be applied to the affected area or a desensitizing toothpaste prescribed. Dental caries and faulty restorations should be removed and replaced with a sedative dressing (**12.1**). Where necessary, the occlusion should be relieved.

Persistent symptoms indicate clinical irreversible pulpitis. The pain tends to increase in duration and intensity. Heat can become more reactive than cold, which may actually have a relieving influence. The pain is often spontaneous and lasts from several minutes to hours. The tooth may be difficult to locate until the periodontal ligament becomes inflamed, when it becomes tender to bite on. Early radiographic changes may be evident (**12.2**). Symptoms of irreversible pulpitis occasionally occur in teeth with primary periodontal lesions. Pain relief is achieved by root treatment but the long-term prognosis for the tooth depends on the periodontal status of the tooth.

The ideal emergency treatment for irreversible pulpitis is to remove the diseased pulp completely and to clean and prepare the pulp canal system. Irrigating the pulp chamber with a 2.5–5.0% solution of sodium hypochlorite ensures disinfection before canal instrumentation. If time does not allow this, removal of pulp tissue from the pulp chamber and coronal part of the root canals is often effective. The use of corticosteroid preparations has been advocated in situations where complete instrumentation of the canals is inconvenient or impossible because profound anaesthesia cannot be secured.

The 'hot tooth' may be dealt with at a subsequent appointment once the inflammation has settled. Difficulties encountered in trying to secure anaesthesia in irreversibly inflamed pulps may be overcome by administering additional local anaesthetic, and using intraligamental, intraosseous and intrapulpal anaesthetic techniques (**12.3**).

If symptoms continue following pulpal extirpation, the presence of infected or inflamed pulpal tissue should be investigated, the occlusal contacts of the tooth should be checked, and if necessary the pulp chamber and root canals should be thoroughly irrigated with 2.5% sodium hypochlorite.

Teeth with undiagnosed fractures may cause symptoms of reversible and irreversible pulpitis. The degree of pain may vary considerably, depending on the extent of the fracture: from momentary pain on encountering heat and cold to spontaneous pain or pain on biting. If reversible pulpitis is diagnosed, restorations should be removed from the suspected tooth, the dentinal fracture sought and the pulp protected from further insult by providing a restoration which reduces microleakage to a minimum and prevents the fracture propagating. Modern dentine

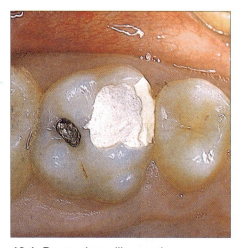

12.1 Dressed maxillary molar

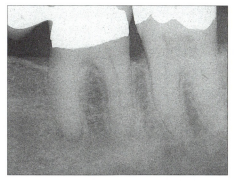

12.2 Thickening of periodontal ligament space

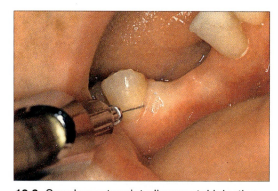

12.3 Supplementary intraligamental injection

bonding materials are useful in small cavities as an interim restoration before constructing a restoration giving occlusal protection (**12.4**). It is impossible to predict long-term events in this situation.

Where a fracture involves the pulp and symptoms suggest an irreversible pulpitis, all restorations should be removed from the tooth and the extent of the fracture examined. If the fractured portion of the tooth is mobile (**12.5**) it should be removed, examined, and the possibility of restoring the remaining tooth substance established. If the tooth is saveable root treatment may commence.

In cases where the tooth is fractured but the fracture has not parted the crown should be supported with a metal band (**12.6**) and root treatment commenced. The long-term prognosis of posterior teeth with oblique fractures above the alveolar crest and involving only the roof of the pulp chamber is higher than vertical fractures involving the floor of the chamber. A fibreoptic light is useful in locating and examining the extent of these fractures.

Emergencies of periodontal origin

Inflammation and infection of the periodontal tissues may cause pain. It is important to establish whether the pain and swelling involving the supporting tissues is of periodontal or pulpal origin. The cause is usually established by carrying out vitality tests.

When dealing with a periodontal abscess emergency treatment will involve instituting drainage, prescribing antibiotics when required and debriding the pocket with ultrasound. Endodontic treatment should not be required.

Acute apical periodontitis is an acute inflammation of the periodontal ligament, generally related to pulpal inflammation but occasionally resulting directly from trauma. When endodontic treatment is initiated in a non-vital tooth with acute apical periodontitis the canal system should be cleaned thoroughly to remove all periodontal irritation and care must be exercised to prevent further insult to the periodontal tissues by over-instrumentation. Corticosteroid preparations are often very effective in relieving the acute phase. Occlusal adjustment to remove contacts is also helpful.

An acute apical abscess (**12.7**) may develop from apical periodontitis. The tooth involved becomes exquisitely painful to touch. The tooth may be extruded from the socket and mobile. To relieve pain the priority is to establish drainage by opening up the pulp chamber of the tooth (**12.8**). The tooth, if tender, should be stabilized while the access cavity is being cut. Any fluctuant swelling should be incised to establish drainage. The pulp chamber should be irrigated with 2.5% sodium hypochlorite to remove superficial organic debris before commencing canal preparation. Following thorough cleaning of the canal system the tooth is sealed to prevent reinfection. Only when there is profuse, uncontrollable drainage should a tooth be left open to drain for a maximum period of 24 hours. When patients have toxic systemic effects and a raised temperature antibiotics should be prescribed. It is advisable to review all patients within 24 hours.

Emergencies resulting from trauma

Traumatic incidents may result in luxation and avulsion injuries and fractures of the crowns and roots of teeth. The endodontic problems arising from these incidents can be managed successfully only after the following questions are answered.

- *What is the nature of the injury?* It is important to assess the extent of both bony and soft tissue injuries. The examination of lacerations and fractures should take precedence over the dental examination. The need for anti-tetanus cover and referral to specialist colleagues should be established.
- *Are the injured teeth preservable and restorable?* The extent of dental damage should be assessed and the efforts required to retain the teeth should be considered, in the light of the patient's overall treatment needs, in order to reach a balanced decision regarding the future of the teeth.
- *Has the vascular/nutritive supply of the pulp been impaired? What is the degree of this impairment?* The assessment of vascular damage becomes particularly important if there is evidence of concussion and intrusive, extrusive, and lateral luxation of teeth.

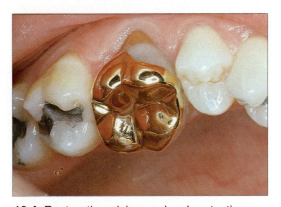

12.4 Restoration giving occlusal protection

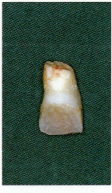

12.5 Removed fractured portion of tooth

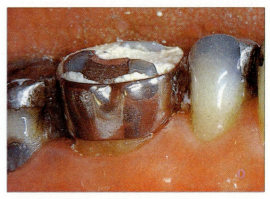

12.6 Mandibular molar supported by an orthodontic band

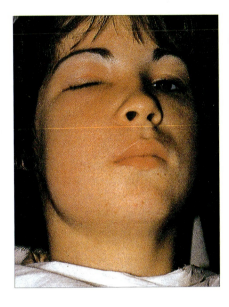

12.7 Acute apical abscess producing a facial swelling

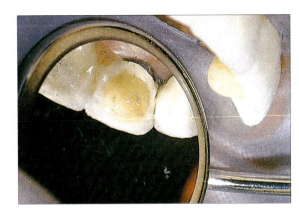

12.8 Tooth drainage of an apical abscess

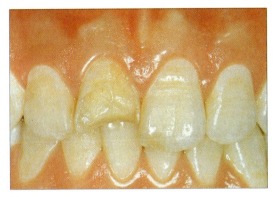

12.9 Fractured incisor crown

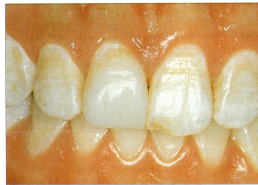

12.10 Restoration of fractured incisor crown

- *To what extent have the pulps of the teeth been contaminated with microorganisms? What is the potential for future contamination?* The endodontic penetration, and potential for further penetration, of bacteria and their toxins will have a profound influence on the immediate and long-term prognosis of fractured teeth.
- *How mature is each tooth and is the root completely formed?* Immature teeth with large pulp spaces are structurally more difficult to restore and need long-term endodontic treatment.

Treatment of fractured teeth

Crown fractures

Crown fractures may involve only the enamel or both the enamel and the dentine (**12.9**). The damaged tooth should be radiographed and vitality tested before protecting the exposed dentine with a liner and a bonded composite (**12.10**). It may be possible to use the fractured portion of the tooth as the restoration.

If injury to a mature tooth results in pulpal exposure root canal treatment is usually indicated; however, partial removal of the pulp may be possible. When the tooth involved is not fully formed and it is desirable to preserve the vital pulp, the treatment options are pulp capping or pulpotomy.

Pulp capping

Pulp capping is usually carried out only on very small and recent exposures; however, the size of the exposure has been shown in healthy pulps to be of little consequence. The tooth should be isolated and the exposure washed with saline. After the bleeding has stopped the area should be covered with calcium hydroxide and the tooth restored. The tooth should be reviewed clinically and radiographically 6 months later.

Pulpotomy

Pulpotomy procedures are performed in immature teeth with large exposures. The tooth is isolated with a rubber dam after administering local anaesthesia. A small portion of the coronal pulp is removed using a high-speed diamond bur under a cooling spray. The pulp stump is washed with saline and after bleeding ceases it is covered with calcium hydroxide and a zinc oxide preparation and the tooth is restored. The tooth should be reviewed initially at 6–12 weeks and then at an interval of 6 months and annually until the root formation is considered complete. The tooth should be observed to establish the presence of a hard tissue barrier without abnormal calcification. If there is radiographic evidence of internal resorption root treatment should be commenced.

Crown–root fractures

The treatment of crown–root fractures depends largely on their position and the degree of mobility of the coronal portion. Fractures involving the gingival crevice usually necessitate root treatment to stem the bacterial contamination that is likely to occur along the fracture line (**12.11**). Before root canal treatment is commenced it is wise to consider whether the fractured portion of the tooth is to be removed and how the tooth will be finally restored. The need for surgery to expose the margins of the fracture, orthodontic extrusion of the root to facilitate restorative procedures, and space maintenance to avoid later restorative problems should be borne in mind.

Root fractures

Mobile root fractures below the level of the alveolar crest should be splinted for up to 12 weeks to secure union of the fragments. The tooth should then be reviewed clinically and radiographically. Vitality testing may be unreliable for a period of 2–6 months.

If the tooth remains firm and is vital no further treatment is necessary. Many undiagnosed fractures remain symptomless and cause no problems (**12.12**).

If vitality is lost, generally the coronal segment becomes necrotic. Root treatment is performed to the fracture line. Calcium hydroxide is used as a long-term medicament (**12.13**) to encourage calcification and formation of a hard tissue barrier against which the root filling can be condensed (**12.14**). Root treatment of both fragments should be attempted rarely, when the whole pulp becomes necrotic; surgical removal of the apical portion may be a more manageable option (**12.15, 12.16**).

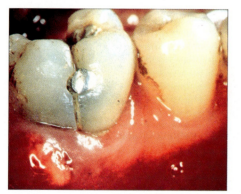

12.11 Fractured tooth requiring root canal treatment

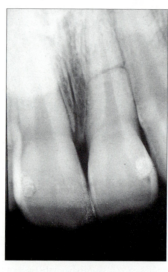

12.12 Untreated undiagnosed fractures

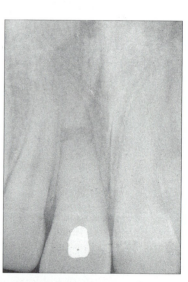

12.13 Calcium hydroxide placed to fracture line

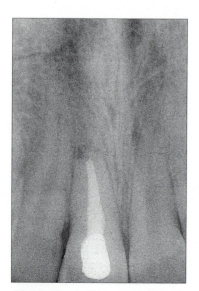

12.14 Root filling placed to fracture line

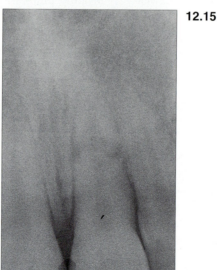

12.15

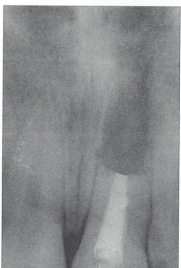

12.16

12.15, 12.16 Surgical removal of apical portion of fractured root

Treatment of unfractured teeth

If there is evidence to suggest that the pulp of a luxated tooth has become necrotic root treatment should be performed.

Completely avulsed teeth that have been replanted should undergo root canal treatment 7–10 days following replantation. There is some evidence to suggest that these teeth benefit from being dressed with calcium hydroxide for 3–6 months before being obturated to reduce the possibility of replacement resorption (**12.17**).

Many types of splint are available for stabilizing replanted and fractured teeth. Vacuum-formed polyvinyl splints (**12.18**) are inconvenient, require laboratory facilities (which delays their fitting) and tend to look rather bulky (**12.19**). The use of etched enamel retained composite (**12.20**), and polymethacrylate reinforced with wire or nylon has also been advocated. Intentionally replanted teeth need to be splinted for 1 week; avulsed and replanted teeth should be splinted for 1–4 weeks depending on the degree of damage to supporting alveolar bone. On average the usual splinting time is 7–10 days.

Emergencies during endodontic treatment

Patients may experience pain after canal preparation and cleaning or following obturation of the root canals.

Acute apical periodontitis occurs quite often following canal preparation. The common causes of this are over-instrumentation, leaving the tooth in traumatic occlusion and over-medication. Patients usually complain of a continuous dull ache and the tooth is very tender to touch. Irrigation of the canals with 2.5% sodium hypochlorite and relieving the occlusion are usually all that is required to offer relief.

Teeth with pre-existing chronic lesions without sinus formation or symptoms can be particularly troublesome. It is as if the bacterial flora within the tooth react to the opening up of the tooth and an exacerbation of the chronic condition ensues, producing an acute apical abscess. Treatment is as for an acute apical abscess.

Inter-appointment discomfort is also encountered with leaking restorations, which allow re-contamination of the canal system. The area of leakage must be found and the problem dealt with.

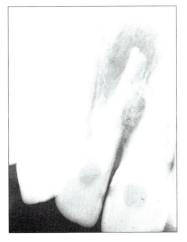

12.17 Replacement resorption

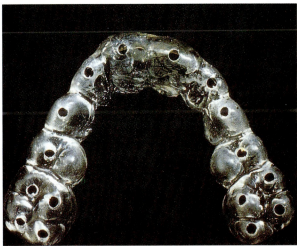

12.18 Polyvinyl splint

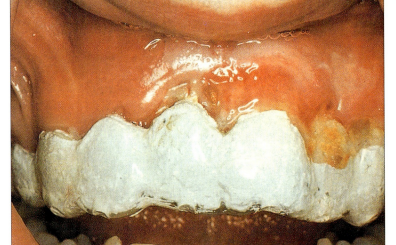

12.19 Polyvinyl splint in place

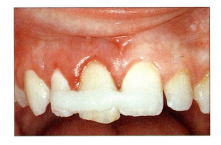

12.20 Composite splint

The probable causes of pain occurring following obturation of the root canal system are traumatic occlusion, an overextended root filling (**12.21**), inadequate cleaning of the root canal system and root fracture precipitated by the filling procedure (**12.22**).

Treatment may involve reassurance, prescription of analgesics (and possibly antibiotics), removal of the root filling and repreparation of the root canals, and surgical endodontics to remove overfilled material or resection of the tooth or root.

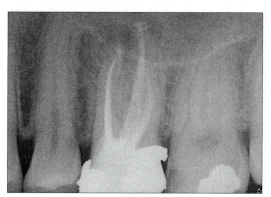

12.21 Overextended root filling

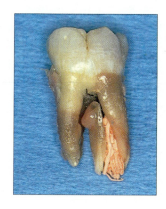

12.22 Root fracture induced during obturation

13 Tooth resorption

Tooth resorption is a physiological or pathological process causing loss of either cementum or cementum and dentine. Tronstad[1] states that

> 'If the predentine or precementum becomes mineralised or in the case of the precementum is mechanically damaged or scraped off, multinucleated cells will colonise the mineralised or denuded surfaces and resorption will ensue.'

Several different clinical types of root resorption are known but they are indistinguishable at a histological level. **13.1** shows multinucleated cells lying in a lacuna. Resorption is considered to be *external* if the original site of the resorption is the periodontal ligament and *internal* if it starts in the pulp.

The aetiology of tooth resorption is unknown, although much is known about the histological process, and much work is needed before all types of resorption can be treated effectively.

Internal resorption

Internal resorption results from a chronic pulpitis, although why some teeth are affected more dramatically than others is not known. Trauma and infection are important aetiological factors.

The typical appearance is a smooth widening of the root canal walls (**13.2**). On rare occasions (when the pulp chamber is affected) it may appear as a 'pink spot' as the enlarged pulp is visible through the thin wall of the crown. Any tooth may be affected but the incidence is highest in incisors. The destruction of dentine may take years or may be very rapid. The pulp usually remains vital and symptomless until the wall of the root is perforated, when it may become necrotic.

Diagnosis

In most cases diagnosis is simple but occasionally it may be difficult to differentiate between internal and external resorption. The diagram and radiograph (**13.3, 13.4**) show external resorption as an irregular radiolucent area overlying the root canal; the canal outline remains visible and intact. A case of external resorption is shown in **13.5**, but it is not easy to diagnose from the radiograph as the canal outline is indistinct. In internal resorption the outline of the canal is interrupted and usually appears as a smooth bulge. Resorption is often difficult to detect in posterior teeth and may be seen only after root treatment has been completed (**13.6, 13.7**).

Treatment

Prompt root canal treatment is necessary in all diagnosed cases: the resorption ceases as soon as the chronically inflamed pulp is removed.

Access cavity

An access cavity is cut in the usual manner but it is not necessary to enlarge the access as this could weaken the tooth.

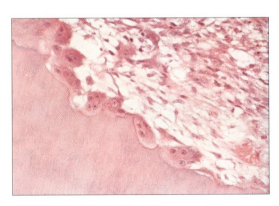

13.1 Multinucleated cells lying in a lacuna

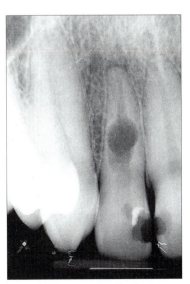

13.2 Internal resorption showing smooth widening of the walls of the root canal

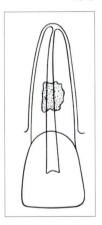
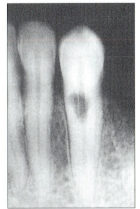

13.3, 13.4 External resorption of an irregular radiolucent area overlying the root canal

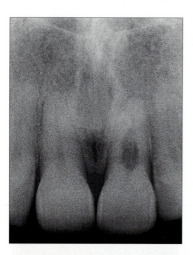

13.5 External root resorption

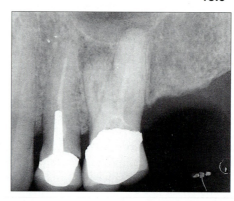 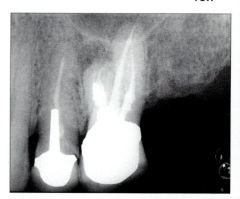

13.6, 13.7 Internal root resorption

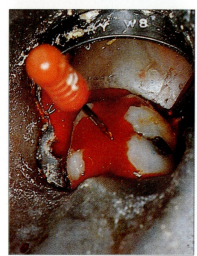

13.8 Haemorrhage of internal resorptive tissue

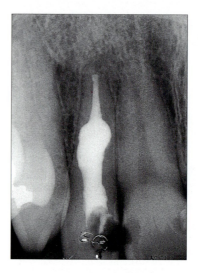

13.9 Gutta percha condensed into defect

Debridement

Debridement is carried out using copious amounts of 5% sodium hypochlorite, which will dissolve organic material inaccessible to instrumentation. Ultrasonic agitation of the solution will improve the result. Haemorrhage is a feature of internal resorptive tissue and may be difficult to control (**13.8**). Ledermix or aluminium chloride will act as a haemostat but complete haemostasis will be achieved only after all the pulp tissue has been removed.

Perforation

The canal should be checked for perforation. An electronic measuring device will help to explore the walls of the canal using a file with a curve placed near the tip. The position of any perforation on the root wall should be noted, which will aid in deciding whether the perforation is accessible for surgery.

Canal medication

A root canal dressing of calcium hydroxide should be used between appointments as a bactericide and to help dissolve any remaining organic debris. If there is no (or only a small) perforation the root may be filled at the second visit, after the canal has been fully prepared.

If a large inaccessible perforation is present long-term calcium hydroxide therapy should be instituted (see Chapter 8). The perforation will not heal completely, but the area of bone loss should heal enough to ensure minimum extrusion of filling material.

Root filling

A number of techniques may be used to fill the irregular root canal spaces: warm lateral condensation may be used but a warm gutta percha injection technique should ensure that the defect is well condensed (**13.9**). Both methods are described in Chapter 9.

Surgery

A surgical approach is preferred if the perforation is large or the bleeding is uncontrollable. The root canal is cleaned, prepared and filled and a flap reflected to expose the defect. The perforation is then sealed with a suitable restorative material. The defect shown in **13.10** and **13.11** was situated buccally providing easy access for surgery. Occasionally it may be better to reflect the flap first, carry out the root treatment, and then seal the perforation.

External resorption

The most common external resorption is the normal physiological process in primary teeth during eruption of the permanent dentition. Pathological resorption of the root surface following damage to the cementum has many causes, including

- impaction of teeth;
- luxation injuries;
- periapical inflammation due to a necrotic pulp;
- periodontal disease;
- excessive mechanical or occlusal forces;
- bleaching endodontically treated teeth;
- tumours and cysts;
- certain systemic diseases;
- radiation therapy.

Classification

External resorption may be classified into five groups.

Inflammatory resorption

Inflammatory resorption is thought to be caused by the presence of infected or necrotic pulp tissue in the root canal (**13.12**). It may occur in dentine surrounding the apical foramen or lateral canal of any tooth. The resorption is sustained by pulpal infection and may progress rapidly.

Root canal treatment in cases of inflammatory resorption carries a good prognosis, the only problem that may be encountered being difficulty in producing an apical stop because the apical constriction is missing. However, a stop can be achieved over time with calcium hydroxide or the chloroform dip technique may be used to provide a good fit in the apical 2–3 mm of the canal (which helps to prevent extrusion of filling material into the periapical tissues (**13.13, 13.14**; see Chapter 9).

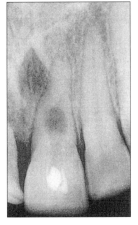
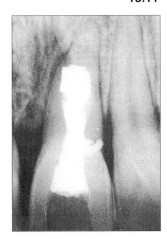

13.10, 13.11 Surgical repair of resorption

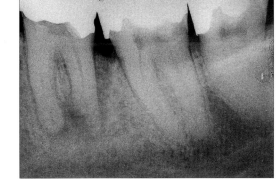

13.12 Inflammatory resorption of distal root of the first mandibular molar

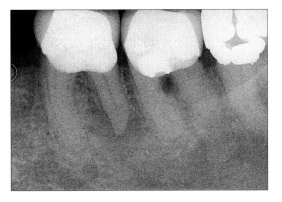
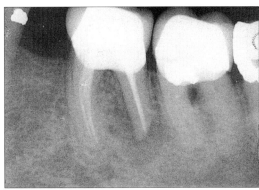

13.13, 13.14 Extrusion of gutta percha prevented by the chloroform dip technique

Surface resorption

This occurs commonly in a mild form as a response to localized injury to the periodontal ligament or cementum. The condition is self-limiting and shows spontaneous repair. It is not usually visible on radiographs. A more destructive type of surface resorption may be caused by acute or chronic pressure, for example an erupting or impacted tooth (**13.15**), orthodontic treatment (**13.16**), or a tumour or cyst. Several systemic diseases (such as hypoparathyroidism, hyperparathyroidism, calcinosis, Gaucher's disease, Turner's syndrome or Paget's disease (**13.17**)) may also cause resorption.

Treatment consists of removing the cause: in the case of systemic disease the patient should be referred to a physician. The condition should be reviewed regularly.

Cervical resorption

Cervical resorption is caused by inflammation within the periodontal ligament, possibly following trauma to the ligament. It is sited in the cervical area of the tooth and may present clinically in two different forms: a wide shallow crater (**13.18, 13.19**) or a burrowing type of resorption (**13.20**). Single, rather than multiple, teeth are affected and the process tends to be slow. Cervical resorption is usually asymptomatic and found on routine radiographic examination. The pulp is not involved until the condition is well advanced. In **13.21** a canine with a subgingival buccal defect is shown; radiolucencies are present in the mid-root area (**13.22**). The extent of the defect with a flap reflected and the pulp exposed is shown in **13.23**. Cervical resorption may follow bleaching of a root filled tooth. 'Pink spot' is more likely to be

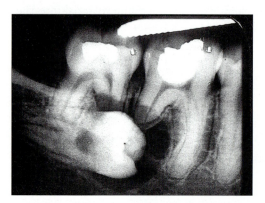

13.15 Resorption due to impacted third molar

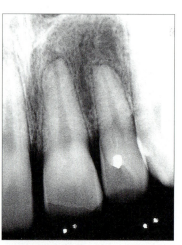

13.16 Resorption as a result of orthodontic treatment

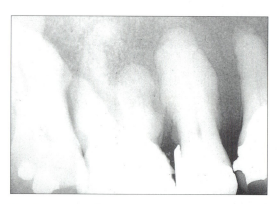

13.17 Paget's disease

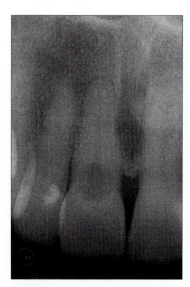

13.18

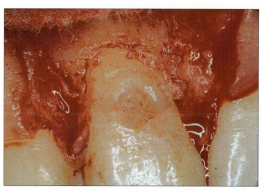

13.19

13.18, 13.19 Cervical resorption

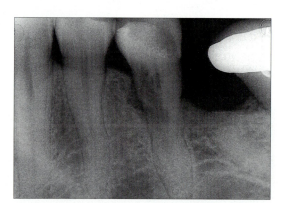

13.20 Burrowing type of resorption

due to this type of burrowing cervical resorption than to internal resorption: **13.24** shows a pink spot on the palatal aspect of a maxillary central.

Treatment involves exposing the lesion, removing the resorptive tissue and inserting a restoration. Severe cases may require orthodontic extrusion or extraction. It is often difficult to decide whether the defect is fully accessible to surgery before a flap is raised. A confident decision can be made only with experience and by taking radiographs using the parallel technique from different angles.

As a rule the pulp is not involved in the early stages. When a flap is raised and the extent of the defect can be seen the decision whether to carry out root canal treatment or not can be made.

Replacement resorption

This is the slow replacement of the root by surrounding bone, which leads to ankylosis (**13.25**). It is the result of damage to cells covering the cementum in luxation injuries. The case illustrated in **13.26–13.29** shows the results of two separate incidents of trauma. The maxillary left central crown of the patient was fractured in a fall at 7 years of age. The tooth subsequently became abscessed and was root treated. Follow-up radiographs over 3 years show no evidence of breakdown (**13.27, 13.28**). The maxillary right central was avulsed at age 8 years and replanted 2 hours later. The tooth was then root filled and a postoperative radiograph taken (**13.26**). A check radiograph (**13.27**) was taken 2.5 years later. Note the onset of replacement resorption in the mid-root portion of the right central incisor. The tooth became infraoccluded by 2.0 mm. The final radiograph (**13.28**) was taken 3 years after replantation. The tooth was extracted and is seen with almost no root substance remaining (**13.29**). The incidence of replacement resorption following avulsion, according to Andreasen,[2] is 80–96%. The condition may be transient if the damage is limited, but in more extensive cases it is progressive. If the pulp is necrotic an overlying inflammatory resorption may be present. Placing calcium hydroxide in the canal may aid bony repair (**13.30, 13.31**).

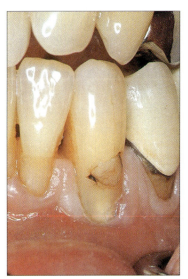

13.21 Subgingival defect

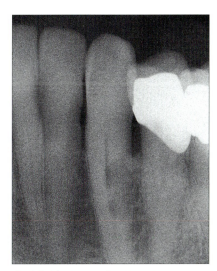

13.22 Radiograph of canine

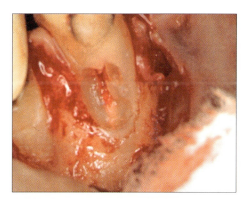

13.23 Extent of defect with flap reflected

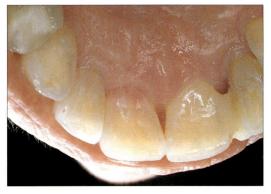

13.24 Pink spot

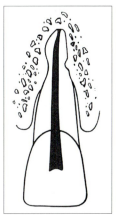

13.25 Replacement resorption. Note the absence of periodontal ligament

Diagnosis is confirmed with a history of trauma, particularly avulsion with a prolonged extraoral time. Radiographically the periodontal ligament space is absent, and the root has a moth-eaten appearance. The tooth has a ringing tone when tapped, and in young patients may not be in occlusion.

Replacement resorption is preventable but not treatable. Extraction should be considered to prevent interference with alveolar growth. In avulsion cases the tooth should be replanted as soon as possible or transported in milk to a healthcare worker. The pulp should be removed 10 days after the trauma if the apex is mature, and root treatment carried out. The pulp of an immature root apex should be monitored with radiographs and pulp testing.

13.26–13.29 Case illustrating two separate incidents of trauma. See text for details

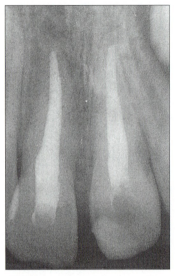
13.26

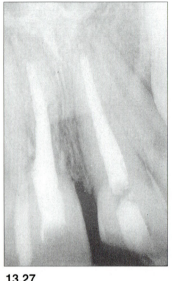
13.27

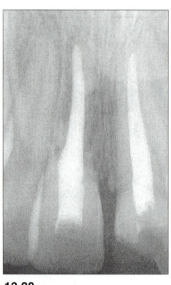
13.28

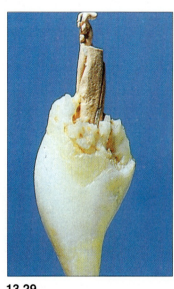
13.29

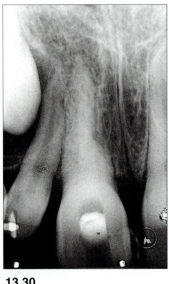
13.30

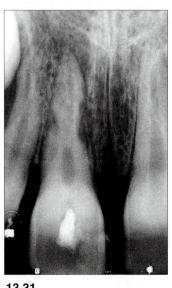
13.31

13.30, 30.31 Bony repair following calcium hydroxide therapy

13.32–13.34 Idiopathic root resorption

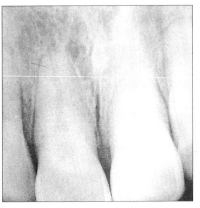

13.32

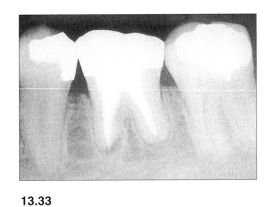

13.33

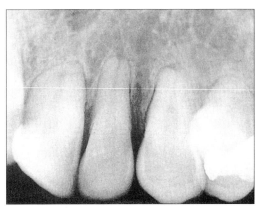

13.34

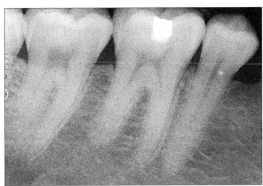

13.35

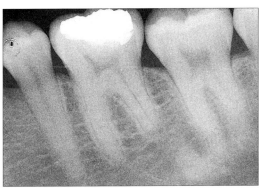

13.36

13.35–13.36 Idiopathic root resorption affecting mandibular first molars

Idiopathic resorption

Some cases of external resorption involving multiple teeth but with no systemic disease do not fit into any of the above categories.

The first case illustrated (**13.32–13.34**) is a 40-year-old Caucasian woman who presented with generalized shortening of the roots but had no symptoms other than some loosening of the teeth. Her blood picture was normal and she had no systemic disease. The patient had never had any orthodontic treatment. The reduction in root length was progressive but slow.

Figures **13.35** and **13.36** show the case of a 32-year-old Caucasian woman with no symptoms, no systemic disease and a normal blood picture. The only teeth affected were the mandibular first molars.

The third patient (**13.37–13.39**) has an aggressive type of generalized cervical resorption. There was no systemic disease present and the blood picture was normal. Crown lengthening was carried out, soft tissue was curetted from the lesions and the defects restored. Damage to the mandibular incisors was so great that the teeth were treated by decoronating, root treatment and post crowning. The disease process was again evident 1 year after treatment.

13.37–13.39 Aggressive generalized cervical resorption. Note that the right side has not been affected

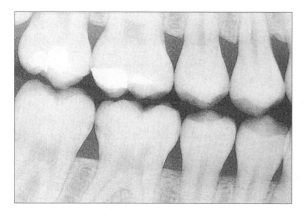

13.37

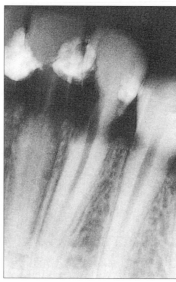

13.38

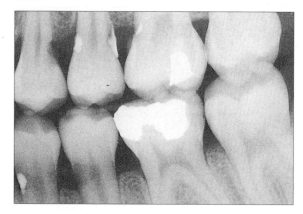

13.39

14 Endodontic problems

Endodontics requires skill and patience and, despite the many claims from dental manufacturers, there are no shortcuts or easy options. Problems will inevitably occur when delicate instruments are used in confined spaces. The increase in demand for molar endodontics, particularly from the older patient, often tests our skills to their limits. Some of the problems that may arise are discussed in this chapter with tips on how to overcome them; however there is no doubt that the best way is to exercise care and patience so that the problems do not occur.

Analgesia

Difficulty in obtaining adequate analgesia is common in root canal treatment, particularly when the patient attends with a painful pulpitis (a condition often described as a 'hot tooth'). Pulpitis can lower the pain threshold in these teeth. A procedure to remove most, if not all, of the pain from these teeth is described below.

Maxillary teeth

Difficulty with analgesia is usually experienced in the premolar and molar regions. Following buccal infiltration a palatal injection should be given over the root apex of the painful tooth. The routine use of a topical analgesic helps to reduce the patient's discomfort of the injection provided that the paste or liquid is left on the site for 30 s before injecting. The palatal injection may still be painful, even after topical has been applied so the operator should apply firm finger pressure to the injection site for several seconds, then roll the finger away, insert the needle down to the bone, and apply further pressure over the needle tip.

Mandibular teeth

The mandibular second premolar and molar teeth are the most difficult in which to produce adequate analgesia. Initially a mandibular block and a long buccal infiltration are given. When the lip and tongue are affected an intraligamental injection is given on the mesial and distal aspects of the tooth slowly, with the bevel of the needle inserted pointing outwards away from the tooth (**2.36**). This procedure allows the operator to start access into the tooth without discomfort; however, pain may be felt as the bur approaches the pulp. A small exposure is made into the pulp and an intrapulpal injection given by inserting the needle into the pulp through the exposure and the injection given quickly to generate a sudden increase in pulpal pressure. It is thought that the resultant deep analgesia of the pulp tissue is due to pressure analgesia. The roof of the pulp chamber is removed and the pulp extirpated as fast as possible because the intrapulpal analgesia lasts only for a few minutes. Another method that may be effective is to inject local analgesic directly into the medullary space around the tooth roots. A special depth limiting bur is used to cut through the cortical plate and directed between the roots to avoid damage. A short needle is then inserted through the hole in the cortical plate and the analgesic injected.

Rubber dam

Difficulties are occasionally experienced with the placement of rubber dam, but in most cases the problem may be overcome.

The broken down tooth

Although it is possible to restore broken down teeth with a pinned amalgam, this prolongs the treatment and makes the construction of the final restoration difficult. The broken down tooth can be isolated in a simpler way that gives better visibility during root treatment. Often it is possible to place a retentive clamp (such as a W8a) directly onto the broken down tooth (**14.1**).

In the case shown in **14.2** the palatal wall of the maxillary first molar is missing, making it difficult to place a clamp. To overcome this problem, holes are punched in the dam from the canine to the second molar and a slit cut with scissors from the second molar to the second premolar. The second molar is clamped and the dam fitted; it is retained mesially with a rubber wedge. Good access is obtained (**14.3**).

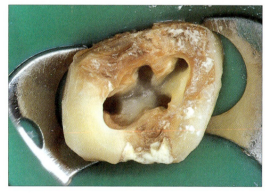

14.1 Retentive clamp on broken down tooth

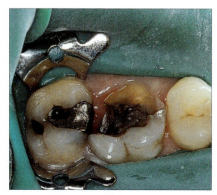

14.2 Palatal wall missing clamp applied to second molar

Saliva leaking beneath the dam may be controlled using a zinc oxide paste or a silicone material specially designed for the purpose (oro-seal, Ultradent products Inc., Salt Lake City, Utah, USA) (**14.4**). The silicone is easy to inject directly and does not set.

Electrosurgery can be used to remove excess gingival tissue (**5.6–5.10**): proliferation of gingival tissue around the root face of a lateral incisor may make isolation and access impossible unless the tissue is removed.

An adhesive restorative material (for example light-cured composite) may be added in small increments to provide a foothold for the jaws of the clamp. A broken down mandibular molar that has been built up with material designed specifically for the purpose is shown in **14.5**.

Metal bands, or crown forms, which may be cemented around the tooth with zinc phosphate, are shown in **14.6**.

Care must be taken to trim the band to fit and smooth any sharp edges (**14.7, 14.8**) which may otherwise lacerate the tongue.

Bridges do not present a problem of isolation. A suitable winged clamp is selected and placed over the abutment tooth to be treated, and the dam is stretched over the clamp (**14.9, 14.10**). Any small gaps may be sealed with a zinc oxide paste or silicone.

Access

Limited opening

Poor access, particularly to the posterior part of the mouth, can make root canal treatment almost impossible. A suggested guide to assess the degree of difficulty is to place two fingers between the patient's incisors; if this is not possible (**14.11**) the degree of difficulty is high and serious consideration should be given to extraction.

Unsupported walls

Cutting an access cavity into the tooth that is heavily restored can weaken the remaining tooth structure, risking an enamel fracture between visits. Any undermined or weakened tooth structure should be removed when the access cavity is cut. These large cavities may be restored temporarily using an adhesive restorative material and not rebuilding to the original contours. Care must be taken not to delay the final restoration because the opposing or proximal teeth could move.

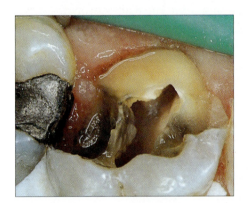

14.3 Good access obtained

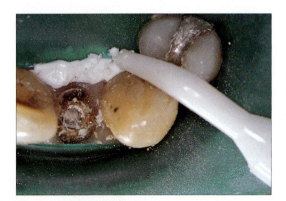

14.4 Sealing rubber dam

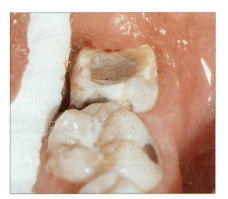

14.5 Broken down tooth built up to allow placement of rubber dam

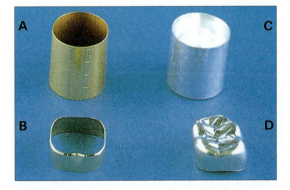

14.6 Metal bands or crown forms used to provide temporary restorations. A, Copper ring; B, orthodontic band; C, aluminium crown form; D, isoform temporary crown

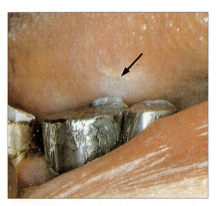

14.7 Tongue lacerated by the sharp edge of a copper ring

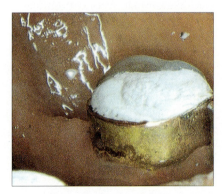

14.8 Sharp edges smoothed

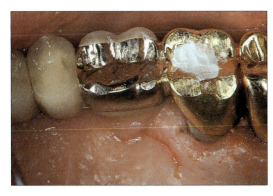

14.9 Bridge requiring root treatment of abutment tooth

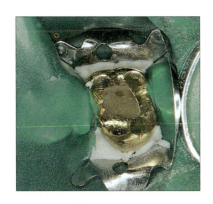

14.10 Dam placed over bridge and sealed

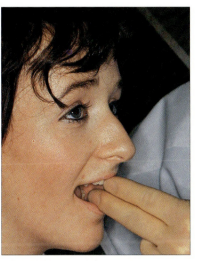

14.11 Restricted opening

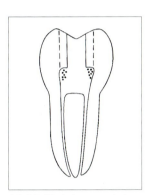

14.12 Debris remaining in pulp chamber

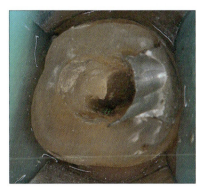

14.13 Part of pulp chamber roof remains

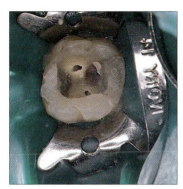

14.14 Access showing roof of pulp chamber

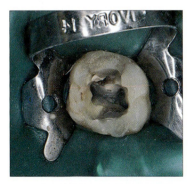

14.15 Access showing pulp chamber floor

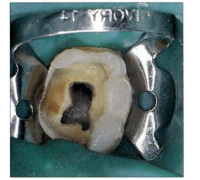

14.16 Floor darker than walls

Roof of pulp chamber

If the roof is not removed organic debris, which may be infected, can remain trapped in the pulp chamber and contribute to failure of the root treatment (**14.12, 14.13**). On occasions inability to locate the canal entrances is caused by failure to remove the roof of the pulp chamber (**14.14**); the canals are clearly visible (**14.15**) when the roof is removed. The floor of the pulp chamber is darker than the walls and a canal entrance may be found in each corner (**14.16**).

Shape of access cavity

The temporary restoration placed in the access cavity should maintain the seal between appointments and so prevent contamination of the root system. If the access is cut without regard to resistance form the dressing may be pushed into the cavity and the seal broken (**7.11, 7.12**). A tapered diamond bur with a non end-cutting tip is used to flare the access cavity, provide resistance form, and avoid damaging the floor of the pulp chamber.

Perforation of the chamber floor

As a last resort a bur may be used to locate sclerosed canal entrances, but there is a danger during this procedure of perforating the floor of the pulp chamber (**14.17, 14.18**) or the wall of the root. If the perforation becomes infected the failure rate is high and the tooth may need to be extracted. Immediate sealing of the perforation with a suitable restorative material is essential. If the perforation is dry a glass ionomer may be used, for the small defect amalgam or cavit is effective. However, it is best to prevent perforation, and several tips for doing this are given below.

- Learn canal morphology so that you know the expected site of the canal entrance.
- Do not place the rubber dam until the canal is located so that the anatomy of the tooth is not masked.
- Mark the outer surface of the tooth with a pencil mark parallel to the bur shank so that the angle of the bur can be adjusted from the radiograph (**14.19**).
- Use a small round bur with a long shank which allows better visibility and accuracy (**14.20**).
- Take radiographs to monitor the depth and direction of the bur (**14.21**) and having located the canal complete the treatment (**14.22, 14.23**).
- Remove any artificial crown if it is suspected that the tooth may be rotated and the canals difficult to find.

Location of canals

Location of canals requires a knowledge of tooth and pulp anatomy. The canal orifices generally tend to be located below the cusp tips or incisal edges (**14.24**). In young teeth the pulp horn may be located coronal to the cemento-enamel junction; in older teeth it may be located at or below the junction (**14.25**). The dimensions of the pulp chamber reduce by calcification, which tends to be greater on the roof of the pulp chamber and the axial walls than on the floor of the pulp chamber (**14.24, 14.25**). The cross-sectional shape of the pulp chamber follows that of the tooth or root at that level (**14.26–14.38**).

When not affected by calcification, the floor of the pulp cham-

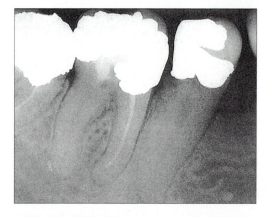

14.17, 14.18 Perforation of floor of pulp chamber

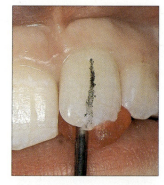

14.19 Pencil line on tooth

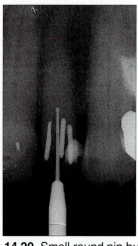
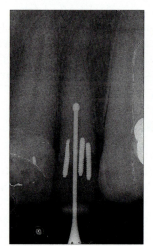

14.20 Small round pin bur

14.21 Checking direction with radiograph. In this case it was necessary to change to a goose-necked bur

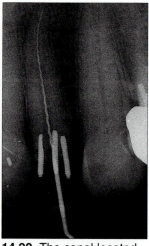

14.22 The canal located

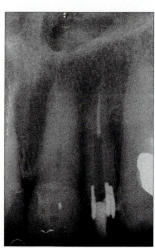

14.23 Completed root treatment

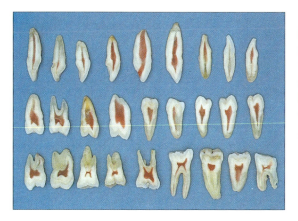

14.24 Longitudinal section of teeth showing the relationship between pulp and external surface

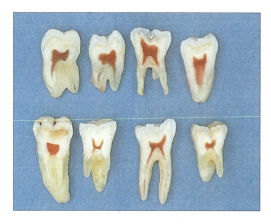

14.25 Relationship between pulp horns and cemento-enamel junction in teeth of various ages

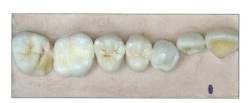

14.26–14.38 Cross-sections of teeth showing relationship between pulp and external surface. This series of photographs shows teeth which have been horizontally sectioned at intervals of 1–3 mm, commencing at the crowns and working towards the apices, demonstrating the relationship of the pulp chamber and root canals to the external contour of the teeth

14.26

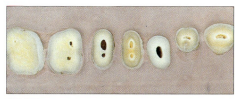

14.27

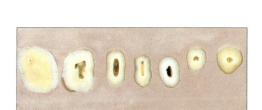

14.28

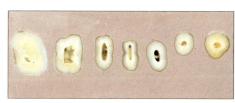

14.29

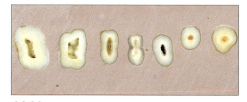

14.30

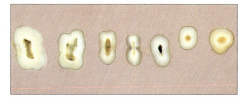

14.31

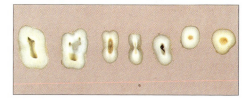

14.32

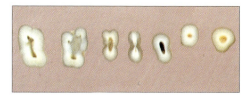

14.33

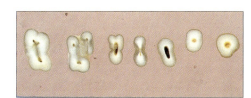

14.34

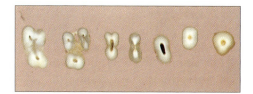

14.35

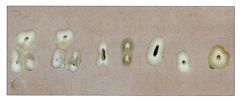

14.36

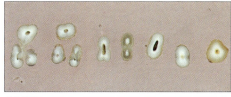

14.37

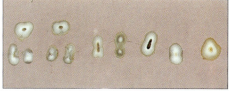

14.38

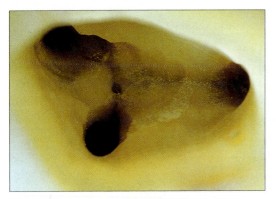

14.39 Floor of pulp chamber

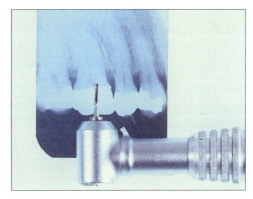

14.40 Judging depth of penetration of bur

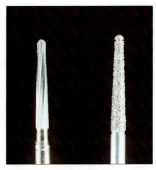

14.41 Safe-ended burs

14.42–14.45 Pulp stones

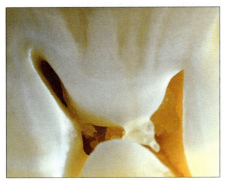

14.42

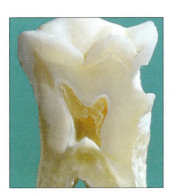

14.43

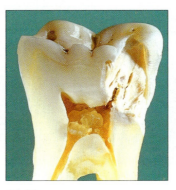

14.44

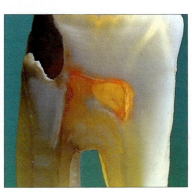

14.45

ber is dark and has a smooth convex form which leads into the root canals (**14.39**). Location of canals is therefore facilitated by proper siting, direction and extent of the access cavity. In addition, the procedure of cutting the access cavity should leave the floor of the pulp chamber intact. To prevent instrumentation of the pulp chamber floor the preoperative radiograph may be used to judge the position and distance of the roof of the pulp chamber from the occlusal entry or other landmark (**14.40**). The use of safe-ended burs in an increasing speed handpiece may also help to maintain the integrity of the floor (**14.41**).

Location of canals is more difficult in the presence of pulp calcification. Pulp stones may be single or multiple, loose or attached and of variable size (**14.42–14.45**). Initial entry to the pulp chamber is made towards obvious pulp space (**14.46**, **14.47**). Loose stones may be removed with a DG16 probe (**14.48**, **14.49**) or using long-shanked excavators (**14.50**, **14.51**). The DG16 probe is an invaluable instrument for locating canals because of its sharp tip. Calcification attached to the chamber or canal walls may need to be drilled away. The direction and extent of drilling should be guided by knowledge of anatomy and radiographic information: long-shanked or goose-neck burs may be appropriate for this purpose (**14.52**).

Location of the second mesiobuccal canal in an upper molar may require removal of a spur of dentine overlying the canal orifices (**14.53–14.55**). In some instances drilling a narrow channel about 0.5 mm deep along the groove from the first mesiobuccal canal to the palatal canal may increase the chances of finding the second canal: **14.56–14.61** show the relationship between the

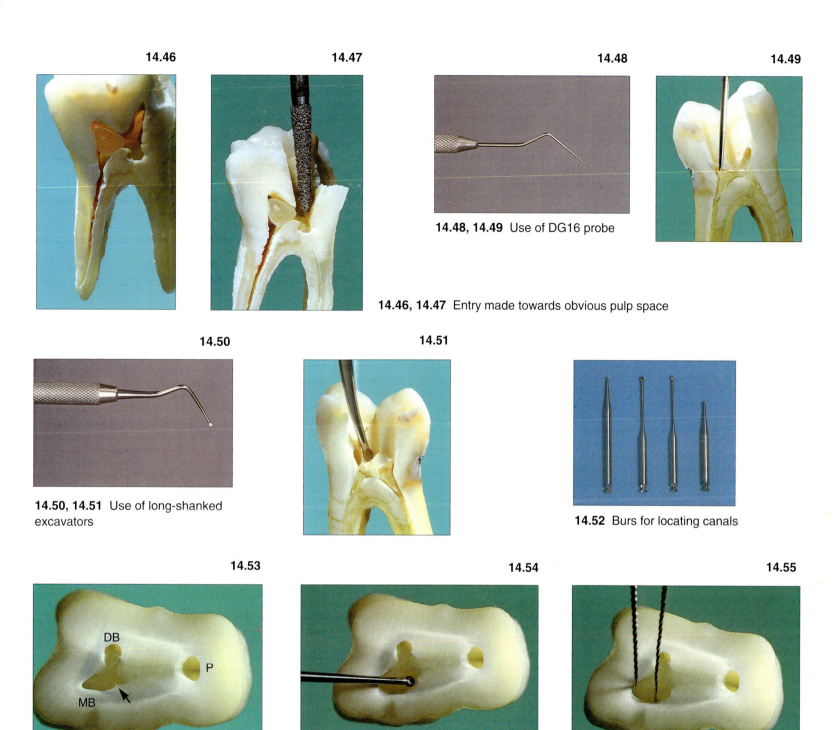

14.46, 14.47 Entry made towards obvious pulp space

14.48, 14.49 Use of DG16 probe

14.50, 14.51 Use of long-shanked excavators

14.52 Burs for locating canals

14.53–14.55 Removal of spur of dentine overlying 2nd mesiobuccal canal (arrowed). MB = mesiobuccal canal; DB = distobuccal canal; P = palatal canal

mesiobuccal, distobuccal and palatal canals at the level of the pulp chamber and 3 mm apically in three maxillary molars. In some instances, a single orifice divides into two, in which case location is aided by a precurved file (**14.62, 14.63**). Transillumination of the tooth or root at the level of the gingival margin using a fibre-optic light may help in locating canals, which show up as dark spots highlighted by illuminated dentine (**14.64**).

Occasionally root canals may be so sclerosed that they are not apparent on a radiograph (**14.65, 14.66**), but this does not always mean that the canals cannot be located. A periapical radiolucency indicates the existence of a canal. In many cases the canals can be located but it is necessary to drill centrally along the long axis of single-rooted teeth (**14.67, 14.68**) or in the appropriate direction of canals in multirooted teeth (**14.69, 14.70**). The burs described above are useful but reference to normal anatomy of the tooth is helpful. Crowned teeth pose greater diffi-

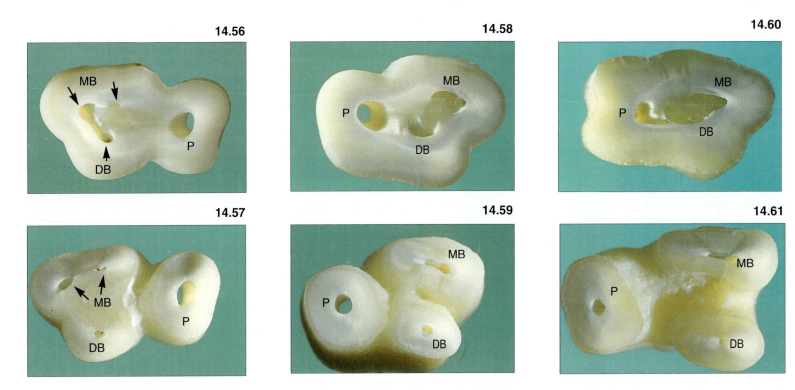

14.56–14.61 Relationship of the two mesiobuccal and palatal canals at the pulp chamber and 3 mm apically

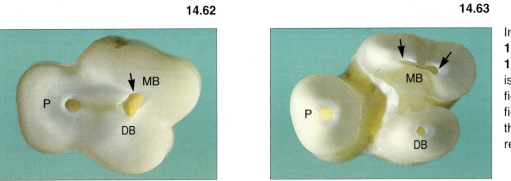

In the pairs of figs shown here (**14.56** and **14.57**, **14.58** and **14.59**, **14.60** and **14.61**, **14.62** and **14.63**) the transverse tooth section is shown from the occlusal aspect in the first fig. and from the apical aspect in the second fig. The apical image has been inversed so that the MB and DB canals appear in the same relationship in each pair of figs

14.62, 14.63 Single orifice at pulp chamber (**14.62**) divides into two 3 mm apically (**14.63**)

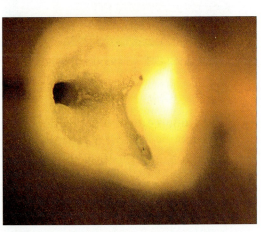

14.64 Transillumination to locate canals

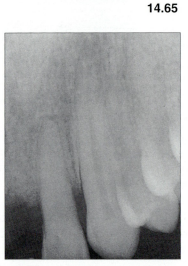
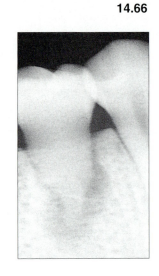

14.65, 14.66 Sclerosed root canals

14.67, 14.68 Drilling to locate canals

14.69, 14.70 A sclerosed pulp chamber and canals in multirooted teeth requires drilling in the appropriate direction

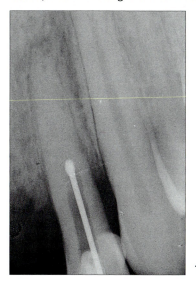

14.67

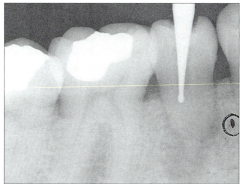

14.68

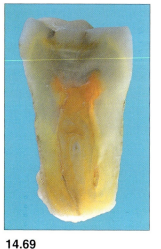

14.69

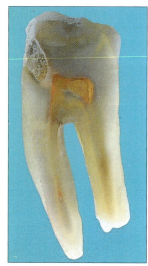

14.70

14.71, 14.72 With care, canals may be located in many instances

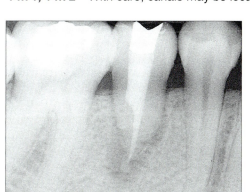

14.72

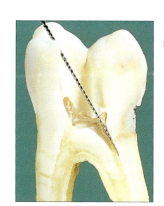

14.73 Negotiation of sclerosed canals

14.71

14.74, 14.75 Canal calcification may be adherent or loose

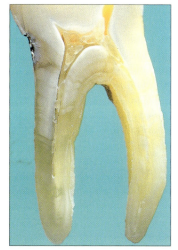

14.74

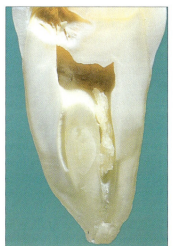

14.75

culty and it is best to cut the access cavity without a rubber dam to aid orientation. It is also important to take check radiographs with the bur in place if there is any doubt about the direction of drilling. The bur angulation can be corrected and a line drawn in pencil parallel to it on the crown. With care, the canals may be located in many instances (**14.71, 14.72**).

Negotiation of calcified canals

Negotiation of all canals should initially be carried out using a small file used as an explorer to investigate its anatomy. When the canals are calcified (**14.73**), negotiation becomes difficult and occasionally is impossible. Calcification of canals is usually irregular, the calcifications being adherent or loose (**14.74, 14.75**). Negotiation of such canals depends on fine instruments, such as the 06, 08 and 10 files (**14.76**), but the tip of the 06 file is prone to damage: use of pathfinder files may help to avoid this problem (**14.77**). Pathfinder files are available in two sizes: K1 (between 06 and 08) (**14.78–14.80**), and K2 (between 08 and 10) (**17.81–14.83**). They are made of stainless steel or carbon steel, the latter being more rigid. The taper of these instruments is reduced to give the tip greater rigidity so that more apical pressure can be applied without the risk of the tip bending. Damage to the tip of small instruments may be due to a relatively abrupt change in the direction of the canal. These can be negotiated by the use of a watch-winding motion for small instruments with some apical pressure. Precurving the tip of the file may be helpful. This motion also helps to advance the file further into the canal. In some canals (**14.84–14.86**), particularly distal canals in mandibular molars, several fine canal orifices may be found initially; gradual instrumentation with a fine instrument will loosen the calcification within the canal. The use of Hedstroem files will help to remove these, enabling the full negotiation of a single canal of relatively normal proportions. Canal negotiation may be facilitated by lubricants such as EDTA preparations (**14.87**) and detergents. The EDTA not only aids the passage of files but also helps to soften the highly calcified deposits and speed initial enlargement.

If canals cannot be located or negotiated, periradicular surgery or extraction should be considered if there is pathology and symptoms; if there are no symptoms or pathology the tooth may be left on review with a dressing of zinc oxide/eugenol over the chamber floor.

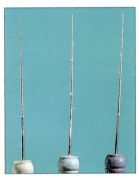

14.76 Use small files (06, 08 or 10) to negotiate calcified canals

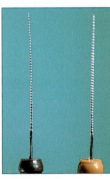

14.77 Kerr pathfinders

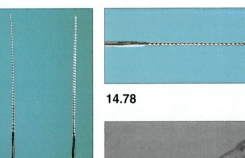

14.78

14.80

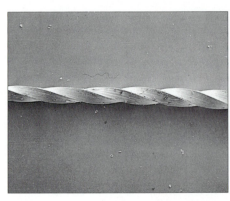

14.79

14.78–14.80 K1 pathfinder

14.81–14.83 K2 pathfinder

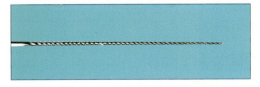

14.81

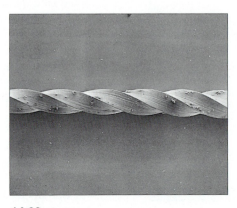

14.82

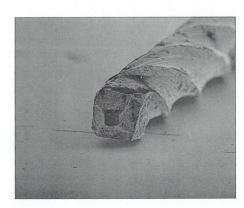

14.83

14.84–14.86 Gradual removal of calcifications from the distal canal of a mandibular molar

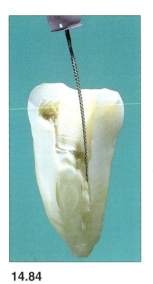
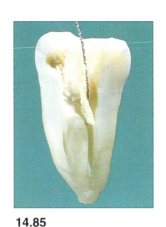
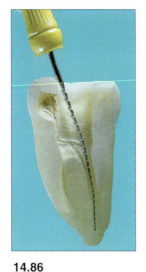

14.84 14.85 14.86

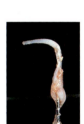

14.87 Canal lubricants: A = RC-prep; B = file-eze; C = gly-oxide

14.88 Extirpated pulp (usually mildly to moderately fibrosed)

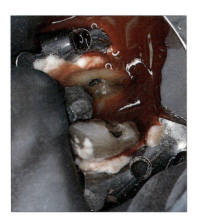

14.89 Hyperaemic pulp

Canal preparation

Cleaning

Removal of pulp tissue

Removal of fibrosed pulp tissue is usually easy – the whole pulp can be removed in one piece on a barbed broach (**14.88**). Occasionally, the pulp tissue is torn short of the apical foramen, leaving a fibrous portion behind. Further instrumentation of such a canal may elicit a spongy sensation in the apical part. Unless the canal is wide the tissue cannot be reached with a barbed broach. The use of large files may compact the tissue and cause a blockage, which may be removed with sodium hypochlorite and small Hedstroem files.

When extirpating a hyperaemic pulp profuse bleeding (**14.89**) may occur, which does not abate, usually because of residual vital tissue in the canal. The scenario may be confused with a perforation. It may be useful to dress such a pulp canal with a corticosteroid preparation and defer treatment to another visit when bleeding due to residual pulp tissue will have subsided.

Elimination of microorganisms

This is usually gauged clinically by the disappearance of signs and symptoms of periapical disease. When a tooth fails to settle, persistent infection either in the canal or in the periradicular tissues, should be suspected. Persistent infection of the periradicular tissues is rare and should be dealt with by surgery. Emphasis should initially be placed on treating residual intracanal infection as follows:

1. Check for recontamination of the canal through a defective or leaking restoration (**14.90–14.92**): it is often signalled by contamination of the cotton wool in the pulp chamber (**14.93**).
2. Re-evaluate morphology of the canal system: have any canals been missed (**14.94**)?
3. Re-evaluate canal preparation: is it complete and adequate? If so, it does not usually need to be filed any wider.
4. Re-irrigate, ensuring adequate penetration of 5% sodium hypochlorite solution. If the lesion still fails to resolve, use irrigants with different antibacterial spectra, such as chlorhexidine.
5. Redress the canal with calcium hydroxide or other alternatives (as discussed in Chapter 8).
6. If there is still no resolution but the canal is dry and clean, obturate the canal(s) and re-evaluate.
7. In the absence of resolution after (6), consider periapical surgery, biopsy and extraction. The cause may be intraradicular infection that is not accessible to conventional cleaning (**14.95, 14.96**) or extraradicular infection. In the case shown (**14.97–14.100**), an apical delta prevented adequate cleaning (**14.97, 14.98**). The tooth failed to settle following conventional treatment. After apical surgery, involving curettage and cleaning of the root apex and three canal exits with an ultrasonic scaler and obturation with amalgam (**14.99**), almost complete healing was evident in 6 months (**14.100**).

14.90–14.92 Check for a leaking restoration

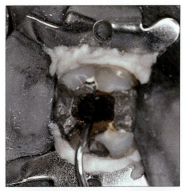

14.91

14.90

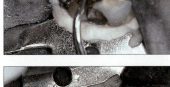

14.93 Contaminated cotton wool removed from a pulp chamber

14.94 Missed lingual canal in mandibular incisor leading to failure

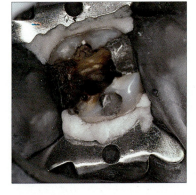

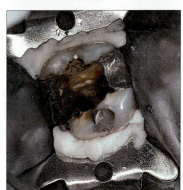

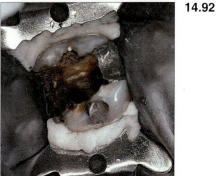

14.92

14.97–14.100 Infected root canal system with apical delta

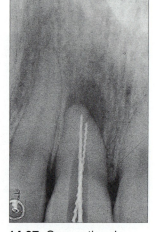

14.95

14.97 Conventional debridement

14.95, 14.96 Inaccessible accessory anatomy may contain residual infection

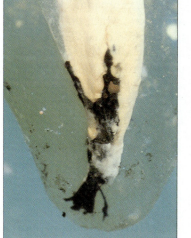

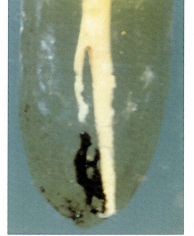

14.96

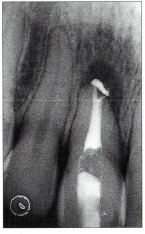

14.98 Root canal obturation with thermoplasticized gutta percha

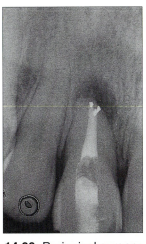

14.99 Periapical surgery was required as sinus reappeared

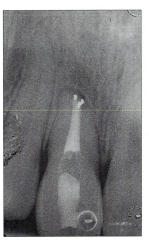

14.100 Healing 6 months postoperatively

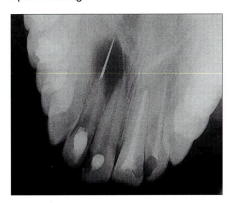

14.101–14.105 Consequences of open drainage

14.101 Needle broken in the tooth by a patient trying to keep the access cavity clean

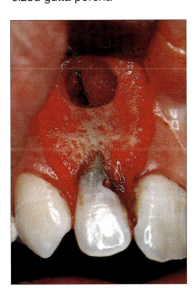

14.102 Surgical removal of needle

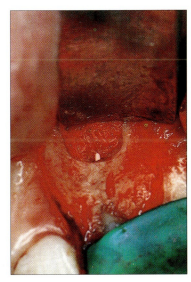

14.103 Through and through obturation following canal debridement

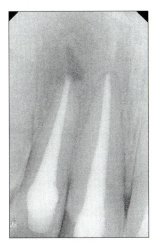

14.104 Immediate postoperative radiograph

14.105 Healing after 6 months

Persistently weeping canal

Sometimes a canal may 'weep' persistently following adequate canal preparation. The exudate is clear and straw-coloured, and may be mixed with blood or pus. Severe weeping is usually due to an infected cyst. Ideally the tooth should be left alone to drain through the canal(s) until the seepage stops and dressing is possible but drainage may be so persistent that the tooth cannot be closed without risking an acute swelling. In these rare instances the tooth may be left on open drainage for no longer than 24 hours. The root canal system of teeth left on open drainage for prolonged periods may become severely contaminated, reducing the chances of success. Attempts to maintain patency of the canals with needles risks further damage, and patients should not be instructed to do this. In the case shown in **14.101–14.105**, the lateral and central incisors were on open drainage and the patient was instructed to keep the access cavities patent with a sterile needle. A heated sewing needle, which had penetrated beyond the apex (**14.101**), then broke in the canal. Further management involved removing the needle (**14.102**), orthograde cleaning of the canal and 'through and through' obturation (**14.103**). The immediate postoperative radiograph is shown in **14.104** and healing six months later in **14.105**.

When the fluid seepage reduces following drainage, the canal(s) should be dressed with a stiff paste of calcium hydroxide to the full working length (see Chapter 8). The dressing should be removed at about 2 weeks and if there is persistent exudation, the canal should be reirrigated and redressed. In cases of infected cysts, it may not be possible to stop exudation using a conventional approach and a combined orthograde/retrograde surgical approach ('through and through') may be required to clean and fill the canal.

Shaping

Difficulty in determining apical termination of canal

Open apex

Determination of the length of incompletely formed roots can be difficult: apex locators do not give accurate readings. Tactile sense may reveal vital tissue short of the radiographic apex (**14.106**), damage to which may delay healing. It may be tempting to clean to the root apex in order to maximize root length, but where there is doubt the shorter length compatible with periapical healing should be selected in the first instance (**14.107**). If this fails to resolve, instrumentation at a longer working length should be attempted (**14.108, 14.109**).

Sensitivity in the root canal at the second visit following canal preparation

Sensitivity to instrumentation short of the working length occasionally occurs and raises suspicion about the accuracy of working length or possibility of perforation. Possible explanations for this include

- proliferation of residual pulp tissue;
- ingrowth of periapical granulation tissue, especially when the apical foramina are wide;
- presence of a lateral canal;
- perforation.

The working length should be confirmed, together with the position of the file relative to the root contour. If deviation or inaccurate length is not suspected, the tissue should be filed away.

Roots not easily deciphered on radiographs

The roots most commonly difficult to see on radiographs are those of upper premolars, especially on an angled view (**14.110**). Accessory roots may also be difficult to see. Length determination may be aided by apex locators.

Loss of control over instrumentation to apical foramen

File short of determined length

This problem may occur in several situations.

Change of reference point

The reference point used should always be noted for later visits. Use of a different reference point will result in inaccurate instrumentation. Apex locators can help to reconfirm length without exposing the patient to additional radiation.

Change in marked length of file

Accidental displacement of the rubber stop is a cause of inaccurate instrumentation: a firmly fitting rubber or alternative stop should be selected.

14.106, 14.107 Vital tissue short of radiographic apex

14.108, 14.109 Instrumentation to radiographic apex

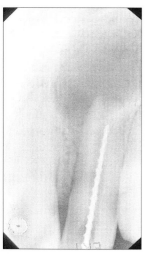
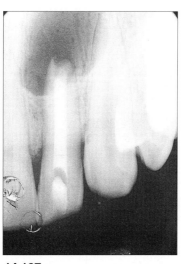
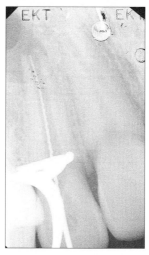
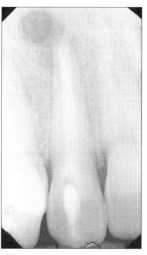

14.106   14.107   14.108   14.109

Canal blockage

This may be caused by dentine debris, calcified tissue particles, organic tissue or restorative material in the canal (**14.111, 14.112**). Inadequate irrigation and recapitulation may cause canal blockage, usually in the apical portion. Successful bypass depends on how compacted the material is. Loose material may be removed by filing with small instruments, good irrigation and/or the use of endosonics.

Canal ledging

Ledges are usually produced by using rigid, end-cutting instruments forcefully, without precurving them, or using automated instruments. Ledges may prevent the smooth passage of instruments and root filling material. They are usually bypassed by precurving the tip of the file and using a watch-winding motion to slip the file past the ledge (**14.113**). Once the file has slipped beyond the ledge a 'catch' is felt as the file binds in the canal. A watch-winding motion is used to negotiate the canal. The canal is then filed until the instrument is loose. Ideally the ledge should be filed away until smooth passage for the rest of the instruments is achieved

Alteration in effective canal length

Preparation of curved canals usually shortens them (Chapter 7). A combination of determining the working length before this change and an apical dentine stop may give the clinical impression of loss of working length (**14.114**).

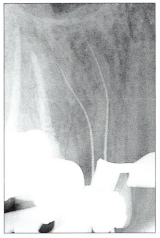

14.110 Difficulty in deciphering premolar roots

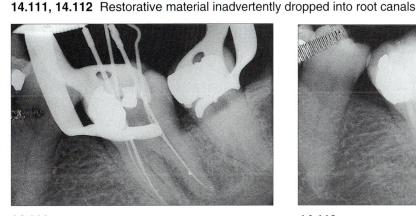

14.111

14.112

14.111, 14.112 Restorative material inadvertently dropped into root canals

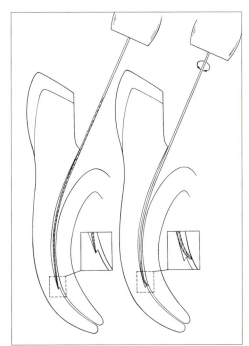

14.113 Bypassing a ledge

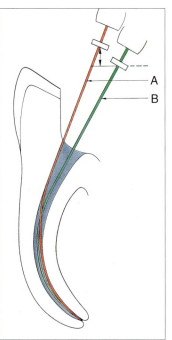

14.114 Apparent loss of working length due to canal preparation and an apical dentine plug. A = position of file after preparation; B = position of file before preparation. File A follows a shorter path in the canal than file B

File longer than determined length

Many of the factors mentioned above may have the opposite effect, so that the file extends beyond the determined length. Causes include displacement of rubber stop, loss of height of the reference point and alteration in length of canal combined with no apical blockage/stop (**14.115**).

Shaping severely curved canals

The principles of preparing curved canals were described in Chapter 7. All of these factors are important in preparing the severely curved canal – except that the potential for canal deviation is greater because of the increased moment of force in canals of greater curvature. Small, precurved flexible files should be used without force in preflared canals. Controlled preparation requires patience and time, and instruments such as Flex R, Canal Master, Flexofile and Flexogates may be useful.

Shaping long, narrow, calcified canals

Preparation of such canals is often time-consuming and frustrating. Unfortunately there are no shortcuts; these canals require patient enlargement to the required size. Use of EDTA lubricants and intermediate files may expedite shaping of these highly mineralized canals.

Deviation of prepared canal from original canal form

Uncontrolled dentine removal results from a variety of factors and causes canal preparation errors such as ledge formation (**14.116**), apical widening/elbow formation (**14.117**) and perforations (**14.118**). Perforations may occur apically on the outer curve and more coronally on the inner curve (**14.119–14.122**). Minor strip perforation may not be apparent radiographically because of the shape of the root (**14.123–14.125**). Prevention of these procedural errors is described in Chapter 7. Apical widening and elbow formation are usually only apparent on the postobturation radiograph (**14.126, 14.127**) and usually result from overfiling with large instruments.

Perforations are characterized by continuous bleeding from the canal and sharp pain if the effect of local anaesthetic is absent. A dry paper point placed in the canal after initial moisture control will usually indicate the level of perforation in the canal (**14.128**). Perforations apical to the alveolar margin have a better prognosis than those more coronal, which may communicate with the oral

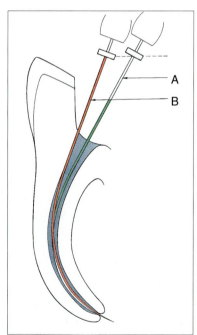

14.115 Overextension of file due to canal preparation and absence of an apical stop. A = position of file before preparation; B = position of file after preparation

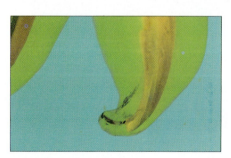

14.116 Ledge formation

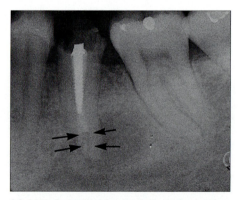

14.117 Apical widening/elbow formation

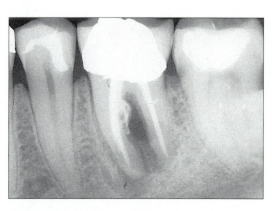

14.118 Severe strip perforation

14.119–14.122 Apical and mid root perforation–clinical and radiographic pictures before and after are shown together with the extracted tooth

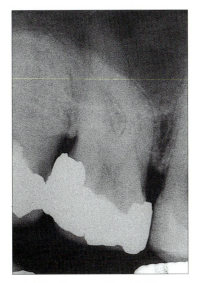

14.119 Preoperative view

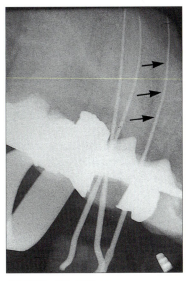

14.120 After filing

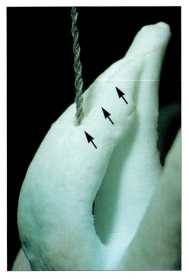

14.121 Apical perforation (mesial view)

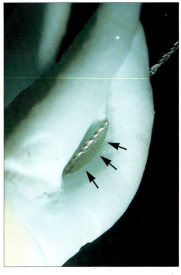

14.122 Mid root strip perforation (furcal view)

14.123–14.125 Minor strip perforation

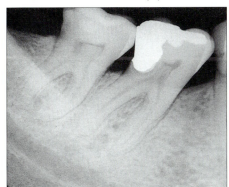

14.123

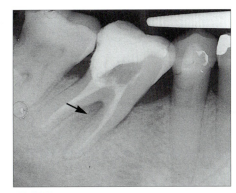

14.124

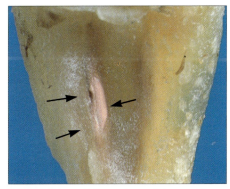

14.125 Furcal view of mesial root of extracted tooth

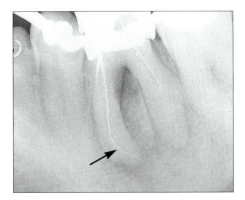

14.126 Before preparation

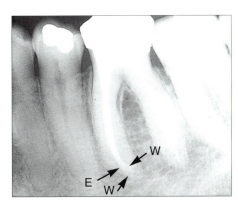

14.127 After obturation showing elbow (E) and apical widening (W) (arrowed)

14.126, 14.127 Apical widening and elbow formation

14.128 Using a paper point to determine site of perforation

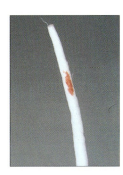

environment and become infected. It is important to prevent infection and to seal as soon as a calcific barrier has formed after dressing with calcium hydroxide. A barrier may not always be apparent, but absence of bleeding and radiographic radiolucency combined with a dry canal are favourable signs. If perforation does not resolve, surgical repair, root resection or extraction may be necessary.

Problems in canal obturation

Technical problems

Technical difficulties may cause a variety of obturation defects. The root filling may have one or all of the following defects:

- it may be long or short of the determined canal length (**14.129**, **14.130**);
- poor adaptation to the canal wall (**14.131**);
- voids may be present in the body of the root filling (**14.132**).

Errors in length and quality of root filling

Many factors causing aberrations in length of canal preparation also result in poor length of the root filling. Poor manipulation of the filling material can also produce an inadequate length of root filling. The cause of such errors depends on the material and technique used, but sometimes apical root resorption may be a contributing factor.

Cold lateral condensation

During lateral condensation, problems in length control may be traced to several factors. Selecting master points that are too large or too small may result in incorrect length: if too small, they may be displaced during compaction (**14.133**). Displacement may also result from the spreader impaling the gutta percha point. Placement of gutta percha points to the correct length may be difficult if the canal preparation is inadequately tapered and not smooth. Accessory points may be pushed through the apical foramen if it is not blocked by the master point. Customizing the master point using the chloroform dip technique may render the tip too soft and cause it to fold over (**14.134**, **14.135**).

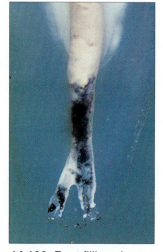

14.129 Root filling longer than the working length

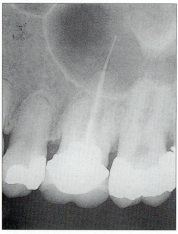

14.130 Root filling short of the working length

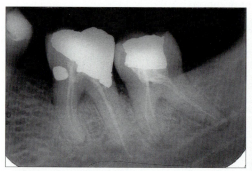

14.131 Poorly adapted root fillings

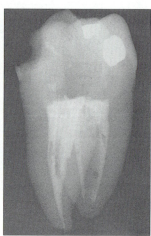

14.132 Root filling with voids

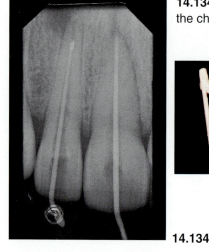

14.133 Extrusion of gutta percha point through apical foramen

14.134

14.134, 14.135 Error in using the chloroform dip technique

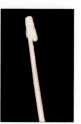

14.135

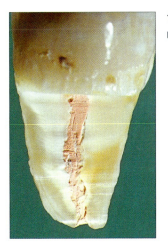

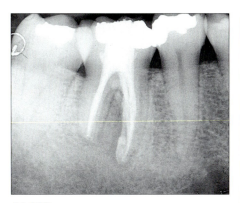

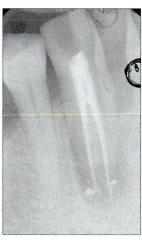

14.136 Inadequate obturation of irregular root canal with cold lateral condensation

14.137

14.138

14.137, 14.138 Extrusion of sealer (**14.138**) and gutta percha (**14.137**) during obturation with Thermafil

Poor adaptation and voids may result from mismatch in taper of accessory points, canal and spreader. Irregularity in the canal walls may cause the tips of the accessory points to fold up against them, resulting in poor obturation. Irregularly tapered canals are difficult to fill satisfactorily using cold lateral condensation (**14.136**).

Techniques using heated gutta percha

The problems inherent in manipulating heated gutta percha depend to some extent on the mode of delivery of the gutta percha: placing cold gutta percha points in the canal and then heating them; injecting molten gutta percha; delivering molten gutta percha on a solid core. The common factor to all of these is the sticky consistency of heated gutta percha. Compaction of such material depends on the degree of plasticity and stickiness, which results in the withdrawal of variable amounts with the plugger. This can be avoided by allowing the gutta percha to cool sufficiently before withdrawing the plugger. Cleaning the plugger with alcohol before insertion and dipping it in sealer powder also help to avoid the problem.

Other problems resulting in poor adaptation and length control of root filling material are unique to the method of delivery but are invariably related to the control of softened gutta percha.

Heating gutta percha in the canal

Length control in these cases is initially determined by placement of gutta percha points but is subsequently affected by the amount of heat reaching the apical gutta percha, its degree of softening and pressure applied to compact it. Its adaptation and presence of voids are dictated by attention to detail in heating and compaction, as described in Chapter 9.

Injecting molten gutta percha into the canal

Length control in these cases is compromised by lack of control in apical placement of gutta percha. The material should be sufficiently heated to give it adequate flow characteristics. The tip of the delivery needle should be placed to within 3–5 mm of the determined working length. There should be an adequate apical barrier to prevent extrusion: this may be cold compacted gutta percha in the apical section, a plug of calcium hydroxide or dentine chips. Good adaptation and avoidance of voids depend on an incremental technique with cold vertical or lateral compaction, the latter accompanied by the use of accessory points.

Delivery of softened gutta percha on a solid core

The technical problems associated with this range of new techniques are not yet well established. The technique is easy and effective but may also be unpredictable mainly in the matter of length control (**14.137, 14.138**).

The effect of sealer on obturation

The consistency and setting characteristics of the sealer may also cause poor obturation: a viscous sealer may have poor flow characteristics; one that is too thin may be difficult to manipulate. A sealer with adequate working time should be mixed to a proper consistency before obturation (see Chapter 9).

Root fractures and cracking sounds during obturation

Lateral condensation is commonly associated with potential for root fracture. A cracking sound during lateral condensation may denote one of several problems. If it is accompanied by the spreader suddenly 'giving' and the ability to condense numerous more gutta percha points, it is likely to be caused by a vertical root fracture. Fractures are more likely if the taper of canal and spreader do not match. Roots that are denuded of bone support may also be more likely to fracture (**14.139**). Use of finger spreaders allows more controlled compaction and reduces the chances of root fracture. Root fracture is not always apparent at the time of obturation but separation occurs over a period of time (**14.140, 14.141**). Roots with narrow mesiodistal dimensions (such as lower incisors, upper lateral incisors, mesial roots of molars and upper premolars) are more prone to fracture (**14.142, 14.143**). The fractures may be invisible on a radiograph if they are superim-

14.140, 14.141 Late presentation of root fracture following cold lateral condensation

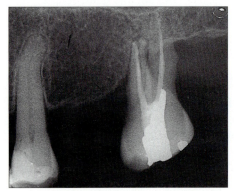

14.139 Vertical root fracture of periodontally involved tooth during cold lateral condensation

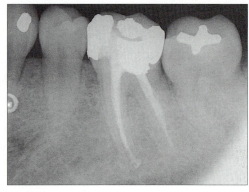

14.140

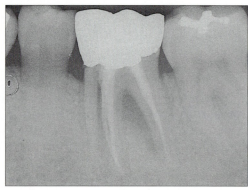

14.141

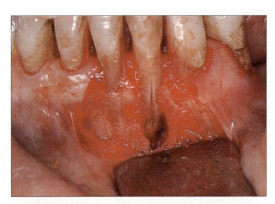

14.142 This vertical root fracture of mandibular incisor was not apparent radiographically as it was superimposed on the root filling

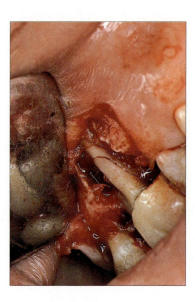

14.143 Oblique root fracture of a molar root in mesiodistal plane which was not visible radiographically

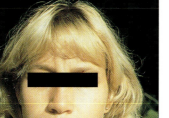

14.144, 14.145 Angioneurotic oedema following an allergic response

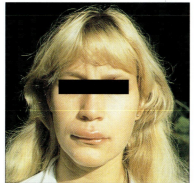

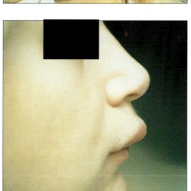

posed on the root filling (**14.142**) or are not in a plane coincident with the beam (**14.143**). Vertical compaction also carries a high risk of root fracture. It is important to prefit the pluggers so that they do not engage dentine walls during condensation.

A cracking sound in a root with two canals, accompanied by the ability to condense more gutta percha into one canal and less or none in the other, is usually due to a septum between the two canals fracturing. This septum should be removed before proceeding with obturation.

Sometimes the cracking sound is caused by the spreader tip slipping off a ledge in the canal or a pre-existing horizontal root fracture.

Adverse response to root filling material

Rarely a patient may be hypersensitive to root filling material. This hypersensitivity may become apparent shortly after filling, an angioneurotic oedema developing (**14.144, 14.145**). Severe local damage with necrosis of tissues may also occur (**14.146**). The root filling material should be removed as soon as possible. Prevention of hypersensitivity is better than treating it, and all patients should be screened for possible allergies to contents of root filling material before treatment commences – for example allergy to adhesive plaster is often due to a reaction to zinc oxide, a major component of gutta percha points. Other well documented adverse responses have been related to extrusion of materials containing paraformaldehyde, which should not be used (**14.147, 14.148, 14.151**). It is very difficult to remove extrud-

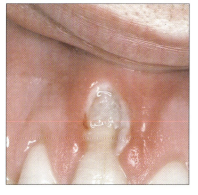

14.146 Severe local necrosis following root filling with a toxic material

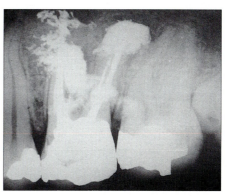

14.147–14.150 Extrusion of toxic root filling materials causes local damage to tissues and nerves

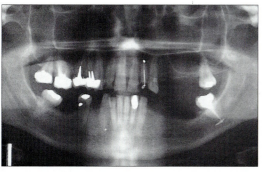

14.148, 14.149 Sagittal splitting of mandible, removal of filling material from inferior dental canal, retrograde placement and pinning of mandible

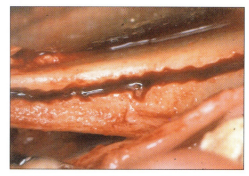

14.150 Sagittal splitting and isolation of inferior dental nerve

ed material from the inferior dental canal and attempting to do so may damage the nerve further. A sagittal splitting of the mandible (**14.148–14.152**) or buccal decortication technique may be used. The mandible may be fixed with a plate (**14.148, 14.149**) or wires (**14.151, 14.152**). Recovery from paraesthesia/anaesthesia is less likely when the material contains paraformaldehyde.

Recontamination of root canals caused by loss of coronal seal

Recementation of an uncemented post crown is known to lead to a flare-up or at least the re-emergence of a periapical radiolucency (**14.153, 14.154**), probably due to recontamination by microorganisms. There is a case to be made for elective replacement of root fillings which have been left open to oral contamination for prolonged periods.

Non-resolution of a periapical radiolucent area

Persistence of a periapical radiolucent area associated with a tooth with a technically satisfactory root filling may be caused by

- persistent periapical granuloma associated with intra or extraradicular infection with bacteria or fungi (**14.155**);
- persistence of a cyst (**14.156–14.158**);
- foreign body reaction (giant cell lesion: **14.159, 14.160**);
- healing by fibrous tissue formation (**1.163**);
- non-endodontic lesion (**14.161**).

If the quality of the root canal treatment is satisfactory, further management should involve surgery and biopsy (see Chapter 10).

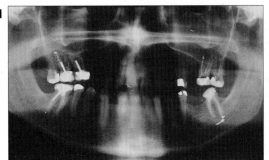
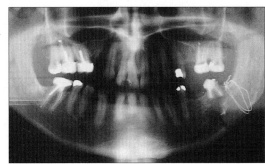

14.151, 14.152 Sagittal splitting of mandible, removal of filling material from inferior dental canal, apicectomy of mandibular molar and wiring of mandible. (**14.148–14.152** courtesy of Dr C. Hopper)

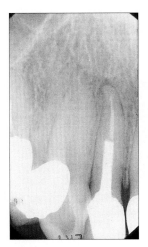
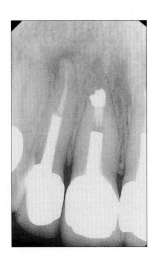

14.153, 14.154 Re-emergence of periapical radiolucency following recementation of a post crown

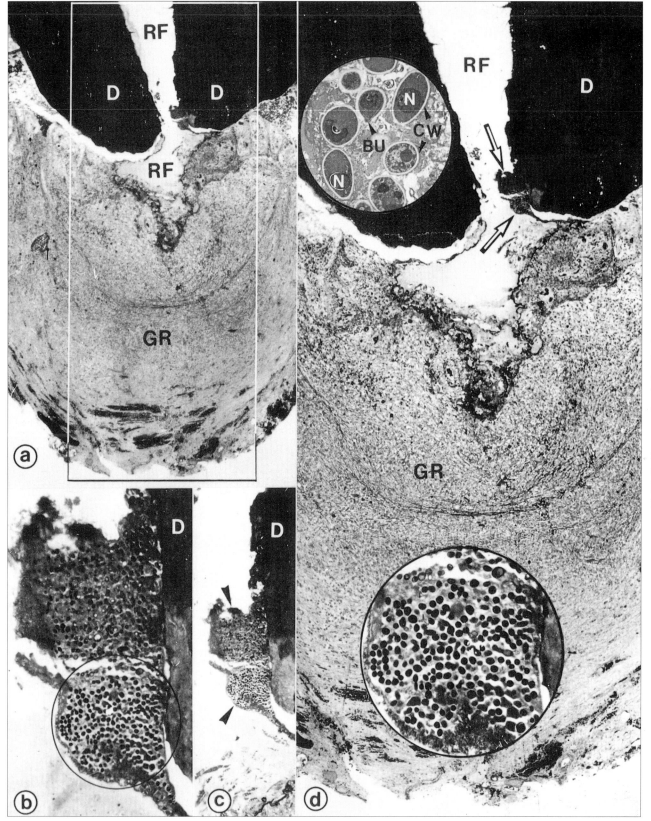

14.155 Fungus in the root canal and apical foramen of a root filled (RF in **a** and **d**) tooth with a therapy-resistant periapical lesion (GR in **a** and **d**). The rectangular demarcated area in **a** is magnified in **d**. Note the two clusters of microorganisms located between the dentinal wall (D) and the root filling (arrows in **d**). those microbial clusters are stepwise magnified in **c** and **d**. The circular demarcated area in **b** is further magnified in the lower inset in **d**. The upper inset is an electron microscopic view of the organisms. They are about 3–4 μm in diameter and reveal distinct cell wall (CW), nuclei (N) and budding forms (BU). Original magnifications: **a** × 33; **b** × 330; **c** × 132; **d** × 59; lower inset × 530; upper inset × 3400 (courtesy of Dr Ramachandran Nair)

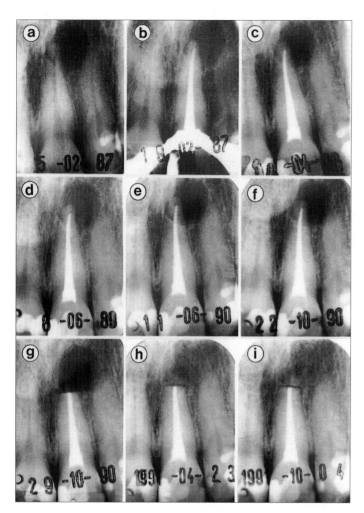

14.156 Longitudinal radiographs of a periapically affected left central incisor of a 37-year-old woman over a period of 4 years and 9 months of clinical management. Note the large eccentrically located apical radiolucency observed before (**a**) and immediately after (**b**) root filling. The lesion did not show any reduction in size in control radiographs taken 14, 28, 40 and 44 months (**c–f**) after endodontics. Apical surgery was performed (**g**) and the periapical area shows distinct bone healing (**h**, **i**) within 1 year of surgery (courtesy of Dr Ramachandran Nair)

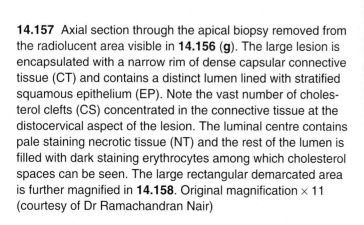

14.157 Axial section through the apical biopsy removed from the radiolucent area visible in **14.156** (**g**). The large lesion is encapsulated with a narrow rim of dense capsular connective tissue (CT) and contains a distinct lumen lined with stratified squamous epithelium (EP). Note the vast number of cholesterol clefts (CS) concentrated in the connective tissue at the distocervical aspect of the lesion. The luminal centre contains pale staining necrotic tissue (NT) and the rest of the lumen is filled with dark staining erythrocytes among which cholesterol spaces can be seen. The large rectangular demarcated area is further magnified in **14.158**. Original magnification × 11 (courtesy of Dr Ramachandran Nair)

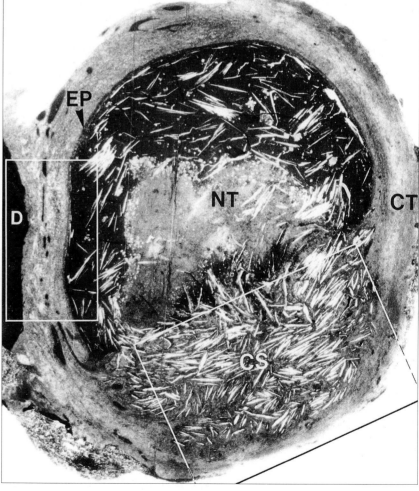

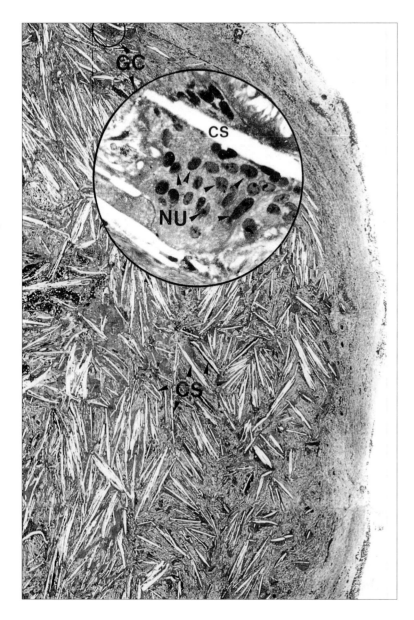

14.158 Presence of vast numbers of cholesterol clefts (CS) in the lesion. The cholesterol spaces are surrounded by multinucleated giant cells (GC), of which a selected one is magnified in the inset. Note the large number of nuclei (NU). Original magnification × 98 (inset × 322) (courtesy of Dr Ramachandran Nair)

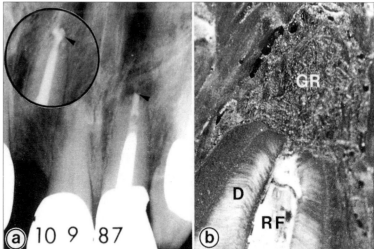

14.159 Two longitudinal radiographs (inset and **a**) of a root filled and periapically affected central maxillary incisor of a 54-year-old man. The first radiograph (inset) taken immediately after root filling in 1977 shows a small excess filling that protrudes into the periapex (arrowhead in inset). Note that the excess filling has disappeared in the radiograph taken 10 years later (arrowhead in **a**) and shortly before surgery was performed. The apical biopsy taken during surgery does not show any excess filling as is evident from the macrophotograph of the decalcified and axially subdivided piece of the biopsy (**b**). RF, root filling; D dentine; GR granuloma. Original magnification of **b** × 10 (courtesy of Dr Ramachandran Nair)

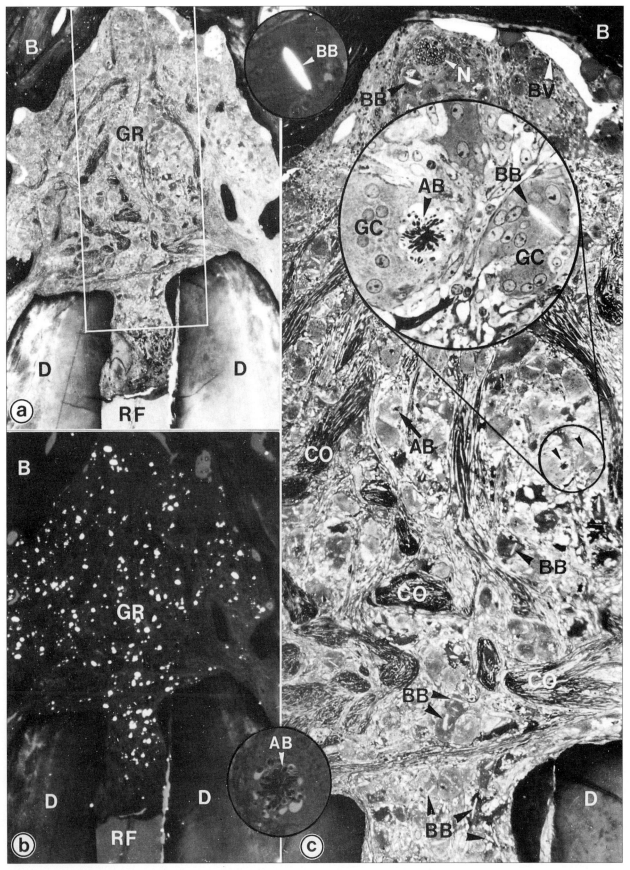

14.160 A semithin section of the apical area shown in **14.159** (**b**) when photographed in conventional light (**a**). The demarcated area in a is magnified in **c**. Note the multinucleated giant cells (GC, inset in **c**) and collagen bundles (CO in **c**) which form the major components of the lesion. Most of the giant cells contain slit-like inclusion bodies which appear as empty spaces in conventional light (BB, in **c** and inset in **c**) but reveals birefringence in polarized light (BB, upper inset in **a/c**). **b** represents the same microscopic field as a when viewed in polarized light. Note the birefringent bodies which are distributed throughout the lesion. Asteroid bodies (AB in **c** and inset in **c**) are non-birefringent in polarized light (AB, lower inset, in **b/c**). BV, blood vessels; B, bone; RF, root filling. Original magnifications: **a/b** × 36; **c** × 115; insets × 460 (courtesy of Dr Ramachandran Nair)

Retreatment

Removal of the root filling material

Gutta percha, silver, titanium or plastic points, paste or cement may be used as root filling materials. The operator should be familiar with the radiographic appearance of these filling materials (**14.162, 14.163**). It is not possible to tell the difference between titanium and gutta percha.

Gutta percha is not difficult to remove from the root canal. The procedure recommended is to start with a suitable sized Gates Glidden bur and enter 2–3 mm into the orifice of the canal. A Hedstroem file, small enough so that it will not bind against the walls, is screwed into the gutta percha. The file handle is then pulled slowly until slight movement is felt, then the file is screwed further into the canal and pulled again. This is repeated until a piece of gutta percha can be removed. The movement should be repeated using a larger Hedstroem file. In **14.164** a mandibular molar with a gutta percha point through the apex into the inferior dental canal is shown; the patient had numbness and pain in the lip (**14.165**). The gutta percha point was removed (**14.166**) and the symptoms subsided over a period of weeks.

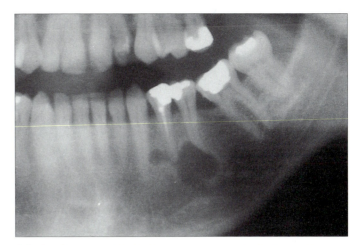

14.161 Non-endodontic lesion–lateral periodontal cyst

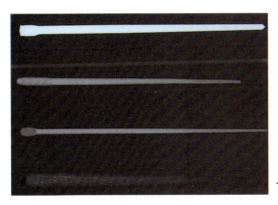

14.162

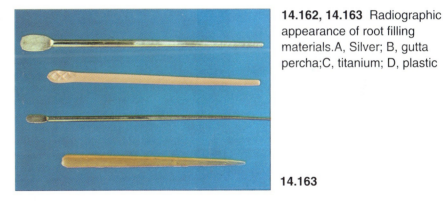

14.162, 14.163 Radiographic appearance of root filling materials. A, Silver; B, gutta percha; C, titanium; D, plastic

14.163

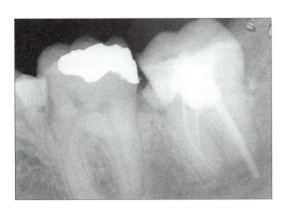

14.164 Gutta percha extruded through apex

14.165 Point removed with Hedstroem file

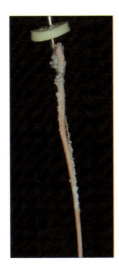

14.166 All gutta percha removed

Another method is to soften the gutta percha with a solvent: chloroform has been used for this purpose but rectified turpentine oil may be less cytotoxic. The problems with using solvent are that removal of all the liquefied gutta percha is time consuming and that any material pushed through the apex cannot be retrieved.

An instrument specifically designed to remove gutta percha from the canal is available. The design is similar to compactors except that it works in reverse, removing gutta percha from the walls rather than condensing it (**14.167, 14.168**). The gutta percha extractor is used in a slow-running standard handpiece.

Silver or titanium points are simple to remove, providing there is sufficient length of point to grip with a pair of pliers. The end of the point is gripped firmly with Steiglitz forceps or other suitable pliers (**14.169**); the pliers are then tapped with a mirror handle to gradually ease the point from the canal. Figure **14.170** shows a maxillary first molar with silver points in the buccal canals; the silver points were tapped out and the canals retreated (**14.171**).

Corroded silver points are easy to remove but great care must be taken to avoid pushing any of the corrosion products through the apex, as this may cause a flare-up.

If the end of the point cannot be gripped several other methods may be applied:

1. Insert a small-diameter hand file between the point and the wall of the canal and attempt to work alongside the point, perhaps using a lubricant containing a chelating agent. A Hedstroem file may pull out the point.
2. Insert a fine ultrasonically operated file between the canal wall and the point and work down. It is important to use a light touch to avoid the instrument tip becoming wedged and breaking. The point is easily loosened and removed in this way.
3. The Masserann kit (**14.172**) is helpful in difficult cases. A

14.167

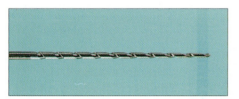

14.168

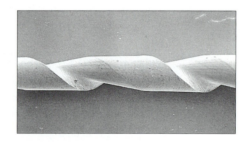

14.167, 14.168 Instrument used to remove gutta percha

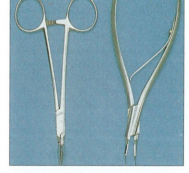

14.169 Steiglitz forceps (left) and fine-beaked pliers (right)

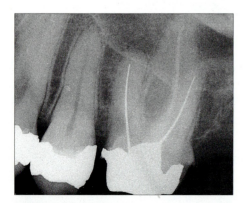

14.170 Silver points in the buccal canals of the maxillary first molar

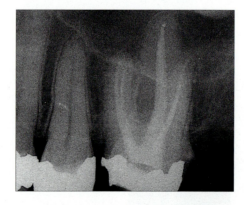

14.171 Tooth retreated with gutta percha and a fourth canal located and filled

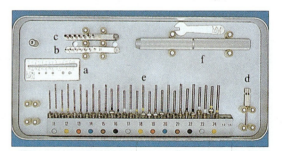

14.172 Masserann kit

trepan bur (**14.173**) is selected, using the feeler gauge, which has a slightly larger internal diameter than the point. The trepan is placed over the end of the point and a trough is cut by hand to a depth of about half the length of the point (**14.174, 14.175**). A trepan one size smaller is then wedged over the end of the point to grip it so that it can be eased out of the canal. The disadvantage of the Masserann method is that it requires the removal of a large amount of dentine, which leaves a weakened root that is liable to fracture. The trepan burs are fragile and easily damaged but are easily sharpened using the manufacturer's instructions.

Removal of fractured instruments

In most cases breaking an instrument in the canal can be avoided. Broken instruments cause aggravation to both patient and operator. If the following three simple rules are followed the risk of instrument separation will be reduced to a minimum.

1. Never use an instrument with damaged flutes or a sharp bend in the shank.
2. Do not force instruments into the canal.
3. Use sequential sizes.

A broken instrument that projects into the pulp chamber can usually be gripped and removed with pliers. If the fractured instrument lies within the canal the methods described above for removing metal points can be tried.

The Masserann kit also contains an extractor for small fragments (**14.176, 14.177**) consisting of a rod which is screwed into a tube. Close to the end of the tube, internally, is a ridge against which the rod engages. The extractor is pushed over the coronal end of the fragment and the rod is screwed home, gripping the end of the fragment against the ridge and permitting removal. In **14.178** the palatal root of the premolar contains a fractured instrument; the extractor was inserted into the canal and the fragment gripped and removed (**14.179**). The extractor is ideal for removing small instruments or spiral root canal fillers: larger instruments require the trepan burs.

If the fractured instrument cannot be removed it may be bypassed in the canal and the filling completed by incorporating the instrument into the gutta percha mass. It is useful to remember that any pain experienced by a patient who has a fractured instrument in a tooth is caused by any micro-organisms that may be lying beyond or around the instrument, not by the instrument itself. It is not negligent to fracture an instrument but the operator is negligent if he or she fails to inform the patient.

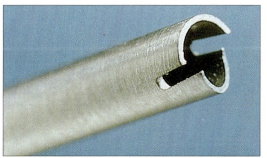

14.173 Trepan bur

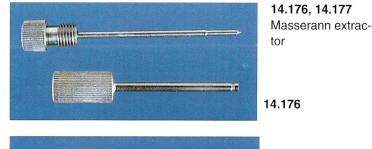

14.176, 14.177 Masserann extractor

14.176

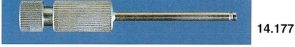

14.177

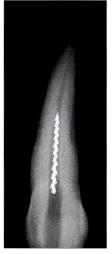
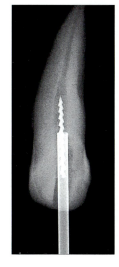

14.175 Trepan bur around end of a file

14.174 Fractured instrument in an extracted tooth

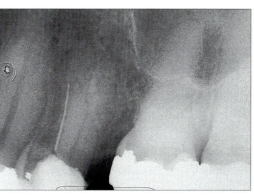

14.178 Fractured instrument in palatal root of a premolar

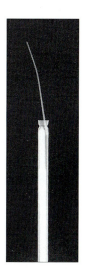

14.179 Instrument gripped and removed by extractor

Removing posts

A post may need to be removed either because the tooth needs retreating or because the post has fractured. The danger in attempting to remove the post is that the root could fracture.

A parallel preoperative radiograph will show the type and length of post in place: a cast post with tapered sides, a manufactured post with parallel smooth sides or a threaded manufactured post.

Threaded posts that lie well within the canal may be removed by cutting a groove in the post end and unscrewing it. If this is not possible threaded posts may be removed with the Masserann kit using a large trepan bur.

Smooth-sided and well fitting posts may be removed using an ultrasonic unit (**14.180, 14.181**). Ultrasonic scalers may be used or special tips (**14.182, 14.183**). The point is held lightly against the end of the post for several minutes, until the cement lute is broken by the vibration and the post loosens. The advantage of this method is that no dentine is removed. Most posts can be removed in this way.

Long retentive smooth-sided posts may have to be removed by a post extractor, provided at least part of the core is present. There are several types: the Eggler (**14.184**) is one example. The Eggler consists of two claws that grip the core and two feet that rest against the shoulders of the prepared root end. The core must be shaped with a bur to ensure the sides are parallel. The mesial and distal shoulders of the crown preparation must be cut to the same height so there is no torsional force. The Eggler is placed over the core and the claws tightened; the feet are then lowered onto the shoulders of the preparation by turning the end knob. Several more turns will ease the post from the post hole (**14.185–14.187**).

When the post is fractured at or beneath the root face either ultrasound or the Masserann kit should be used. Figure **14.188** shows a short threaded post fractured below the root face (**14.189**). A trepan bur (**14.190, 14.191**) was used to remove the post (**14.192, 14.193**).

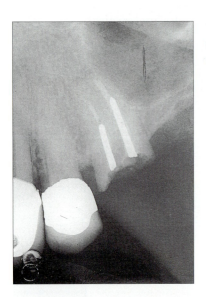

14.180 Fractured posts in both canals of maxillary second premolar

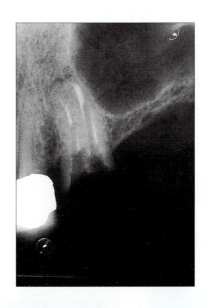

14.181 Posts removed using ultrasound

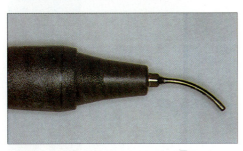

14.182 Special ultrasonic piezoelectric handpiece and tip

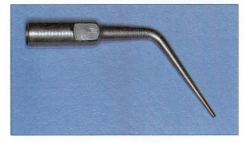

14.183 Ultrasonically activated tip designed to remove metal objects

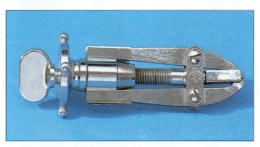

14.184 Post remover (Eggler)

14.185 **14.186** **14.187**

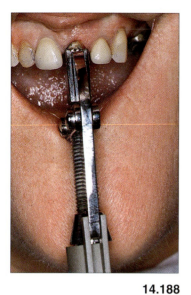
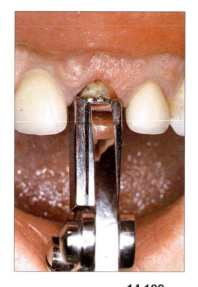
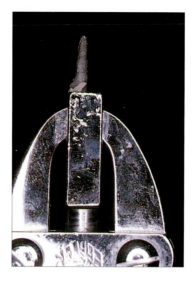

14.185–14.187 The claws are tightened around the core, the end knob rotated and the post forced out against the shoulders of the root face

14.188 **14.189** **14.190** **14.191**

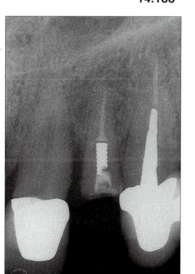
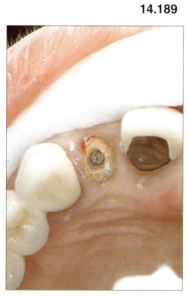
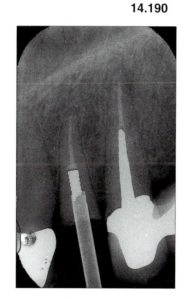
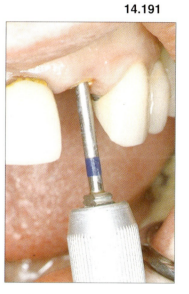

14.188, 14.189 Threaded post fractured within the canal

14.190, 14.191 Trepan around the end of the post

14.192 **14.193**

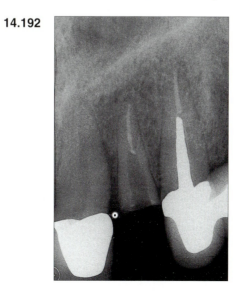
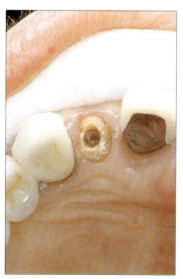

14.192, 14.193 Post removed

239

15 Restoration of the root-filled tooth

Much has been written about restoration of the root-filled tooth, in part because root-treated teeth are often severely damaged and require novel and ingenious ways of restoration. A very wide range of dowel or retention systems is available to aid restoration but significant research to support the claims of the manufacturers of these systems is lacking. It has been a long held clinical impression that root-treated teeth are more susceptible to fracture and therefore may require different considerations when restoring them than vital teeth. The high fracture rate of endodontically treated teeth restored with MOD amalgams has been documented[1] (15.1, 15.2). The three main reasons advanced to explain this high fracture rate are given below.

Altered physical properties of tooth tissue

The idea that root-treated teeth are brittle has long been propagated as an explanation for the apparently higher fracture rate of such teeth but no convincing evidence has been found to support this theory.

Weakening due to loss of tooth tissue

Many studies have evaluated the effect of pattern of tooth tissue loss as a cause of tooth weakening. The loss of marginal ridge integrity is probably one of the most important factors. The width of occlusal isthmus and depth of cavities compound the situation. Loss of roof of the pulp chamber has been considered to be an important contributory factor in the weakening effect but there is no research to support this theory. Its importance probably lies in its contribution to the increased depth of the cavity, making the cusps more susceptible to flexure (15.3, 15.4). Loading on such cusps may lead to unfavourable stresses at the cervical region, making the cusps prone to fracture (15.5, 15.6).

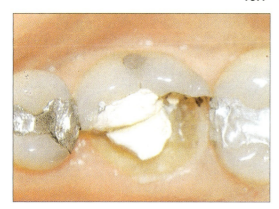

15.1, 15.2 Fractured root-filled teeth

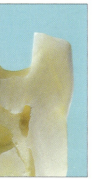

15.3, 15.4 Deeper proximal boxes and lack of roof of pulp chamber render cusps more prone to fracture

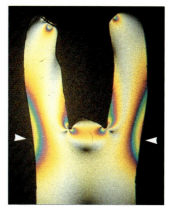

15.5, 15.6 Photoelastic models showing concentration of stress increases at the base of the cusps (arrowed) when the roof of the pulp chamber is removed (courtesy of Mr P. O'Neilly)

Loss of proprioception

Loss of the dental pulp may deprive the tooth of some of its mechanoreceptive properties. Teeth without pulps have a higher 'load perception' threshold and may take up to twice the load of a tooth with vital pulp before registering its application. Despite lack of clear evidence, this concept, together with tooth weakening, offers an attractive explanation for the high rate of mechanical failure of root-treated teeth (**15.7–15.9**).

Principles of restoration of root-treated teeth

The principles governing restoration of all teeth also apply to root-treated teeth; however, in view of the discussion above it is important to pay special attention to two factors:

1. preservation of remaining tooth tissue, and
2. reduction of stress and its favourable distribution within remaining tooth tissue.

The most conservative restoration design compatible with acceptable aesthetics and function should therefore be selected. Occlusal loads can only be assessed subjectively from the history: breaking restorations or teeth, occlusal tooth tissue loss due to attrition, mobility and drifting and the size and activity of the muscles of mastication are indicators of high loads. A young individual with a thick-set jaw, well developed muscles of mastication and marked faceting on occlusal contact areas is likely to exert greater occlusal loads. Restoration design is dictated not only by the pattern of residual tooth tissue but also by the properties of the restorative materials used. Consideration of these and the occlusal demands of the individual case, together with meticulous execution of the clinical procedures should lead to a successful restoration.

Restorability of tooth

The restorability of the tooth should be determined before endodontic treatment as part of a restorative treatment plan. Space available should be sufficient to place an aesthetic, functional restoration with cleansable contours which will optimize the health of the periodontal tissues and adjacent teeth. Often the tooth requiring endodontic therapy is severely broken down and movement of neighbouring teeth may result in occlusal (**15.10**) and proximal (**15.11, 15.12**) loss of space, which may occasionally be corrected by orthodontic movement but this is not always a practical solution. Even when the tooth is not to be restored but used as an overdenture abutment, an assessment of the space for a denture is important (**15.13, 15.14**). A denture with thin metal framework may fracture (**15.15**).

An adequate amount of remaining tooth tissue is necessary in addition to space. Although it is difficult to describe strict limits, a cast restoration encompassing at least 2 mm of sound dentine around the circumference would make longevity of the restoration more predictable (**15.16**).

In the absence of sufficient coronal tooth tissue it may be possible to gain retention from the root. Under such circumstances it is critical to evaluate the length, width, shape and curvature of the root, to assess the potential use of a dowel. If the amount of coronal dentine is inadequate it may, under exceptional circumstances, be possible to extrude the tooth orthodontically. Alveolar bone is extruded with it, which then must be recontoured surgically before restoration (**15.17–15.20**).

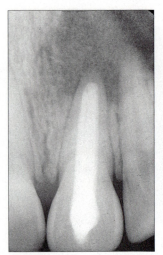

15.7 Before

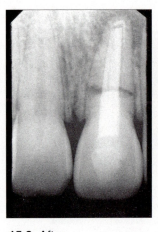

15.8 After

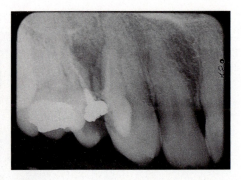

15.9

15.7–15.9 Root-filled teeth are prone to fracture

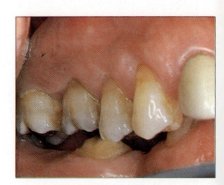

15.10 Occlusal loss of space

15.11, 15.12 Proximal loss of space

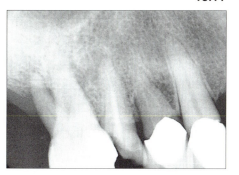
15.11

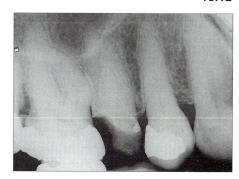
15.12

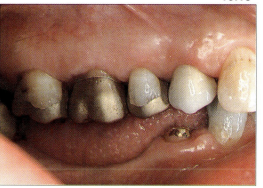
15.13

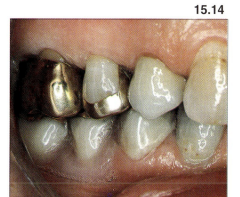
15.14

15.13, 15.14 Occlusal space considerations for overdenture situation (arrowed)

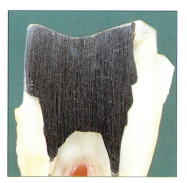

15.16 The margins should be finished on sound tooth tissue

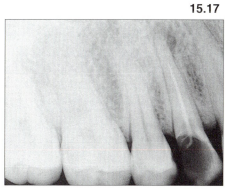

15.15 Fracture of denture due to thinness of framework

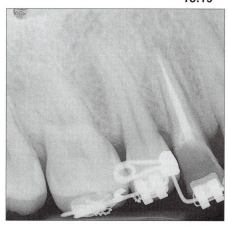
15.17

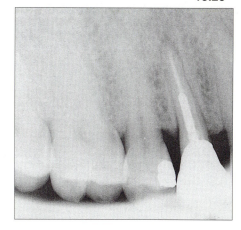
15.18

15.19

15.20

15.17–15.20 Orthodontic extrusion and periodontal surgery are necessary to make tooth tissue supragingival for restoration

When to restore after endodontic treatment

The decision to place expensive restorations on teeth immediately after completion of root canal treatment may be difficult because of the uncertainty of success of the canal treatment. It may take several years for a periapical lesion to heal but it is not practical to wait this long before a permanent restoration is placed: indeed, an early permanent coronal seal is an important final stage in the completion of endodontic treatment to prevent recontamination of the root canal system and ensure success. Fortunately, the success rate of root canal treatment is relatively high (80–95%),[2] so it is not necessary to review the tooth for longer than an arbitrary period of a couple of weeks before providing the permanent restoration. During this time there should be no sinus and no tenderness to palpation of the soft tissues over the apices or to percussion of the tooth. Any tooth with an uncertain postoperative endodontic status may require a longer review period before restoration.

Anterior teeth

Unfortunately, severely broken down anterior teeth require immediate restoration for aesthetics and provision of predictable function. Three options may be considered to achieve this:

1. A temporary post crown may be suitable if the post has adequate length and is well fitting. Otherwise its decementation not only causes inconvenience but also allows coronal leakage, further compromising the prognosis.

2. If there is a risk of losing the temporary post crown (**15.21**), a compromise is to construct the permanent post and core and to cement it permanently, then place a temporary crown (**15.22**). This reduces the chances of coronal leakage and, should periapical surgery be required (**15.23**), allows modification of the margin for a permanent crown once the gingival margin has stabilized (**15.24**).

3. Another alternative is to use a temporary overdenture, allowing the temporary seal to remain intact (**15.25, 15.26**). If the root ultimately needs to be extracted, this overdenture will also serve as an immediate replacement. The disadvantages include additional cost, time and acceptability to the patient.

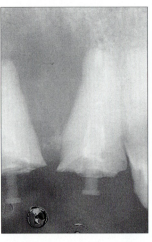

15.21 The use of temporary post crowns may be complicated by recontamination of the root canal system

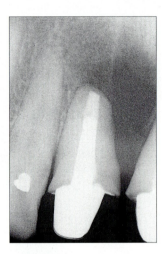

15.22 Permanently cemented post, core and temporary crown

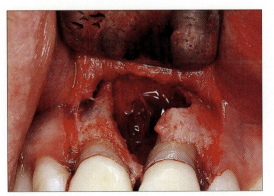

15.23

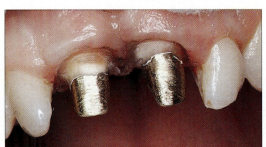

15.24

15.23, 15.24 If surgery is required, the preparation margins may be modified after healing to avoid exposure of the crown/tooth junction

Posterior teeth

In posterior teeth the amalgam core can serve as the temporary occlusal surface. The cores should have adequate proximal and occlusal contacts (**15.27, 15.28**).

Restoration of the root-treated tooth should achieve satisfactory aesthetics, form and function while preserving and protecting the maximum amount of tooth tissue. In any given situation a number of design options are available. The choice depends on the structural integrity of tooth, aesthetic and protective requirements. In order to place these in perspective a number of clinical cases will be used to illustrate the application of these principles.

Teeth with adequate tooth tissue for retention without auxiliary aids

Posterior teeth

Relatively intact teeth

Endodontic treatment is sometimes necessary on a tooth that has not been restored before or that does not have caries. The pulp may be compromised by periodontal disease (**15.29**), trauma (**15.30**) or accidental severance of the blood supply during surgery (**15.31**). Following root canal treatment, restoration of

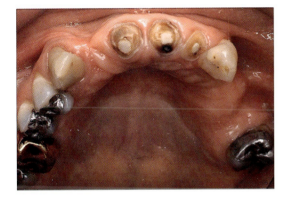
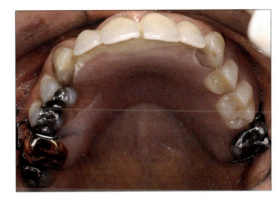

15.25, 15.26 Use of temporary overdenture over abutments

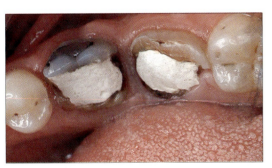
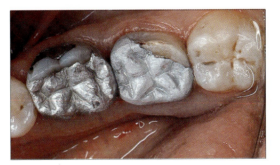

15.27, 15.28 Use of amalgam cores as interim restorations

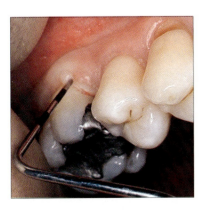

15.30 Trauma to the first molar caused by a cricket ball resulting in root fracture

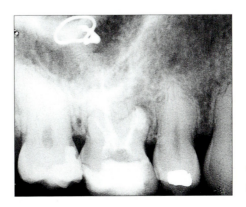

15.29 Pulp death caused by periodontal disease

15.31 Pulp compromised by orthognathic surgery

the access cavity may be carried out with a plastic restorative material such as amalgam or posterior composite, provided there is no evidence of cracks in the tooth or signs of heavy occlusal loading (**15.32, 15.33**).

The presence of cracks across marginal ridges or cusps (**15.34, 15.35**) and signs of heavy occlusal loading indicate the need for cuspal protection – in the short term using a cemented orthodontic band (**15.36**) and in the long term preferably using a cast partial veneer gold restoration (**15.37, 15.38**). The design of such a restoration may be challenging: the problem is to provide adequate retention and resistance form and to maintain the margins in the proximal areas away from contact areas to enable direct examination and access for cleaning. The nature of proximal contact (**15.37–15.39**) dictates whether it is possible to maintain the margin above the contact or below it: the latter effectively means cutting a minimal proximal box (**15.37, 15.38, 15.40**).

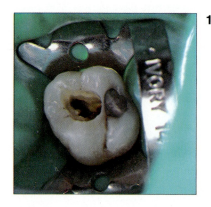
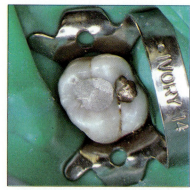

15.32, 15.33 Simple restoration of access cavity

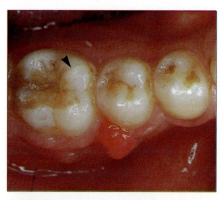

15.34 Fracture line–mesiolingual cusp (arrowed)

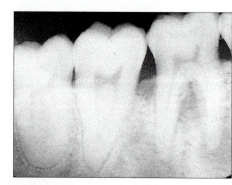

15.35

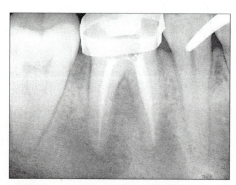

15.36 Cemented orthodontic band

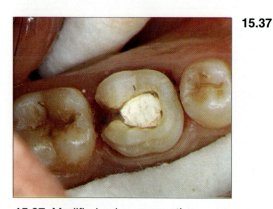

15.37 Modified onlay preparation

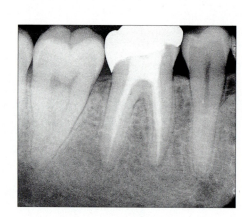

15.38

15.34–15.38 Intact tooth with crack requires cast restoration with occlusal coverage

Provided that a sufficient wraparound effect is achieved and the preparation is minimally tapered, a satisfactory degree of retention and resistance form may be obtained. Where it is considered to be insufficient, cast pins may be employed to increase retention (**15.41, 15.42**).

Recent suggestions include the use of adhesive techniques, retaining the composite materials by acid-etching enamel and using dentine bonding agents to increase the strength of the tooth. Although supported by laboratory studies, the durability of such bonding remains to be clinically proven. The technique has been recommended as a temporary means of reinforcing a tooth after endodontic treatment. Caution should be exercised in restoring large cavities with this technique because of the potential for cusp deformation and fracture caused by curing shrinkage of the composite material (**15.43, 15.44**).

Where cuspal coverage is required it may be possible to bond a base metal alloy to the prepared occlusal surface. The use of a precious metal alloy is made possible by plating or heat treatment (**15.45, 15.46**). In the case shown, occlusal surfaces eroded by acid and attrition were restored by bonding heat-treated gold castings to the occlusal surfaces. Minimal tooth preparation consisted of preparing a bevelled margin of 1 mm depth around the circumference. This technique may be a useful conservative method for restoring relatively intact root-filled teeth.

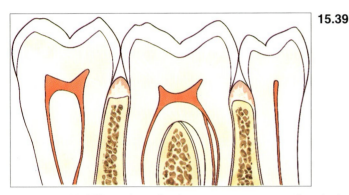
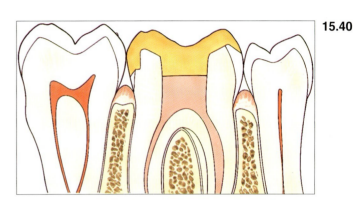

15.39, 15.40 Effect of proximal contacts on preparation design–mesial margin above and distal margin below contact point

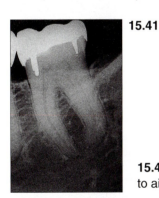
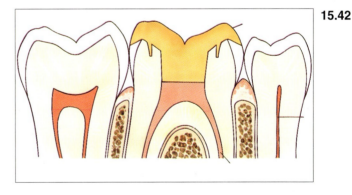

15.41, 15.42 Use of cast pins to aid retention of cast onlay

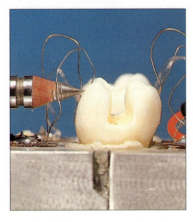

15.43 Experimental measurement of cusp deformation caused by curing composite material in a mesio-occlusal distal cavity, using an adhesive technique (courtesy of Dr N. Meredith)

15.44 Strain in buccal and lingual cusps with time after curing and displacement of the cusps (courtesy of Dr N. Meredith)

Teeth with a proximo-occlusal cavity

The case of a root-treated tooth with an existing proximal box needs different consideration (**15.47**). The restoration in this case will depend on the width and depth of the box and the occlusal loading. In a tooth with a moderately wide, shallow, proximal box and no signs of severe occlusal loading, a plastic restorative material may suffice (**15.48**). A tooth with a similarly sized cavity but with signs of heavy occlusal loading, or which provides lateral excursive guidance that cannot be eliminated, may benefit more from a cast partial veneer metal restoration (**15.49, 15.50**). A plastic restoration would be inadequate in a tooth with a wide, deep box with signs of heavy occlusal loading but a cast metal cuspal coverage restoration would help to reduce such stresses and protect the tooth from fracture (**15.51**, a photoelastic model representation of the situation shown in **15.6**, under identical conditions but with a cuspal coverage restoration). The model remains relatively stress-free even when the load is doubled (**15.52**). Figures **15.53–15.60** illustrate restoration of two cases with plastic restorative material cores followed by cuspal coverage restorations. In **15.53–15.56**, the premolar has been restored initially using composite on the buccal wall of the undermined cusp to prevent discoloration by amalgam and the rest was filled with amalgam (**15.54**). The tooth was then prepared for a partial coverage cast onlay (**15.54, 15.56**). In **15.57–15.60**, a molar with a wide mesial box and part of the mesiolingual cusp tip missing (**15.57**) has been restored with an amalgam core (**15.58**) and prepared for a modified onlay (**15.59, 15.60**). For teeth in a condition intermediate to the extremes described, the choice of restoration is a matter of clinical judgement.

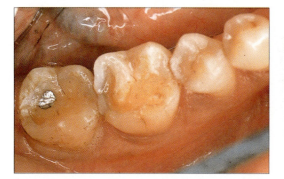

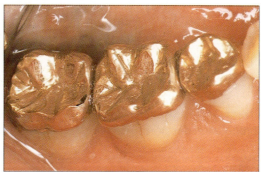

15.45, 15.46 Bonding of conservative cast occlusal onlays to teeth (Courtesy of Ms J. Wickens)

15.47 Root-filled tooth with moderately sized mesio-occlusal amalgam restoration

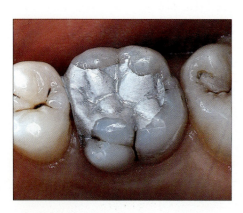

15.48 Restoration of tooth in **15.47** using new amalgam

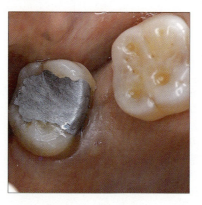

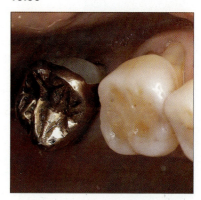

15.49, 15.50 Restoration of a tooth with moderately sized mesio-occlusal amalgam with cast onlay restoration

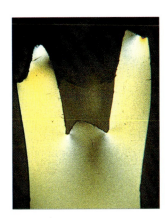

15.51 Photoelastic demonstration of absence of cervical stress concentration due to capped cusp cast onlay restoration (courtesy of Mr P. O'Neilly)

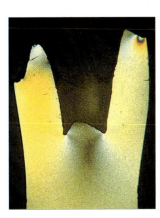

15.52 Even doubling the occlusal load makes little difference to the stress pattern (compare with **15.5** and **15.6**) (courtesy of Mr P. O'Neilly)

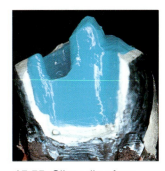

15.55 Silver die of premolar

15.53–15.56 Restoration of root-filled mandibular premolar with capped cusp cast onlay restoration

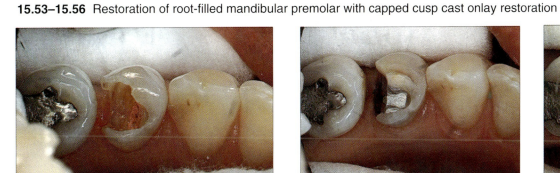

15.53

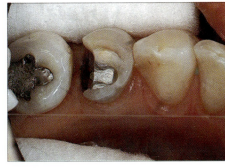

15.54

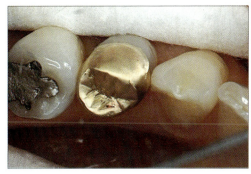

15.56

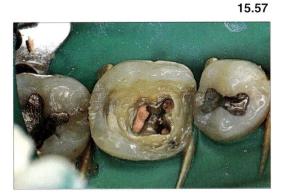

15.57

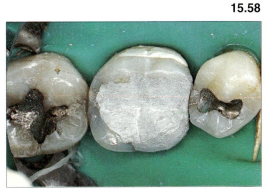

15.58

15.57–15.60 Restoration of root-filled mandibular molar with capped cusp cast onlay restoration

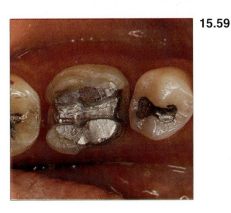

15.59

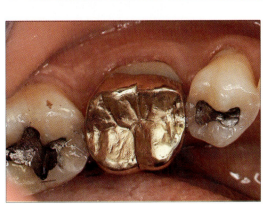

15.60

Teeth with MOD (mesio-occluso-distal) cavities

The presence of two proximal boxes makes it almost mandatory that cuspal protection is used, unless there is no opposing tooth or the tooth occludes against a tissue-borne denture. Treatment options include use of plastic restorative materials or cast restorations.

Amalgam may be used to provide cuspal protection by reducing cusp height and rebuilding the entire occlusal surface. Although this is a relatively cheap method of restoring a compromised tooth it is not always easy to develop correct occlusal contacts, and more occlusal reduction is required to provide adequate strength for the amalgam. The method is suitable for teeth already lacking considerable tooth tissue (**15.61–15.63**).

Composite resin materials suffer from the disadvantages discussed above, particularly when the cavity is large (**15.64, 15.65**). The problem of curing shrinkage and its unfavourable stressing of residual tooth tissue may be partly overcome by using indirect composite or porcelain inlays but these are relatively new

15.61–15.63 Restoration of a severely damaged premolar and molars using capped cusp amalgam restorations

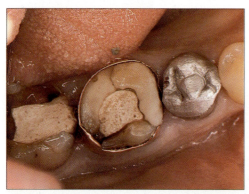
15.61

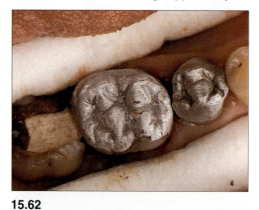
15.62

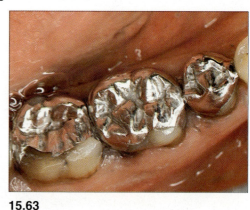
15.63

15.64, 15.65 Use of composite material to restore mesio-occlusal distal cavity in a root-filled tooth

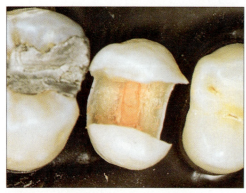
15.64

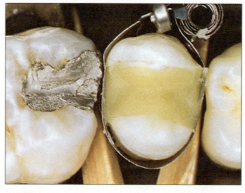
15.65

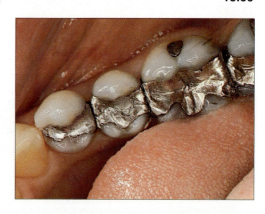
15.66

15.66–15.69 Restoration of a mandibular premolar with a capped cusp cast onlay restoration

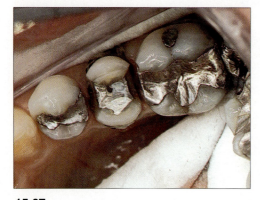
15.67

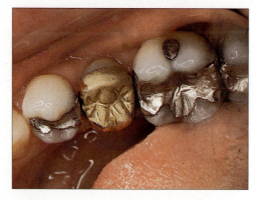
15.68

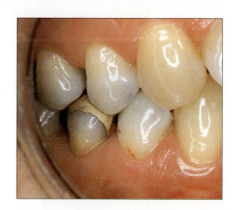
15.69 Buccal view

methods of restoration and no long-term clinical follow-up studies have been undertaken to support their use.

The most conservative treatment option is to consider (where appropriate) the use of partial veneer onlays (**15.66–15.69**), which help to minimize sacrifice of tooth tissue and provide adequate cuspal protection with proper design. On a mandibular tooth the need for a functional cusp bevel and occlusal shoulder on the buccal aspect means greater metal coverage of the buccal surface (**15.69**); on a maxillary tooth, the extent of metal coverage of the buccal cusp may be minimized (**15.70, 15.71**). Aesthetics may be improved by sandblasting the surface to reduce shine. The design may be modified to suit the situation if further tooth tissue is missing (**15.72, 15.73**). However, if the preparation is executed inadequately the restoration will be retained poorly, resistance form will be reduced and the aesthetics unacceptable.

The aesthetics of an extensive gold restoration may not be acceptable to some patients, who may prefer a full-coverage ceramometal restoration. However, before considering such a restoration the amount of tooth tissue likely to be lost in providing space for the dual thickness of metal and porcelain should be considered: the minimum thickness required is 1.3 mm. This may weaken the tooth further but may be an acceptable risk in order to secure the aesthetic requirements. As long as extracoronal tooth tissue loss is minimal the preparation of an access cavity in addition to sacrificing dentine for a ceramometal restoration may leave enough tooth tissue for retention and resistance form (**15.74**). The preparation of the upper premolar shown in **15.75** for a ceramometal crown resulted in a pulp exposure but root canal therapy through the access cavity left enough tooth tissue (**15.76**) for retention and resistance form without resorting to a post/core.

15.70, 15.71 Restoration of a maxillary premolar with a capped cusp cast onlay restoration

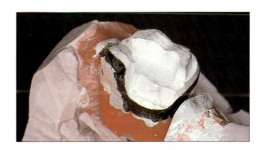

15.72

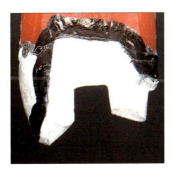

15.70 Silver die of preparation

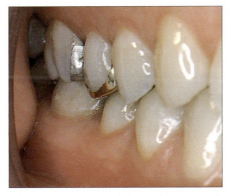

15.71 Anterobuccal view of cemented casting

15.73

15.72, 15.73 Modified cast onlay preparation

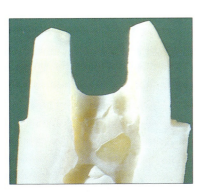

15.74 Following access for root canal treatment and preparation for a ceramometal restoration, remaining tooth tissue must be adequate for retention and resistance form

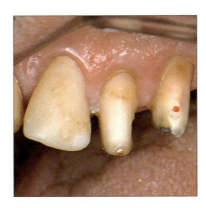

15.75 Pulp exposure following preparation for a ceramometal crown

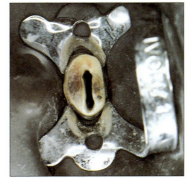

15.76 Adequate tooth tissue remains after access for root canal treatment

Anterior teeth

Relatively intact teeth

Unrestored intact anterior teeth may require endodontic treatment because of pulp necrosis caused by traumatic injury (**15.77**), severance of blood supply during surgery (**15.78**) or transplantation (**15.79**). Restoration of such teeth would normally be confined to the access cavity (**15.80**) and may be achieved satisfactorily with composite restorative material. In such cases 'reinforcement' of the tooth by placement of a post or dowel remains controversial (**15.81**). The rationale for post placement is based on the belief that the root-treated tooth is inherently weak and that the post would provide a degree of reinforcement by distributing some of the stresses to the root but the scientific support for this is equivocal. It appears that whether a tooth is made more resistant to fracture by placement of a dowel depends on the type of loading. It is widely accepted that if a post is not required to aid retention then it should not be placed and if one is placed then it should be at the expense of the minimal amount of tooth tissue. The need for a post is a subjective clinical assessment based on the amount and distribution of dentine remaining after the tooth has been prepared for the selected restoration. In figures **15.82** and **15.83** sufficient dentine cores remained after crown preparation to render post/cores unnecessary; in **15.84**, loss of tissue in the three teeth was variable. Residual dentine cores are supplemented by the

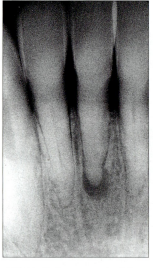

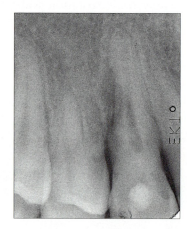

15.78 Pulp necrosis caused by orthognathic surgery

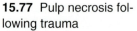

15.79 Pulp damaged by transplantation

15.77 Pulp necrosis following trauma

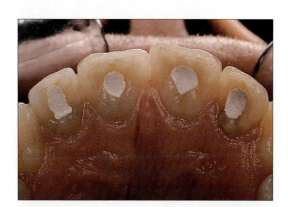

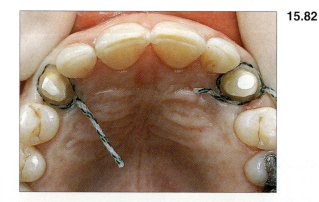

15.82

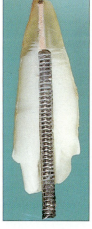

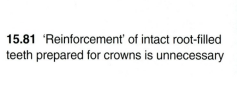

15.80 Intact teeth requiring root canal treatment may be restored with composite material

15.81 'Reinforcement' of intact root-filled teeth prepared for crowns is unnecessary

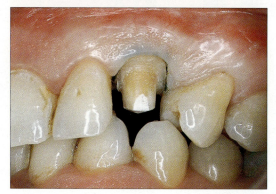

15.83

15.82, 15.83 Adequate dentine cores remaining after crown preparation render posts or cores unnecessary

gold cores. The idea of 'reinforcement' has recently been resurrected with the possibility of using adhesive luting cements to bond posts of materials with physical properties similar to those of dentine but there is as yet no clinical evidence to support their use.

Previously unrestored root-treated teeth may require more extensive restoration than simply access filling; for example, if the crown requires realignment or if its discoloration cannot be eliminated by bleaching alone. The most conservative restoration likely to satisfy aesthetic and functional requirements should be selected, so as not to weaken the tooth further. Such restorations may include composite or porcelain veneers (**15.85, 15.86**), with or without tooth preparation according to the prevailing preoperative condition. The least conservative preparation is for a ceramometal crown but even using this design the tooth should be prepared to review the need for supplementing the retention by a dowel.

Teeth with proximal cavities

A common clinical situation is one in which an anterior tooth has mesial and distal cavities or restorations (**15.87**). The addition of an access cavity leaves such a tooth with a band of missing tissue across the middle of its crown (**15.88**). Provided that the labial enamel plate is intact, relatively strong and unblemished by discoloration or surface deformities such as pitting, the tooth may be satisfactorily restored with composite restorative materials (**15.89**). A crown may give a better aesthetic result, particularly if adjacent teeth also need to be crowned, but will not necessarily confer greater strength or durability on the tooth. The presence of additional cavities/restorations or tooth tissue loss would strengthen the case for full coverage cast restorations (**15.90–15.92**).

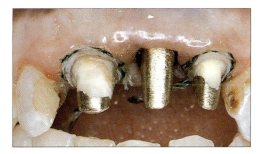

15.84 As much tooth tissue should be retained as possible, supplemented with a metal core as necessary

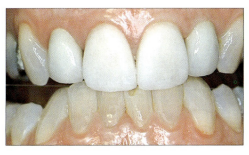

15.85, 15.86 Porcelain veneers

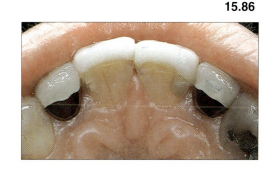

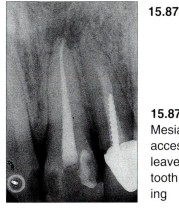

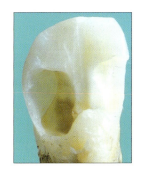

15.87, 15.88 Mesial, distal and access cavities leave a band of tooth tissue missing

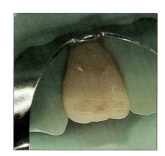

15.89 Restoration of missing tissue with composite restorative material

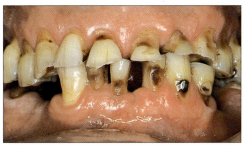

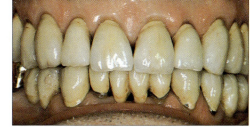

15.90–15.92 Full-coverage ceramometal crowns for restoring teeth with severe tissue loss

Teeth with inadequate tissue for retention without auxiliary aids

Anterior teeth

A full-coverage cast restoration may be desirable if extensive tooth surface has been lost due to erosion, abrasion or attrition. Poor aesthetics due to large restorations and severe discoloration may also make a full crown more desirable. In such circumstances the 'rooftop' preparations once recommended are now considered too destructive. It is considered better to prepare the tooth for the required restoration according to the requisite space demands and make good the tooth tissue deficit for retention and resistance form with a metal core retained by a dowel (**15.93, 15.94**). Spicules of tooth tissue which would not contribute to the strength of the tooth and may jeopardize uncomplicated construction of a core may be sacrificed at this stage (**15.95, 15.96**). In this way a more conservative restoration may be constructed.

Characteristics of dowels

Dowels may be selected from a range of prefabricated designs (**15.97–15.110**), may be custom made (**15.111**) or may be customized from prefabricated designs (**15.112–15.116**). Dowels are selected on their properties of retention, stress distribution, ease of application and cost. The characteristics determining retention and stress distribution include shape, length, diameter, surface configuration and the presence of a diaphragm.

Shape

Dowels may be parallel-sided or tapering (**15.117**). The parallel-sided dowels provide better retention per unit length than the tapered dowels. An increase in taper decreases retention. The stress-distributing characteristics of the two designs differ during installation and functional loading. Tapered dowels generate the least stress during cementation (**15.118**), parallel-sided dowels generate greater stress by virtue of the hydraulic pressure devel-

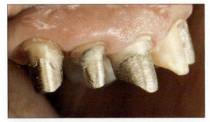

15.93

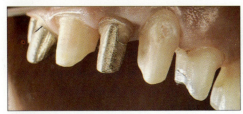

15.94

15.93, 15.94 Use of post cores to supplement retention

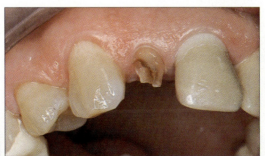

15.95

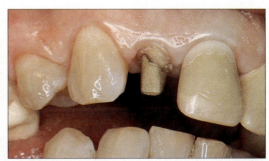

15.96

15.95, 15.96 Following preparation for a crown, spicules of tooth tissue which would not contribute to strength of the tooth should be sacrificed before dowel/core construction

15.97–15.110 Prefabricated post systems

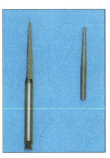
15.97 Filpost (titanium)

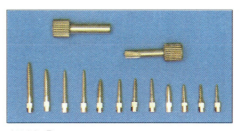
15.98 FKG pivots **15.99** Dentatus

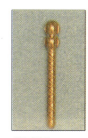
15.100 Post-stud

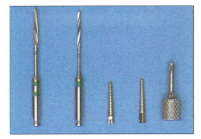
15.101 Maillefer Unimetric (titanium alloy-1mm)

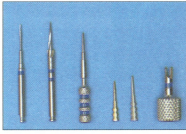
15.102 Maillefer Cytco (titanium alloy)

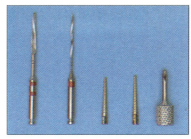
15.103 Maillefer Unimetric (titanium alloy-0.8mm)

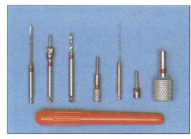
15.104 Maillefer Radix Anker Compact (titanium alloy)

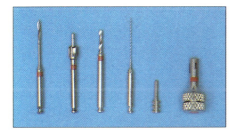
15.105 Maillefer Safix Anker (titanium alloy)

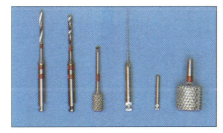
15.106 Maillefer RS Tenons Radiculaires

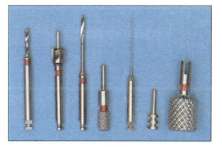
15.107 Radix Anker (titanium alloy)

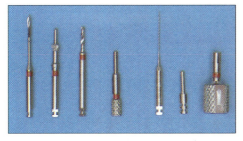
15.108 Maillefer Radix Anker–Long (titanium alloy)

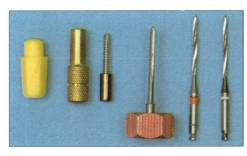
15.109 Kurer STD Anchor

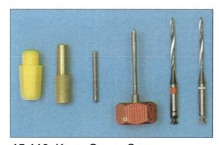
15.110 Kurer Crown Saver

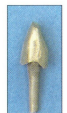
15.111 Custom-made post/core

15.112–15.116 Prefabricated post systems that can be customized

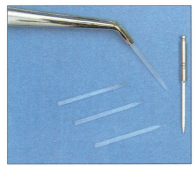
15.112 Dentatus Classic Post System

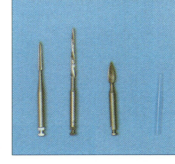
15.113 Mooser System (Burn out plastic posts)

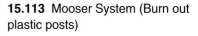

oped (**15.119**). However, the parallel-sided posts perform better in function (**15.120**) because tapered posts generate a wedging force (**15.121**); this may be alleviated if the shoulder rest is firm but this would concentrate stress at the shoulder.

Although parallel-sided dowels are considered more desirable, the natural tapering shape of roots and prepared root canals mitigate against using a dowel parallel along its entire length. Inevitably the dowel will be tapered in the coronal portion and be parallel-sided apically (**15.122**), which carries a danger of apical root perforation (**15.123**). One solution to this problem has been to taper the apical portion (Mooser and Dentatus classic posts: **15.113, 15.112**). Despite its relatively poorer retention and stress distribution characteristics the tapered post has been used successfully in many cases because it can be made to fit the prepared canal, which often makes it a more conservative choice: parallel-sided posts require preparation of the canal to a matching shape, which can render their use less conservative. A compromise is to select the narrowest parallel-sided post compatible with adequate retention and strength of post and root (**15.124**).

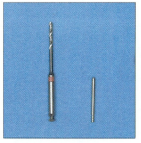
15.114 Optident Parallel Post System

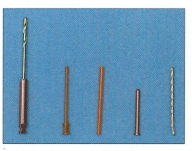
15.115 Parapost System

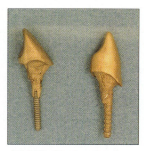
15.116 Customized parapost

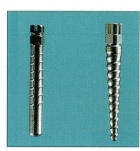
15.117 Parallel-sided or tapering dowels

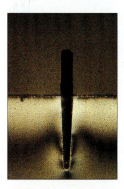
15.118 Tapered dowels generate least stress during cementation (courtesy of Mr P. O'Neilly)

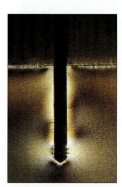
15.119 Parallel dowels generate greater stress during cementation (courtesy of Mr P. O'Neilly)

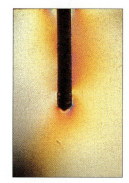
15.120 Parallel dowels provide better stress distribution in function (courtesy of Mr P. O'Neilly)

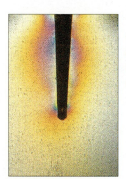
15.121 Tapered dowels generate a wedging force in function (courtesy of Mr P. O'Neilly)

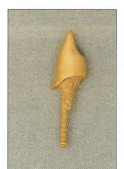
15.122 Dowel tapered coronally but parallel apically

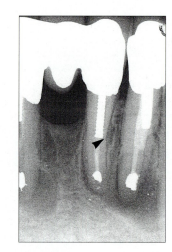
15.123 Root perforation caused by the parallel post in a mandibular incisor (arrowed)

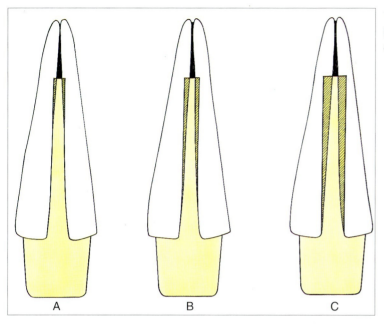

15.124 Selection of appropriate diameter of parallel-sided post: B = optimum for retention and root strength

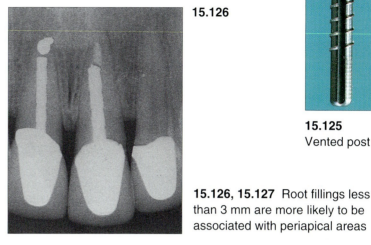

15.126

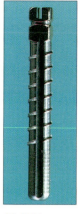

15.125 Vented post

15.126, 15.127 Root fillings less than 3 mm are more likely to be associated with periapical areas

15.128–15.131 Root curvature and cross-sectional anatomy determines the length and diameter of the post to be used

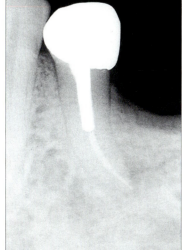

15.127

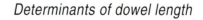

15.128

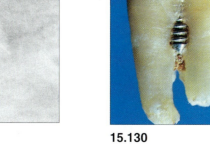

15.129

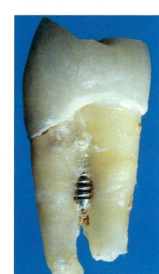

15.130

Length

Length is as important a determinant of post retention as it is for crown preparations. Longer posts provide better retention and stress distribution for all types of posts in function. Unfortunately, an increase in length also leads to greater stresses during installation, particularly of the parallel-sided dowels. This can be eased to an extent by ensuring that the post is vented (**15.125**).

Determinants of dowel length

Although long posts are desirable, their length is usually limited by the need for a minimum length of root filling. There is no common agreement about the minimum length of root filling that should remain in the apical portion of the root: lengths from 3 to 7 mm have been suggested. There is little firm clinical evidence to provide guidance, but what there is indicates that apical filling material of less than 3 mm is more likely to be associated with periapical disease (**15.126, 15.127**). The remaining root filling should be at least 3 mm long, and preferably as long as the minimum acceptable length of post will allow.

Root morphology also influences dowel length. The degree and position of root curvature (**15.128, 15.129**) and the cross-sectional size and shape of the root will limit the length and diameter of the post (**15.130, 15.131**).

Many different clinical yardsticks have been advocated for determining post length, including 'various fractions of root length, 1/3, 1/2 and 2/3' (**15.132**), 'of similar length to the crown', 'in teeth with loss of periodontal support the post should extend apical to the alveolar bone'. Of these guidelines the last two are widely accepted. The required length of post for retention must be weighed against occlusal loading: if the loading is unfavourable, restoration even with long posts may become uncemented (**15.133, 15.134**) but if occlusal loading is minimal, extremely short posts may suffice (**15.135, 15.136**). It is sometimes argued that many roots are not long enough to accommodate optimum lengths of both post and root filling and that the length of one or the other needs to be compromised. The choice of which is more important is a matter of clinical judgement.

Diameter

Posts must be of a minimum diameter to be strong enough not to deform (**15.137**) but the design of the restoration also contributes to the fatiguing of the post and even a wide post will fracture if its design is poor (**15.138**). The diameter of a cast post should be greater than that of a wrought post of the same alloy if it is to be as strong. In narrow roots, posts made of wrought metal should therefore be considered. Wider posts provide only slightly better retention and their use also means thinner and weaker residual root dentine, which may be prone to fracture (**15.139**). If the restoration is badly designed the chances of root fracture increase (**15.140**). The minimum post diameter compatible with adequate strength and retention should be considered.

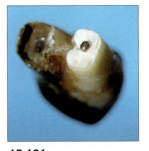

15.131

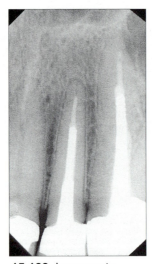

15.132 Long posts

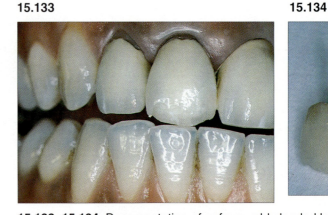

15.133, 15.134 Decementation of unfavourably loaded long posts. Note fractured porcelain on upper right central incisor

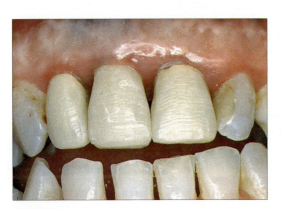

15.135 Anterior open bite

15.135, 15.136 Survival of favourably loaded short posts

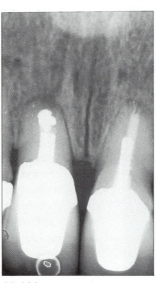

15.136

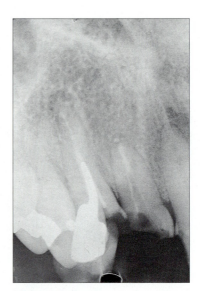

15.137 Deformation of post. Courtesy of Mr P. King

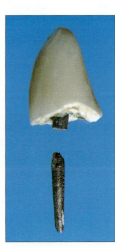

15.138 Fracture of post. Courtesy of Mr P. King

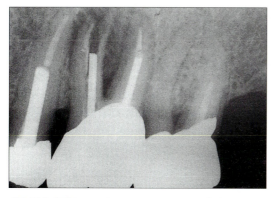

15.139 Wide posts may cause root fracture because of the amount of dentine sacrificed

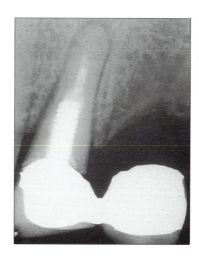

15.140 Unfavourable restoration designs increase the risk of root fracture

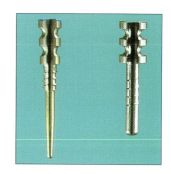

15.141 Serrations on posts increase retention

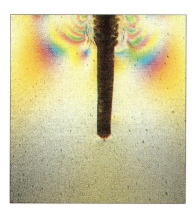

15.142 Higher stresses are associated with threads (courtesy of Mr P. O'Neilly)

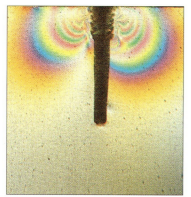

15.143 Further increase in stresses upon loading (courtesy of Mr P. O'Neilly)

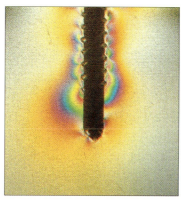

15.144 Stresses caused by placement of a threaded parallel post (courtesy of Mr P. O'Neilly)

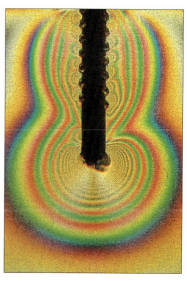

15.145 Increase in stresses if the post is tightened by a quarter turn (courtesy of Mr P. O'Neilly)

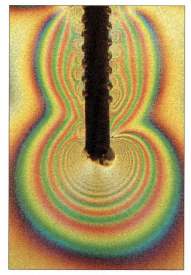

15.146 Loading increases the stresses further (courtesy of Mr P. O'Neilly)

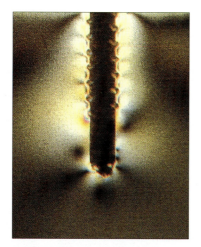

15.147 Removing the post and tapping the threads before replacement decreases the stresses (courtesy of Mr P. O'Neilly)

Surface configuration

The surface of posts may be smooth, roughened, serrated or threaded and may be modified for venting (**15.141**). Surface characteristics influence seating and retention: rough or uneven surfaces increase retentive capacity. Threaded posts have the best retentive properties. Prefabricated posts with a variety of thread designs are available (**15.97–15.110**). They may be threaded along their entire length or along only a restricted portion. Threaded posts generate the greatest stresses, as demonstrated by the concentration of stresses around the threaded portion of the post shown in **15.142**. The stresses increase when the post is loaded (**15.143**). The manner of placement of the post also influences the stress generated. The stress associated with the threads upon conventional placement is shown in **15.144**. If the post is tightened by an extra quarter turn, the stress increases tremendously (**15.145**). Upon loading, the stresses increase further (**15.146**), but are proportionately much lower than those due to overtightening. Removing the post and tapping the threads before replacement decreases the stresses considerably (**15.147**).

Loosening the fit of the post by removing and replacing it, and then cementing it in place, also reduces the stress (**15.148, 15.149**). Serrations on the posts are also associated with increased stresses but not to the same extent as threads (**15.150**): loading once again increases stresses (**15.151**). The improved retention due to serrations and threads should therefore be weighed against the disadvantages of increased stress concentration. The surface of the post may also be modified with cutaway portions or channels, which act as escape routes for luting cement during installation (**15.125**) and allow better seating and improved retention.

Diaphragm

A diaphragm or an apron, usually placed on the palatal aspect, may help to brace the tooth and distribute stresses more favourably (**15.152**). It is also useful for making good lost tooth tissue. When there is inadequate coronal tooth tissue a correctly designed and placed diaphragm prevents concentration of stresses around the apical portion of a post, which can lead to horizontal or oblique fractures of the root (**15.153, 15.154**).

Posterior teeth

Teeth requiring root canal treatment are often broken down to the extent that retention for a restoration is compromised (**15.155**). Restoration then requires installation of a core to replace the lost dentine before a full or partial coverage cast restoration may be placed on the tooth (**15.156**).

Retention for the core may be achieved in a number of ways, including the use of grooves and slots, dentine pins and dowels. Slots and grooves cut into residual dentine require favourable distribution of the remaining dentine (**15.157–15.159**). The depth and size of these retentive devices depend on the physical properties of the core material. Most of the currently available plastic materials require reasonable bulk to provide strength, which limits their clinical application.

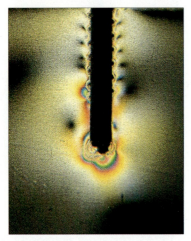

15.148 Loosening the post by tapping and cementing in place also reduces stresses (courtesy of Mr P. O'Neilly)

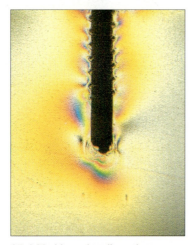

15.149 Upon loading, the stresses are considerably reduced compared to **15.146** (courtesy of Mr P. O'Neilly)

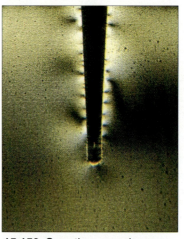

15.150 Serrations are also associated with stress concentration, but less so than the threaded design (courtesy of Mr P. O'Neilly)

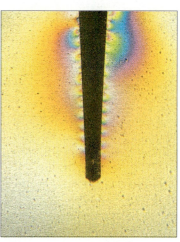

15.151 On loading the stress concentration increases further (courtesy of Mr P. O'Neilly)

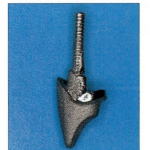

15.152 Diaphragm built into post/core

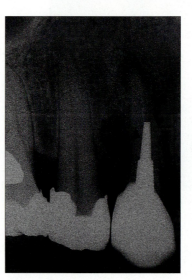
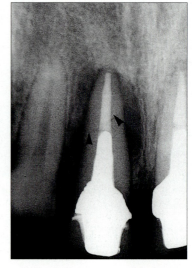

15.153, 15.154 Root fractures associated with apices of posts (arrowed)

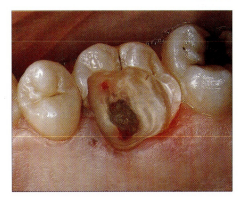
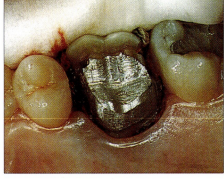

15.155, 15.156 Tooth requiring a core to retain a cast restoration

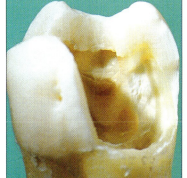
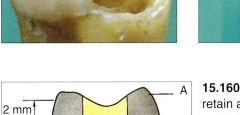

15.157–15.159 Use of slots and grooves for retaining a core

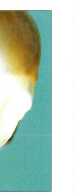

15.160 Use of dentine pins to retain an interim restoration: A = amalgam; B = access restoration; C = Gutta percha; D = cotton wool; E = pin

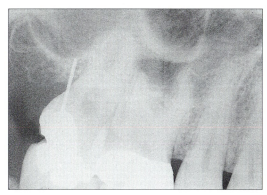

15.161 Pin perforation

The use of dentine pins in root-treated teeth is controversial. The presence of a pulp chamber and root canals should provide adequate retention. Rarely, a pin may be useful to help retain an interim amalgam restoration while root canal treatment is being performed (**15.160**). Placement of dentine pins is associated with complications such as perforation (**15.161**) and induction of stresses in the dentine possibly leading to cracks (**15.162**) and fracture (**15.163, 15.164**). Induced stresses are greatest with threaded (**15.165**) and friction grip pins and least with cemented pins but the latter require greater length for equivalent retention. Stresses due to pins may be reduced by

- pinhole preparation with a sharp drill using a speed-reducing handpiece and minimum number of passes so as not to cut the hole eccentrically (**15.166**);
- using pins with minimal mismatch between size of pinhole and pin;
- inserting the pin using a hand wrench (**15.167**) and unwinding it by at least a quarter turn so as not to engage the bottom

of the pinhole;
- using a threaded pin at least 4 mm long, with 2 mm in dentine, 2 mm in restorative material and with 2 mm of restorative material above the tip of the pin (**15.160**);
- using pins with sharper threads to minimize stresses during installation (however, these potentially increase stresses in function);
- using pins made of alloys softer than dentine, such as titanium, which may induce less stress;
- using only one pin per cusp because pins placed close together result in interaction of stresses and an increased potential for fracture (**15.168**).

The pulp space may be used for retention in a number of ways, the most conservative of which is the Nayyar amalgam/dowel core (**15.169–15.171**). This involves placing amalgam in the pulp chamber and into the root canals to a depth of about 3 mm to retain the coronal amalgam, which may act as the final capped cusp restoration (**15.172**) or the core that may be cut down for placement of a cast restoration (**15.173–15.175**). The shortness of the dowel reduces the disturbance of the root filling. Adequate remaining tooth tissue is essential and should be judged in terms of

- depth of pulp chamber (**15.171, 15.172, 15.176**);
- distance from floor of pulp chamber to furcation (**15.172,**

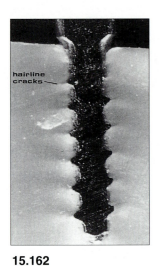

15.162

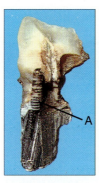

15.163 a = enamel; B = pin channels; c= fracture plane

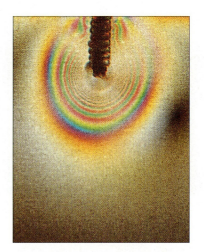

15.164 Fracture of tooth along a pin channel: A = pin

15.165 Threaded pins generate the greatest stress (courtesy of Mr P. O'Neilly)

15.162–15.164 Stresses generated by pins can cause cracks in dentine which can lead to tooth fracture

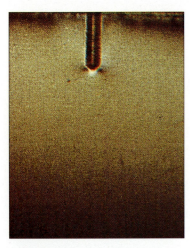

15.166 Pinhole prepared by a sharp drill generates minimal stress (courtesy of Mr P. O'Neilly)

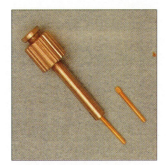

15.167 Hand wrench for insertion of pins

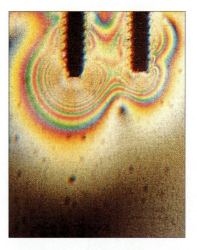

15.168 Pins placed close together cause stresses to accumulate (courtesy of Mr P. O'Neilly)

15.169–15.176 Nayyar amalgam cores

15.169

15.170

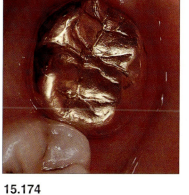
15.171 Case shown in **15.169** and **15.170**

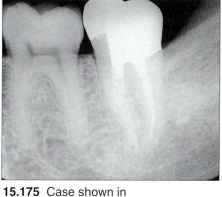

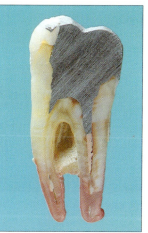
15.172

15.173

15.174

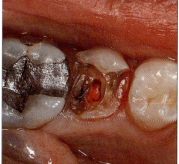
15.175 Case shown in **15.173** and **15.174**

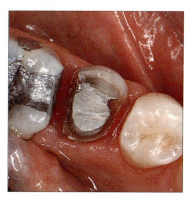
15.176

15.177

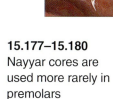
15.178

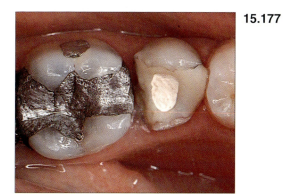

15.179

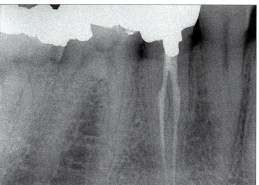
15.180

15.177–15.180 Nayyar cores are used more rarely in premolars

15.176), floor to amelocemental junction (**15.172, 15.176**), floor to alveolar crest (**15.171, 15.175**) and the projected margin of the crown (**15.173–15.175**);
- thickness of dentine at the level of the crown margin (**15.16**).

Nayyar cores are more rarely placed in premolars (**15.177–15.180**). When the remaining coronal dentine is not enough to support such a core, retention may be gained by placing a dowel into one of the canals, usually the one with the

263

15.181, 15.182 Stainless steel posts/amalgam core in maxillary molar

15.183

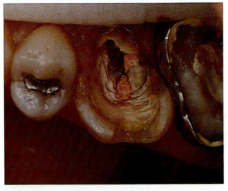

15.181

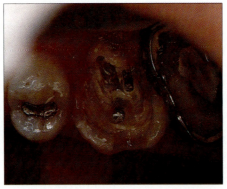

15.182

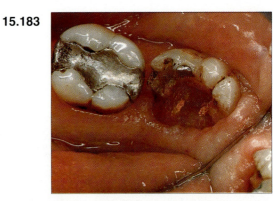

15.183–15.186 Stainless steel post/amalgam core in mandibular molar

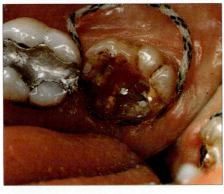

15.184

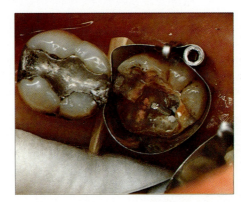

15.185

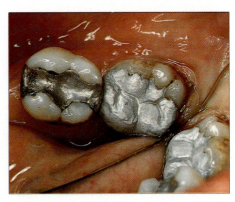

15.186

largest and straightest root (the palatal canal in an upper molar (**15.181, 15.182**) and the distal canal in a lower molar (**15.183–15.186**)). The dowel and the residual coronal dentine will then provide the retention for the core. Multiple roots make it possible to place multiple posts, which do not have to be as long as in single-rooted teeth (**15.187**).

15.187 Multipost/core

Core materials

Amalgam

Amalgam remains the material of choice for cores because of its strength, versatility, availability and dimensional stability. Its one drawback was the slowness of set, making it difficult to prepare the core for a cast restoration at the same visit. However this disadvantage has largely been overcome by new faster setting alloys. Reports of systemic problems caused by amalgam are unfounded.

Composite

Composite cores became popular because they set rapidly and are strong. However, they have largely fallen into disfavour because they tend to absorb moisture and are dimensionally unstable, because eugenol temporary cements tend to soften the core and because moisture in the core affects the physical properties of acid-based permanent luting cements, such as zinc phosphate, glass ionomer or polycarboxylate, unfavourably.

Cermet

Cermets or metal reinforced glass ionomers have also been recommended as core materials, but their strength does not compare with that of amalgam or composites. It is suitable only for use as a space-filler to reduce the amount of metal in the cast restoration. It should not be used as a structural core that provides the principal retention and resistance form.

15.188–15.190 Three-quarter partial veneer preparations preserving tooth tissue

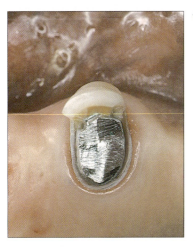

15.188

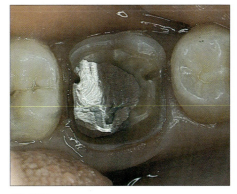

15.189

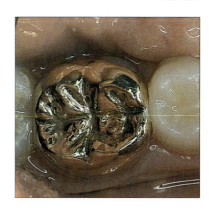

15.190

15.191–15.201 Indirect technique for construction of cast multipost/core

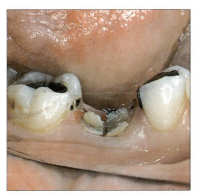

15.191

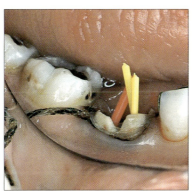

15.192

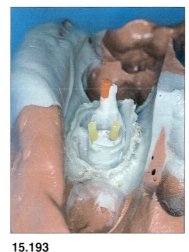

15.193

15.194

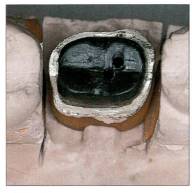

15.195

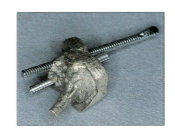

15.196

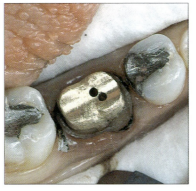

15.197

Once placed, the cores may serve as interim restorations before being prepared for cast restorations. If aesthetic requirements allow, a conservative partial veneer restoration such as a three-quarter crown is preferable (**15.188–15.190**). The margins of the casting should always be placed on sound tooth tissue.

Cast cores

Cast multiple posts or cores may be used in multirooted teeth with little remaining coronal tooth tissue by constructing only one of the posts integral with the core and cementing the remaining post(s) into their respective canals through the core. This method can be applied using indirect or direct techniques.

In the indirect technique an impression of the tooth (**15.191**) and post canals (**15.192**) is taken using preformed plastic patterns and rubber-base impression material (**15.193**). A model with a dye is constructed (**15.194**), on which the post and core is waxed with withdrawable posts in two canals (**15.195, 15.196**). The cast post and core is tried in the mouth for fit (**15.197**) and the removable posts are inserted through their respective channels (**15.198**). The post/core system is cemented with a suitable luting cement (**15.199, 15.200**). The final crown is constructed with margins on sound tooth tissue (**15.201**).

Where some coronal tooth tissue remains (**15.202–15.205**) it may interfere with the path of insertion of the core. The canal providing the path of least resistance may be selected for the principal post to help preserve tooth tissue and place a partial veneer cast restoration. If a substantial amount of tooth tissue needs to be sacrificed to provide a path of insertion for the core, it may be better to cement preformed posts into the canals and build up a core with plastic restorative materials.

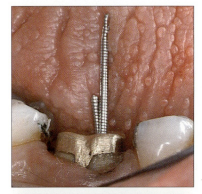
15.198

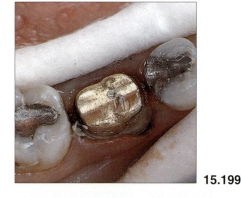
15.199

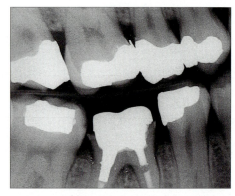
15.200

15.202–15.205 Cast multipost/core method for three-quarter crown

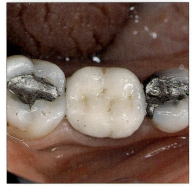
15.201

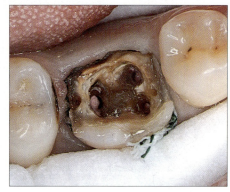
15.202

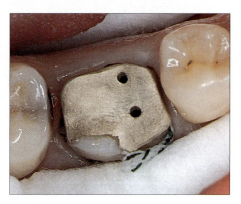
15.203

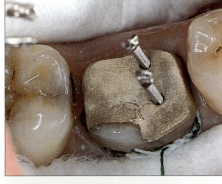
15.204

15.206, 15.207 Direct technique for construction of cast multipost core

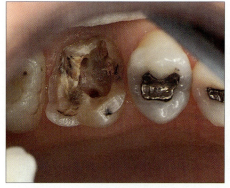
15.206   15.207

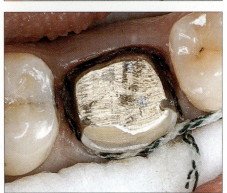
15.205 Tooth prepared for 3/4 crown

The direct technique may also be used to construct a multiple post and core system using preformed plastic patterns and acrylic resin (**15.206, 15.207**). The method is more difficult to perform than the indirect technique but is more suitable in some circumstances.

Root-treated teeth as abutments

It is generally accepted that the stresses on an abutment tooth are different from, and likely to be more severe than, those on a single unit (**15.208**). There may be a higher tendency for root-treated abutment teeth and their restorations to fail mechanically than vital abutments. For this reason many operators avoid using root-treated teeth as abutments. However, it is also documented that such teeth can survive despite acting as abutments (**15.209, 15.210**): the truth probably lies somewhere in between. The potential for failure is a function not only of endodontic status but also of the amount of remaining dentine, restoration design and occlusal loading. The bridge shown in **15.209** and **15.210** would not be expected to survive, yet it has been in place for at least 10 years. Different bridge and denture designs impose different stresses on the teeth and it is important to select a design likely to reduce such stresses. Fixed-fixed bridge designs distribute stresses equally between abutments whereas the minor retainer in a fixed-movable design takes the lower load. The terminal abutment for a free-end saddle design is likely to take greater loads than an abutment for a bounded saddle. Crown: root ratios, bracing, type of retention and rest seat design all influence lateral loading of abutment teeth. The number of remaining teeth and potential for bracing from other teeth and soft tissues may also dictate overall loading. The denture design selected should attempt to minimize stresses on root-treated teeth.

Occlusal loading

Occlusal loading is difficult to control. It depends not only on the occlusal contacts but also on eating and chewing habits, parafunctional activity and the state of the masticatory musculature. There is only limited scope in influencing the nature and magnitude of occlusal forces. This can be achieved by adequately designing the intercuspal, excursive and closure contact relationships of teeth. Lateral forces are often regarded as being the most damaging and therefore designing excursive occlusal contacts to preferentially load adjacent vital and more robust teeth may be useful.

Restoration of a tooth with a resected root

If the crown of a tooth scheduled for root resection is intact, the only restorations required are the amalgam seal in the canal of the root to be resected and the access restoration (**15.211, 15.212**).

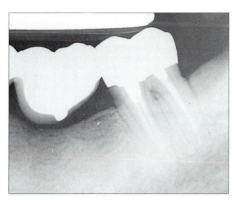

15.208 Stresses are likely to be more severe on an abutment tooth

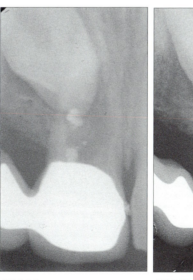

15.209, 15.210 Survival of severely weakened tooth as a bridge abutment

15.209   **15.210**

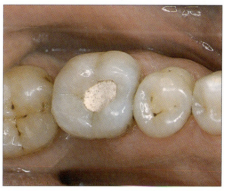

15.211

15.212

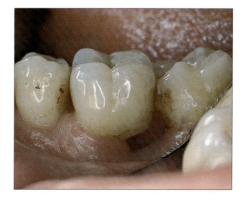

15.211, 15.212 Conservative restoration of tooth with resected root

15.213–15.218 Restoration of hemisected mandibular second molar and first molar

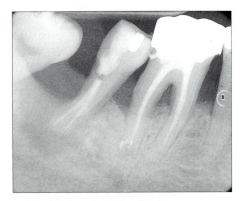

15.213 After endodontic treatment

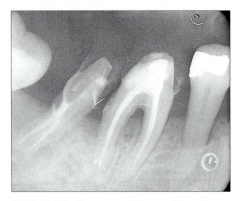

15.214 Tooth preparation and temporization

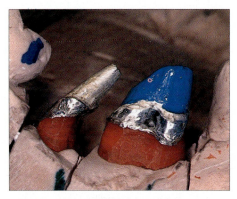

15.215 Silver dies

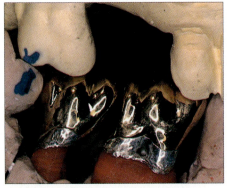

15.216 Constructed crowns

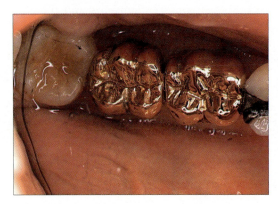

15.217 Immediately post cementation

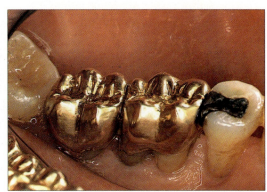

15.218 2 years post cementation

If the tooth already has a restoration with stable interproximal and occlusal contacts no further restoration should be required. In the absence of stable contacts a suitable restoration should be constructed (**15.213–15.218**): **15.218** shows the teeth still functioning at an appointment 2 years after treatment. Potential problems include drifting of the tooth and fracture of the remaining root(s) (**15.219**).

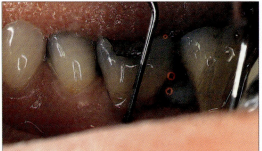

15.219 Root fracture of hemisected molar

Restoration of a hemisected tooth

The reasons for hemisection were discussed in Chapter 11. The procedure may be followed by extracting one of the halves or restoring both halves as premolars (**15.220–15.232**). This

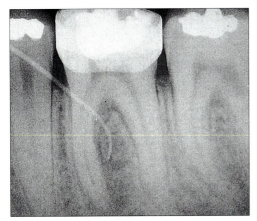

15.220 Fractured mandibular molar with endodontic involvement and sinus tract

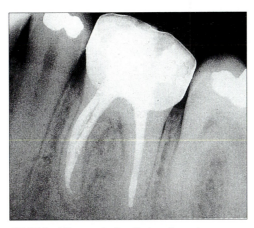

15.221 After endodontic treatment

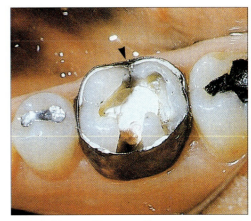

15.222 Lingual fracture line visible (arrowed)

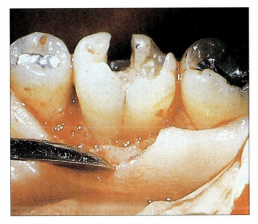

15.223 Lingual flap reflected

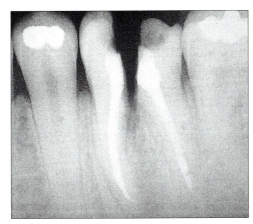

15.224 Crown hemisected

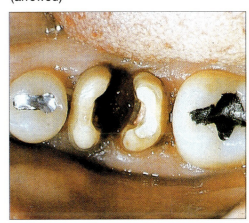

15.225 Mesial and distal portions prepared for crowns. NB furcal shape of roots

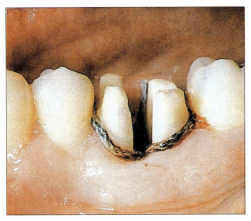

15.226 Cord retraction of gingivae. NB difficulty of retraction in furcal area

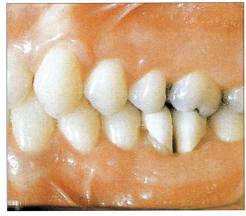

15.227 Buccal view of acrylic temporary restorations

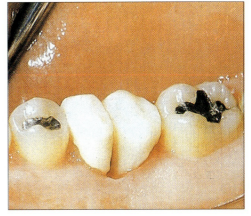

15.228 Lingual view of acrylic temporary restorations

15.220–15.232 Restoration of both halves of a hemisected tooth as premolars (courtesy of Mr A. Croysdill)

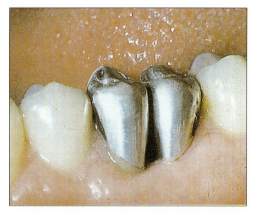

15.229 Silver temporary restorations constructed to allow adequate gingival healing

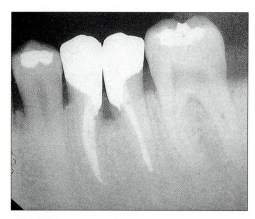

15.230

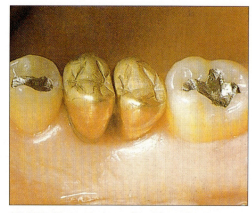

15.231 Lingual view of gold castings

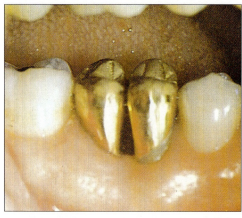

15.232 Buccal view of gold castings. NB wide embrasure

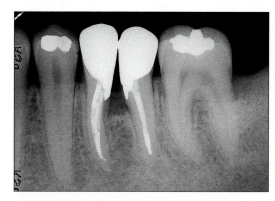

15.233 Difficulties of contouring restorations in the furcation

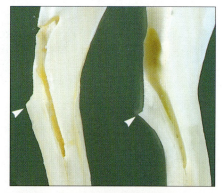

15.234 Margin placement and contouring difficulties caused by the shape of the tooth in the furcal region (arrowed)

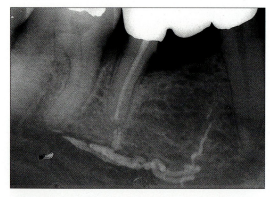

15.235 Use of a hemisected tooth as a bridge abutment. NB this root, incidentally, was one in which a formaldehyde-containing material had been used and had entered the ID canal. The patient suffered permanent paraesthesia

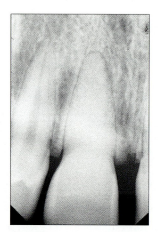

15.236

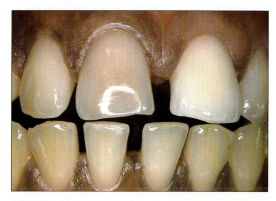

15.237

15.236, 15.237 Dense opaque discoloration due to obliteration of pulp

sequence of photographs shows the restoration of a tooth with a buccolingual vertical fracture but healthy periodontal tissues. When such treatment is carried out because of furcal exposure due to periodontal disease, access may be better. However, the main difficulty lies in margin placement and contouring the furcal aspects of the restorations (**15.233**) due to the shape of the residual tooth in this region (**15.225, 15.234**). Contouring the proximal areas between the two premolars is very difficult. Occasionally the remaining half of a molar may be used as a bridge abutment (**15.235**). If a dowel is needed in either situation, it is better to consider extraction.

Treatment of tooth discoloration

Non-vital teeth may be discoloured by various factors including caries, restorations, secondary calcification and contamination of dentinal tubules by blood or food products. Removal of the cause usually removes the discoloration, except in the case of severe secondary calcification which gives a dense, opaque yellow discoloration (**15.236, 15.237**). Options for treatment include

1. vital bleaching;
2. non-vital bleaching;
3. labial/buccal veneers;
4. crowns.

Vital bleaching is unlikely to be very successful. Use of home-bleaching products is potentially harmful and has been banned in Europe.

Non-vital bleaching (use of bleaching agents in the access cavity under rubber dam isolation) is quite effective (**15.238–15.246**). Bleaching may be performed at the chairside by placing hydrogen peroxide in the pulp chamber, which may be 'activated' with light or heat to enhance its effect. Bleaching is usually used after the pulp chamber has been prepared by removing the root filling material to cervical level (**15.239**) and covering it with a layer of zinc phosphate (**15.240**). The dentine is then etched for an arbitrary period of 30 seconds with phosphoric acid (**15.241**), washed away and the cavity dried. Hydrogen peroxide is flooded into the canal, taking care to ensure that there is no overflow (**15.242**). After 5–10 minutes, the access cavity is gently dried and a paste of sodium perborate mixed with water (**15.243**) is applied. The

15.238–15.246 'Walking bleach' technique

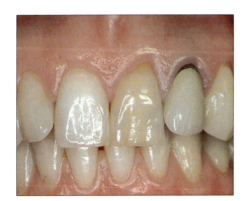

15.238 Preoperative view

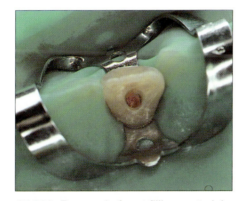

15.239 Removal of root filling material

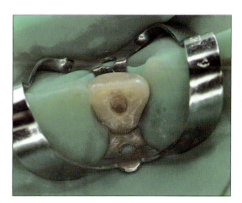

15.240 Zinc phosphate base

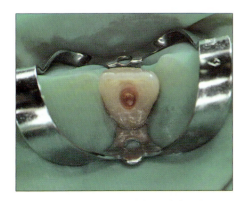

15.241 30 second etching of dentine

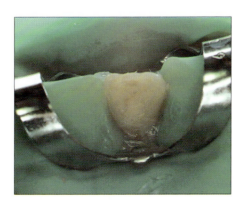

15.242 Hydrogen peroxide placed with cotton pledget

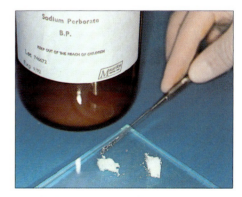

15.243 Mixing paste of sodium perborate

access cavity is properly sealed to prevent loss of dressing in the period between appointments. There may be some improvement at this stage (**15.244**); 1 week later, further improvement is seen due to the 'Walking bleach' technique (**15.245**). Repetition of this procedure may improve the situation further (**15.246**).

Composite or porcelain *veneers* can effectively mask discoloration, provided that it is not severe and that an adequate thickness of masking material is used. A combination of bleaching and veneering may help if neither method alone is sufficient to eliminate discoloration.

Ceramometal or ceramic *crowns* are capable of providing excellent aesthetics but require an adequate thickness of porcelain, which means sacrificing more tissue in an already weakened tooth.

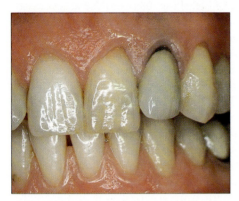

15.244 Mild improvement at end of visit

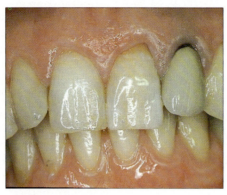

15.245 More significant improvement after one week

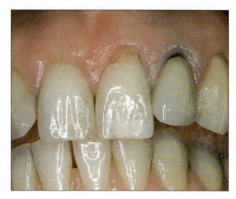

15.246 May be some marginal improvement after repetition of procedure

16 Primary dentition

Endodontic treatment of the primary dentition differs from that of the permanent teeth for two main reasons – pathology and morphology. Even the ultimate aim is different in that primary teeth need be retained only until exfoliation occurs.

Diagnosis of pulp pathology

It has been shown that inflammatory changes in the pulp occur more rapidly in the primary tooth in response to dentine caries than in the permanent tooth. Pathological changes within the pulp become irreversible early after the carious attack, and rapidly extend throughout the coronal pulp. It would be desirable to be able to diagnose the condition at this stage before total pulpitis develops. However, an additional problem is that symptoms resulting from pulpal pathogenesis in the primary teeth may not be severe, and often infection has spread to periradicular tissues before treatment is sought (**16.1, 16.2**).

Diagnosis is also hampered because children are usually poor historians and respond unpredictably to subjective clinical tests. As a result, few useful conclusions concerning the condition of the pulp can be made from clinical findings.

Therefore, the diagnosis of early or partial pulpitis cannot be made with any certainty on clinical grounds, and the techniques chosen on those premises have no rational histological basis.

Morphology of the primary tooth

The morphology is such that the enamel and dentine are thinner and the pulp chamber, with its extended horns, larger in proportion, than in permanent teeth (**16.3**).

The molar teeth have irregularly shaped ribbon-like canals which become narrower with the deposition of secondary dentine, and there are ramifications and lateral branches. In the inter-radicular area the floor of the pulp chamber is thin and there are numerous accessory canals. The resulting permeability of the dentine in this area often leads to inter-radicular rather than periapical bone loss associated with infected primary molars (**16.4**).

The roots of the primary teeth are in close relationship to the developing permanent successor and will, during exfoliation, undergo resorption. This therefore limits the materials which can be used in the canals, resorbable pastes being necessary.

In addition, trauma to or infection of primary teeth may damage the successional teeth, causing enamel defects, arrested development of the permanent tooth germ or cyst formation (**16.5**).

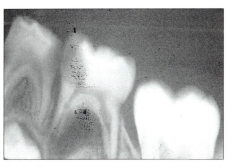

16.1 Gross caries, internal and external root resorption, and bone loss

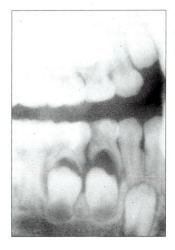

16.2 Extensive caries and periradicular bone loss

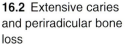

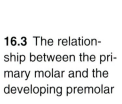

16.4 Inter-radicular bone loss in a primary molar

16.3 The relationship between the primary molar and the developing premolar

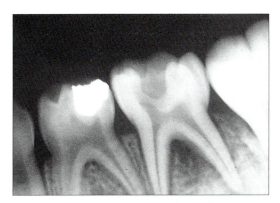

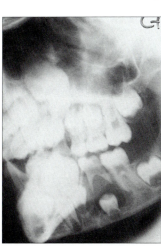

16.5 Infection of primary molar affecting follicle of developing premolar

Techniques of pulp therapy

Indirect pulp capping

The deep carious lesion which is symptomless clinically and without radiographic change may be treated by intermittent excavation and indirect pulp capping. The treatment, which is carried out under local analgesia with good isolation, involves removing all peripheral caries to provide sound cavity margins, and carefully excavating deep soft caries overlying the pulp. A dressing of calcium hydroxide is applied to the remaining carious dentine and sealed effectively to prevent fluid or bacteria leaking into the cavity. The treatment is considered to progress satisfactorily if, after a minimum period of 6 weeks, the tooth is symptomless, and on removal of the dressing there is evidence of arrest of the lesion and reparative dentine formation. The carious dentine will be darker in colour, less moist and harder. Any remaining soft dentine is removed with a large bur or excavator before a further dressing of calcium hydroxide, the insertion of a lining and final restoration.

Direct pulp capping

Due to the rapid progress of pathological changes in the pulp, and its poor healing ability, this has limited effectiveness in the primary dentition. The technique is indicated only in small traumatic exposures arising accidentally during cavity preparation in an area of otherwise sound dentine in a symptomless tooth. The long-term effectiveness of this treatment in other circumstances, such as a carious exposure, compares poorly with pulpotomy procedures.

One-visit formocresol pulpotomy

The rational basis for the use of this technique in the primary dentition is the existence of healthy pulp in the root canals, which is left following removal of the inflamed coronal pulp tissue. The difficulties of diagnosing this situation from available clinical evidence have already been discussed, and have led some clinicians to favour a two-visit devitalizing technique, which makes no assumptions concerning the health of the radicular pulp tissue.

Those authorities who advocate a single-visit method assume that after removal of the inflamed coronal tissue healing may take place at the surface of the radicular pulp, which is essentially normal. However, previously, when calcium hydroxide was used widely in the vital pulpotomy technique in the primary dentition in the belief that healing would occur, internal resorption of the root canals was frequently observed. The use of the one-visit formocresol technique in carefully selected cases is considered by many clinicians as a useful treatment with a very good prognosis.

The procedure is carried out using local analgesia, and isolation is achieved preferably with a rubber dam or with a saliva ejector and cotton wool rolls. Cavity preparation is completed and peripheral caries removed before exposing the pulp by removing deep caries (**16.6, 16.7**).

The entire roof of the pulp chamber is removed along with any overhanging dentine which may hinder removal of fragments of coronal pulp (**16.8**).

The coronal pulp tissue is then removed with either a sharp excavator (**16.9**) or a large round bur at slow speed (**16.10**), to avoid weakening the fragile walls of the tooth or perforating the thin floor of the pulp chamber.

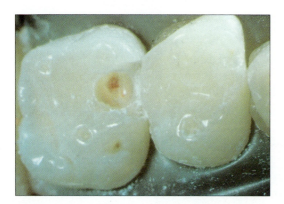

16.6 Cavity preparation with pulpal exposure

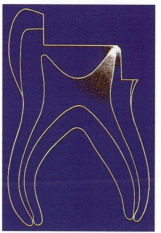

16.7 Cavity preparation completed before pulpotomy

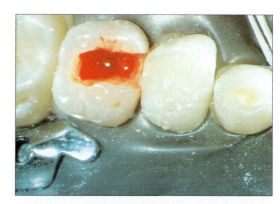

16.8 Removal of pulp chamber roof

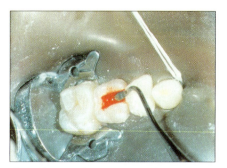

16.9 Excavation of tissue from pulp chamber

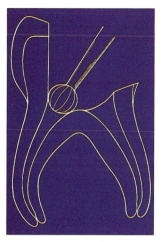

16.10 Removal of pulp tissue with large round burr

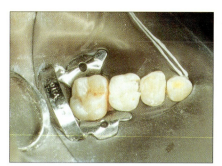

16.11 Haemostasis with cotton wool

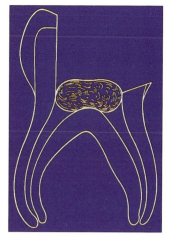

16.12 Formocresol applied on cotton wool pledget

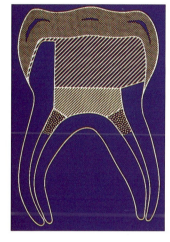

16.13 Restoration with stainless steel crown, cement, zinc oxide and eugenol. Fixed tissue is present in the entrance of the radicular system

Irrigation of the pulp chamber with sterile water or normal saline dislodges the pulp and dentine debris. The cavity is dried with pledgets of cotton wool to allow the haemorrhage to be controlled and the pulp stumps to be identified (**16.11**).

The natural cessation of bleeding of the radicular pulp is taken to indicate the presence of healthy tissue. The openings of the root canals are covered with a cotton wool pledget moistened with Buckley's formocresol (35% cresol, 19% formalin in aqueous glycerine) (**16.12**). After 5 minutes the cotton wool is removed; fixation should have caused the tissue at the entrance to the canals to become dark brown in appearance.

A thick cream of zinc oxide and eugenol is placed in the floor of the chamber and over the radicular pulp. This is followed by a further layer of cement, placed without pressure. The tooth is finally restored, usually with a preformed nickel–chrome crown to prevent later cuspal fracture (**16.13**).

The Buckley's formocresol is used in a 1:5 solution, which has been shown to be as effective as the more concentrated form. However, there is still a risk of damage through spillage on the soft tissues, leakage into the interdental area (where it may cause sloughing of the papilla) and diffusion into the periapical area. More recently, concern has been expressed about possible local and systemic toxicity as well as the mutagenicity and carcinogenicity of formocresol. Therefore 2% glutaraldehyde has been investigated as an alternative medicament. The reactions following glutaraldehyde are irreversible (unlike those of formocresol): it is less likely to penetrate the periapical foramen and less solution is required to fix the tissues. It also appears that more vital tissue remains in the root canal following the use of glutaraldehyde. However, the success rate of pulpotomies using glutaraldehyde may not be as good as with formocresol, and further long-term studies are required. In addition glutaraldehyde may cause hypersensitivity reactions.

If the radicular pulp has undergone some inflammatory change, it will be difficult to control pulpal haemorrhage during the one-visit procedure, and a two-visit technique may be required. In addition, if the patient has experienced pain the two-visit technique should be used to allow for assessment.

Two-visit formocresol pulpotomy/two-visit paraformaldehyde pulpotomy

In both techniques the aim is to fix the remaining radicular pulp tissue to the apex by applying either formocresol or paraformaldehyde devitalizing paste (paraformaldehyde 1.00 g, lignocaine 0.06 g, propylene glycol 0.5 ml, Carbowax 1.3 g and carmine) for a period. The prognosis of these treatments is favourable.

Following cavity preparation and removal of the coronal pulp, a dressing of either medicament is sealed into the pulp chamber for 7–10 days, after which the patient is questioned about any symptoms. The dressings are removed and the tooth is re-examined for signs of periradicular infection. If the radicular pulp appears fixed the tooth is restored as previously described. In addition, if complete anaesthesia cannot be obtained during cavity preparation the devitalizing paste may be applied to the exposure on a cotton wool pledget without amputation of the pulp. This seldom leads to complete pulpal devitalization, but may reduce sensitivity and so permit a pulpotomy or further application of devitalizing paste at the second visit.

However, when the pulp is infected such that there is clinical or radiographic evidence of inter-radicular pathology, or the root canals contain necrotic tissue or pus, different techniques are required either to disinfect the pulp or to remove the radicular tissue.

Disinfection technique

The cavity is prepared and the coronal pulp chamber and access to the canals thoroughly cleaned to allow placement of a dressing of cotton wool moistened with Beechwood creosote, formocresol, or camphorated monochlorophenol. This is sealed in the cavity for 7–10 days, after which the tooth is re-examined for mobility, the presence of a sinus or any tenderness to pressure. If the tooth is satisfactory it is restored as for the previous pulpotomy procedure. If signs of infection persist a further period of disinfection is required.

The prognosis for this technique is much poorer than for the pulpotomy procedures, and recently a pulpectomy technique has been developed.

Pulpectomy

In this method the infected tissue is removed from the canals using mechanical methods and pharmacological agents. Radicular pulp tissue and debris are removed with broaches and the canals prepared with files, using an estimated measurement of length from the diagnostic radiograph, and taking care not to instrument beyond the apex or perforate the root, which may have a marked curvature. Access and the morphology of the root limits the preparation and it may be necessary to use an antimicrobial dressing to aid disinfection. Following irrigation and drying the roots are filled with a resorbable iodoform or zinc oxide and eugenol paste, which is either syringed into the canal or condensed with pluggers (**16.14**).

Pulpectomy is increasingly being used for managing vital primary molars because of the concerns about formocresol and glutaraldehyde. The pulp chamber and canals are cleaned, irrigated, dried and filled in one visit.

Follow up

Any endodontically treated tooth requires regular clinical and radiographic assessment to observe any pathological sequelae which may occur and may effect the developing successional tooth.

The series of photographs in **16.15–16.17** shows the continued premolar development over a 4.5 year period in the absence of pathology, associated with primary molars treated by the one-visit formocresol pulpotomy technique.

An inadequate two-visit devitalizing pulpotomy on a primary second molar shows internal resorption perforating the root, and leading to an area of inter-radicular radiolucency (**16.18**).

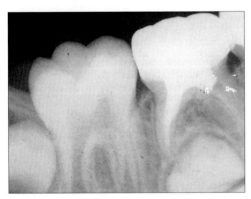

16.14 Post pulpectomy filling and restoration

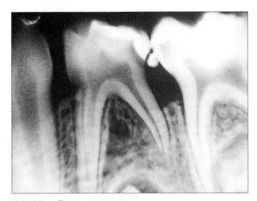

16.15 Pretreatment

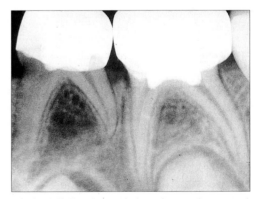

16.16 Following pulpotomies and restoration with stainless steel crowns, 9 months later

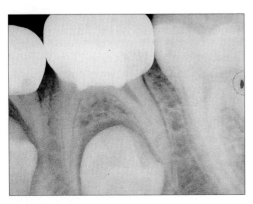

16.17 Follow up 4½ years later, showing absence of pathology and continued premolar development

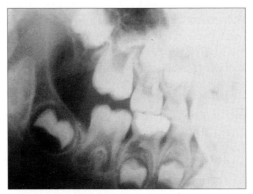

16.18 Failed devitalizing pulpotomy with internal resorption perforating root

16.19 shows the Beechwood creosote disinfection technique used on a primary second molar, which failed because of extensive external and internal resorption of the mesial root.

The primary molar in **16.20** was treated by the pulpectomy technique, but there is evidence of internal resorption around the filling material in the distal root.

Chronic infection of a primary molar, whether pulp-treated or untreated, may cause disturbance of the enamel formation of the developing premolar, resulting in a hypoplastic defect (**16.21**). More seriously there may be gross disturbance or cessation of the development of the underlying tooth germ (**16.22**).

Chronically infected primary teeth, whether pulp treated or untreated, may be occassionally associated with formation of infected follicular cysts around the successional teeth (**16.23**).

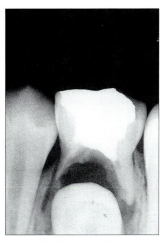

16.19 Failed disinfection pulpotomy with extensive root resorption

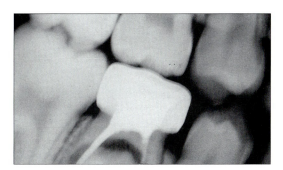

16.20 Failed pulpotomy with root resorption

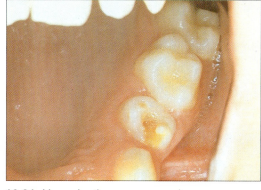

16.21 Hypoplastic upper premolar

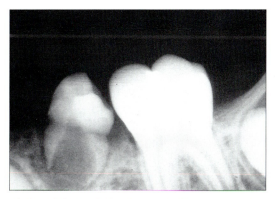

16.22 Disturbed development of lower premolar

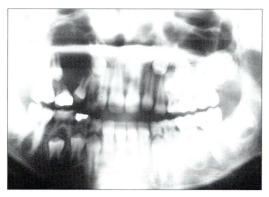

16.23 Infected follicular cyst displacing upper right second premolar

17 Medicolegal aspects

A letter from a solicitor alleging that a patient has been treated negligently has a dramatic effect on any dental practitioner, however experienced or qualified. Unfortunately these letters are arriving with ever-increasing frequency, in line with the increasing frequency of claims against health professionals generally.

Endodontic treatment is responsible for a high proportion of the cases that have to be defended each year.

Good communication and a caring friendly attitude towards the patient would prevent most cases coming to court. If the patient feels that the dentist has done his or her best, even though there is still a problem, it is unlikely that legal action will be taken.

Recording treatment

It is essential to record dental treatment in a way that is accurate, legible and complete. The following should be recorded:

- medical history, including aspects relevant to endodontic treatment;
- dental history;
- history of the present complaint, including presenting symptoms;
- clinical examination, both intraoral and extraoral;
- results of vitality tests;
- radiographs and report;
- diagnosis and treatment planning;
- medication prescribed, including antibiotics;
- use of analgesia;
- method of isolation, particularly if rubber dam was not used;
- working length of root canals and their reference points;
- size to which canals have been prepared;
- intracanal medication used;
- dressing applied to seal access cavity;
- root-filling material and technique used;
- type of sealer used;
- number of radiographs taken.

Any complications or errors that occur during treatment must be explained to the patient and recorded – for example, iatrogenic incidents such as broken instruments, overfilling or underfilling and perforations. The explanation to the patient should provide objective factual information with appropriate clinical reassurance. Adequate explanations by the operator assist in reducing the patient's fear and uncertainty.

Informed consent

The proposed treatment plan should be clearly explained, discussed, and agreed by the patient, particularly when there are alternative treatments or special problems. It should be recorded that the patient has agreed to the treatment and to the cost. The patient should be informed in writing if the treatment plan is complex and likely to demand high fees. The treatment of patients below the age of 16 years must be agreed by a parent or legal guardian, either by completing a form for the purpose or recording the consent on the patient's records.

A patient who is pregnant and requires radiography must give her consent, which should be recorded.

Review

Treatment should be reviewed periodically and recorded. Reassessment and re-evaluation of endodontic treatment is desirable for a minimum period of 4 years after treatment. A tooth that had an area of radiolucency at the time of treatment should be assessed by taking follow-up radiographs using the parallel technique. It is not possible to say that treatment has been successful until there is evidence of bony healing.

Standard of care

Operators who use techniques or materials that are not considered current practice will jeopardize their defence in a court of law. An example would be the extrusion of a paraformaldehyde root canal sealer into the inferior dental canal which has produced paraesthesia; if a sealer had been extruded which did not contain paraformaldehyde but still produced paraesthesia the operator would be in a better position to defend the case. It is the responsibility of dentists to keep themselves up to date with current accepted practice.

References and further reading

Chapter 1

1. European Society of Endodontology: Consensus report of the European Society of Endodontology on quality guidelines for endodontic treatment (1994). *Int. Endodont. J.*, **27**(3): 115–124.
2. Callis PD, Charlton G and Clyde JS (1993). A survey of patients seen in consultant clinics in conservative dentistry at Edinburgh Dental Hospital in 1990. *Brit. Dent. J.*, **174**(3): 106–110.
3. Eriksen HM (1991). Endodontology—epidemiologic considerations. *Endodont. Dent. Traumatol.*, **7**: 189–195.
4. Ray H, Trope M, Buxt P and Switzer S (1993). Abstract #7 — The influence of various factors on the radiographic periapical status of endodontically treated teeth. *J. Endodont.*, **19**(4): 187.
5. Bhaskar SN (1966). Periapical lesions — Types, incidence and clinical features. *Oral Surg., Oral Med., Oral Pathol.*, **21**(5): 657–671.
6. Lalonde ER and Luebke RG (1968). The frequency and distribution of periapical cysts and granulomas. *Oral Surg., Oral Med., Oral Pathol.*, **25**(6): 861–868.
7. Block RM, Bushell A, Rodrigues H, and Langeland K (1976). A histopathologic, histobacteriologic and radiographic study of periapical endodontic surgical specimens. *Oral Surg., Oral Med., Oral Pathol.*, **42**(5): 656–678.

Further Reading

Browne RM and Tobias RS (1986). Microbial microleakage and pulpal inflammation: A review. *Endodont. Dent. Traumatol.*, **2**: 177–183.

Gutmann JL and Harrison JW (1991). Surgical Endodontics. Blackwell Scientific Publications (ISBN # 0-86542-096-3).

Kim S and Trowbridge HO (1994). Pulpal reactions to caries and dental procedures. In *Pathways of the Pulp*, sixth edition, edited by Cohen S and Burns RC,. Mosby, pp. 414–433. ISBN 0-8016-7979-6.

Klevant FJ and Eggink CO (1983). The effect of canal preparation on periapical disease. *Int. Endodont. J.*, **16**(2): 68–75.

Lim KC and Kirk EEJ (1987). Direct pulp capping: a review. *Endodont. Dent. Traumatol.*, **3**: 213–219.

Nair PNR, Sjogren U, Schumacher and Sundqvist G (1993). Radicular cyst affecting a root-filled human tooth: a long term post-treatment follow-up. *Int. J. Endodont.*, **26**: 225–233.

Pitt Ford TR and Rowe AHR (1989). A new root canal sealer based on calcium hydroxide. *J. Endodont.*, **15**: 286–289.

Pitt Ford T, and Roberts G J (1990). Tissue response to glass ionomer retrograde root fillings. *Int. Endodont. J.*, **23**: 233–238.

Ramachandran Nair PN, and Schroeder HE (1984). Periapical actinomycosis. *J. Endodont.*, **10**: 567–570.

Ramachandran Nair PN (1987). Light and electron microscopic studies of root canal flora and periapical lesions. *J. Endodont.*, **13**: 29–39.

Ramachandran Nair PN, Sjogren U, Krey G, Kahnberg KE and Sundqvist G (1990). Intraradicular bacteria and fungi in root filled, asymptomatic human teeth with therapy–resistant periapical lesions: A long-term light and electron microscopic follow up study. *J. Endodont.*, **16**: 580–588.

Ramachandran Nair PN, Sjogren U, Krey G and Sundqvist G. (1990). Therapy-resistant foreign body giant cell granuloma at the periapex of a root filled human tooth. *J. Endodont.*, **16**:589–595.

Simon JHS (1980). Incidence of periapical cysts in relation to the root canal. *J. Endodont.*, **6**: 845–848.

Smith CS, Setchell DJ and Harty FJ (1993). Factors influencing the success of conventional root canal therapy — a five year retrospective study. *Int. Endodont. J.*, **26**: 321–333.

Sundqvist G (1992). Ecology of the root canal flora. *J. Endodont.*, **18**: 427–430.

Chapter 2

Endocarditis Working Party of the British Society for Antimicrobial Chemotherapy (1990). Antibiotic prophylaxis of infective endocarditis. *Lancet*, **335**: 88–89, 1992; **339:** 1292–1293.

FDI. Guidelines for antibiotic prophylaxis of infective endocarditis for dental patients with cardiovascular disease (1987). FDI technical report no.28. *Int. Dent. J.*, **37**: 235 236.

Ingle JI, Taintor JF. In: *Endodontics*, 3rd ed. Philadelphia: Lea and Febiger, 1985; 505–555.

Longman PL, Field EA. Revised guidelines for the prophylaxis of infective endocarditis (1992). *Dent. Pract.*, **30**: 1–2.

Chapter 5

British Dental Association. *Control of Cross Infection in Dentistry*. British Dental Association advice sheet, July 1991.

General Dental Council. (UK) Regulations May 1992, paragraphs 16(a)–22.

Chapter 6

1. Vertucci, FJ (1984). Root canal anatomy of the human permanent teeth. *Oral Surg., Oral Med., Oral Pathol.*, **58**:589–599.
2. Fanibunda, KB (1986). A method of measuring the volume of human dental pulp cavities. *Int. Endodont. J.*, **19**:194–197.
3. Lowman JV, Burke, RS and Pellu, GB (1973). Patent accessory canals: incidence in molar furcation region. *Oral Surg., Oral Med., Oral Pathol.*, **36**: 580–584.
4. Burch, JG and Hulen, S (1974). A study of the presence of accessory foramina and topography of molar furcations. *Oral Surg., Oral Med., Oral Pathol.*, **38**: 451–455.

Chapter 7

1. Inoue N (1977). A clinico-anatomical study for determining root canal length by use of a novelty low frequency oscillation device. *Bull. Tokyo Dent. Coll.*, **18**: 71–90.
2. O'Neill LJ (1974). A clinical evaluation of electronic root canal measurement. *Oral Surg.*, **38**: 469–473.
3. Blank LW, Tenca JI, Pelleu GB (1975). Reliability of electronic measuring devices in endodontic therapy. *J. Endodont.*, **1**: 141–145.
4. Bal CS and Chaudhary M (1989). Evaluation of accuracy of an electric device (Neosono D-SE) for the measurement of tooth length. *Ind. J. Dent. Res.*, **1**: 58–65.
5. Stein JT, Corcoran JF, Zillich RM (1990). The influence of the major and minor foramen diameters on apical electronic probe measurements. *J. Endodont.*, **16**: 520–522.
6. Fouad AF, Krell KV, McKendry DJ, Koorbusch GF, Olson RA (1990). A clinical evaluation of five electronic root canal length measuring instruments. *J. Endodont.*, **16**: 446–449.
7. McDonald NJ, Hovland EJ (1990). An evaluation of the apex locator Endocater. *J. Endodont.*, **16**: 5–8.
8. Keller ME, Brown CE, Newton CW (1991). A clinical evaluation of the Endocater—an electronic apex locator. *J. Endodont.*, **17**: 271–274.
9. Chanan Y, Cergneux M, Ciucchi B, Holz J (1992). Accuracy of electronic assessment of root canal length: an in vivo study. *Int. Endodont. J.*, **25**: 32.
10. Ferrand N (1987). Definition electronique de la longueur de travail lors du catherterisme endodontique. Etude clinique avec le RCM apex locator a partir de 97 cas. Thesis No. 421087 Universitie de Lille, France.11.
11. Ducoin F (1991). Accuracy of 2 electronic canal length measuring instruments. *Rev. Fr. Endodont*, **10**: 27–33.
12. Ricard O, Roux D, Bourdeau L, Woda A (1991). Clinical evaluation of the accuracy of the evident RCM Mark II apex locator. *J. Endodont.*, **17**: 567–569.
13. Lucci A, Nussbacher V, Grosrey J (1993). A novel noninstrumented technique for cleansing the root canal system. *J. Endodont.*, **19**: 549–553.
14. Weine FS (1982). *Endodontic Therapy*, 3rd Edition, Mosby ISBN 0-8016-5380-0.
15. Roane JB (1991). *Clark's Clinical Dentistry*, Vol. 1, edited by Jefferson F. Hardin, J.B. Lippincott.

Further Reading

Baumgartner JC and Cuenin PR (1992). Efficacy of several concentrations of sodium hypochlorite for root canal irrigation. *J. Endodont.*, **18**: 605–612.

Bystrom A and Sundqvist G (1983). Bacteriological evaluation of the effect of 0.5% sodium hypochlorite in endodontic therapy. *Oral Surg., Oral Med., Oral Pathol.*, **55**: 307–312.

Fava LRG (1983). The double-flared technique: an alternative for biomechanical preparation. *J. Endodont.*, **9**: 76–80.

Goerig AC, Michelich RJ and Schultz HH (1982). Instrumentation of root canals in molar teeth using the step down technique. *J. Endodont.*, **8**(12): 550–554.

Lim SS and Stock CJR (1987). The risk of perforation in the curved canal: Anticurvature filing compared with Stepback technique. *Int. Endodont. J.*, **20**(1).

Morgan LF and Montgomery S (1984). An evaluation of the crown-down pressureless technique. *J. Endodont.*, **10**(10): 491–498.

Mullaney TP (1979). Instrumentation of finely curved canals. *Dental Clinics of North America*, **23**: 575.

Stock CJR (1991). Current status of the use of ultrasound in Endodontics. *Int. J. Dent.*, **41**:175–182.

Wildey WL and Senia ES (1989). A new root canal instrument and instrumentation technique: a preliminary report. *Oral Surg., Oral Med., Oral Pathol.*, **67**(2):198–207.

Chapter 9

1. Tagger M, Tagger E (1989). Periapical reactions to calcium hydroxide-containing sealers and AH26® in monkeys. *Endodont. Dent. Traumatol.*, **5**: 139–146.
2. Saunders EM (1990). In vivo findings associated with heat generation during thermomechanical compaction of gutta percha.

Part 1 — Temperature levels at the external surface of the root. *Int. Endodont. J.*, **23**(5): 263–267.

Part 2 — Histological response to temperature elevation on the external surface of the root. *Int. Endodont. J.*, **23**(5): 268–274.

Further Reading

Allison DA, Weber CR and Walton RE (1979). The influence of the method of canal preparation on the quality of apical and coronal obturation. *J. Endodont.*, **5**(10): 298–304.

Gerstein H (1983). *Techniques in Clinical Endodontics*. WB Saunders Company, ISBN 0-7216-4087-7.

Goodman A, Schilder H and Aldrich W (1974). The thermomechanical properties of gutta percha. II. The history and molecular chemistry of gutta percha. *Oral Surg., Oral Med., Oral Pathol.*, **37**(6): 954–961.

Metzer Z, Nissan R, Tagger M and Tamse A (1988). Apical seal by customised versus standardised master cones: A comparative study in flat and round canals. *J. Endodont.*, **14**: 381–384.

Schilder H, Goodman A and Aldrich W (1974). The thermomechanical properties of gutta percha. I. The compressibility of gutta percha. *Oral Surg., Oral Med., Oral Pathol.*, **37**(6): 946–953.

Schilder H, Goodman A, Aldrich W (1974). The thermomechanical properties of gutta percha. III. Determination of phase transition temperatures for gutta percha. *Oral Surg., Oral Med., Oral Pathol.*, **38**(1): 109–114.

Schilder H, Goodman A and Aldrich W (1985). The thermomechanical properties of gutta percha. V. Volume changes as a function of temperature and its relationship to molecular phase transition. *Oral Surg., Oral Med., Oral Pathol.*, **59**: 385–396.

Tagger M, Tamse and Katz A. (1984). Evaluation of the apical seal produced by a hybrid root canal filling method, combining lateral condensation and thermatic compaction. *J. Endodont.*, **10**(7): 299–303.

Chapter 10

Langeland K, Rodrigues H, Dowden W (1974). Periodontal disease, bacteria, and pulpal histopathology. *Oral Surg.*, **37**: 257–270.

Lowman JV, Burke RS, Pelleu GB (1973). Patent accessory canals: incidence in molar furcation region. *Oral Surg.*, **36**: 580.

Simon J, Glick D, Frank A (1972). The relationship of endodontic-periodontic lesions. *J. Periodontol.*, **43**: 202–208.

Tagger M, Smukler N (1977). Microscopic study of the pulps of human teeth following vital root resection. *Oral Surg.*, **44**: 96–105.

Walton R, Torabinejad M. In: *Principles and Practice of Endodontics*. WB Saunders, 1989; 442.

Chapter 13

1. Tronstad L (1988). Root resorption – etiology, terminology and clinical manifestations. *Endodont. Dent. Traumatol.*, **4**: 241.
2. Andreasen JO. In: *Traumatic Injuries of the Teeth*, 2nd ed. Philadelphia: W.B Saunders, 1981; 211.

Further reading

Pindborg JJ. *Pathology of the Dental Hard Tissues*. Copenhagen: Monksgaard, 1970.

Shafer WG, Hine MK, Levy BM. *A Textbook of Oral Pathology*, 3rd ed. Philadelphia: W.B. Saunders, 1974.

Chapter 14

Gutmann, Dumsha, Lovdahl, Hovland (1992). *Problem solving in Endodontics*, 2nd edition, Mosby–Year Book.

Ramachandran Nair PN, Sjogren U, Krey G, Kahnberg, KE and Sundqvist G (1990). Intraradicular bacteria and fungi in root-filled, asymptomatic human teeth with therapy-resistant periapical lesions: Long term light and electron microscopic follow-up study. *J. Endodont.*, **16**(12): 580–588.

Ramachandran Nair PN, Sjogren U, Krey G, Kahnberg, KE and Sundqvist G (1990). Therapy-resistant foreign body giant cell granuloma at the periapex of a root filled human tooth. *J. Endodont.*, **16**(12): 589–595.

Ramachandran Nair PN, Sjogren U, Schumacher E (1993). Radicular cyst affecting a root filled human tooth: a long term post-treatment follow-up. *Int. Endodont. J.*, **26**(4):225–233.

Chapter 15

1. Hansen EK, Asmussen E and Christiansen NC (1990). In vivo fractures of endodontically treated posterior teeth restored with amalgam. *Endodont. Dent. Traumatol.*, **6:** 49–55.
2. Smith CS, Setchell DJ and Harty FJ (1993). Factors influencing the success of conventional root canal therapy – a five year retrospective study. *Int. Endodont. J.*, **26**: 321–333.

Further reading

Hansen EK, Asmussen E (1993). Cusp fracture of endodontically treated posterior teeth restored with amalgam — Teeth restored in Denmark before 1975 versus 1979. *Acta Odontol. Sacnd.*, **51**: 73–77.

Huang TG, Schilder H and Nathanson D (1991). Effects of moisture content and endodontic treatment on some mechanical properties of human dentine. *J. Endodont.*, **18**(5): 209–215.

Randow K and Glantz PO. (1986). On cantilever loading of vital and non-vital teeth—an experimental clinical study. *Acta Odontol. Scand.*, **44**: 271–277.

Sedgeley CM and Messer HH (1992). Are endodontically treated teeth more brittle? *J. Endodont.*, **18**(7): 332–335.

Sorensen JA and Martinoff JT. (1984). Intracoronal reinforcement and coronal coverage: A study of endodontically treated teeth. *J. Prosthet. Dent.*, **51**: 780–784.

Sorensen JA and Martinoff JT. (1984). Clinically significant factors in dowel design. *J. Prosthet. Dent.*, **52**: 28–35.

Sorensen JA and Martinoff JT. (1985). Endodontically treated teeth as abutments. *J. Prosthet. Dent.*, **53**: 631–636.

Chapter 16

Brook AH, Winter, GB (1975). Developmental arrest of permanent tooth germs following pulpal infection of deciduous teeth. *Brit. Dent. J.*, **139**: 9–11.

Ketley CE and Goodman JR (1991). Formocresol toxicity: is there a suitable alternative for pulpotomy of primary molars. *Int. J. Paed. Dent.*, **1**: 67–72.

Shaw WC, Smith DMH and Hill FJ (1980). Inflammatory follicular cyst. *J. Dent. Child.*, **47**: 97–101.

Index

Numbers in bold print refer to illustrations and their captions.

Abscesses
   acute apical 48, 196, 199, **2.43–2.44**, **12.7–12.8**
   acute periradicular 29, **1.118**, **1.120**, **1.129–1.139**
   periodontal 196, **12.7–12.8**
   tooth drainage 196, **12.8**
Abutments 267, **15.208–15.210**
Access
   cavities *see* Access cavities
   problems 210–212, **14.11–14.23**
   for restorations 70, **4.10**
   root canals **7.76–7.77**
   for treatment 41, **2.10**
Access cavities 98–100, **7.5–7.37**
   buccal aspect **7.15–7.17**
   cutting 99, **7.13–7.17**
   heavily restored teeth 210
   internal resorption 201
   judging depth **7.14**
   lingual aspect **7.17**
   restoration 246, **15.32–15.33**, **15.80**
   shape 99–100, 211, **7.11–7.12**, **7.18–7.37**
   temporary seal 149–150, **8.26–8.30**
Accessory canals 89–90, **6.11–6.14**
Actinomyces spp. **1.121**
Adrenaline 190
AH26 153
Aldehydes 145
Alphaseal 171–174, **9.158–9.178**
Altered adaptation syndrome 33
Alveolar bone 10–11, **1.45–1.48**
Alveolar crest fibres **1.34**
Amalgam
   cores 264
   leaking **5.31**
   placing before root resection **10.37–10.38**
   plugger 79
   restoration of root–filled tooth **15.47–15.50**
American probe No 3 **5.6**
Anachoresis 21
Anaesthesia 83–84
   intraligamental 195, **12.3**
   mandibular 190
   maxillary 190, **11.31**
   periodontal ligament 46, **2.36**
   surgical endodontics 190
Analgesia 83–84, 209
   mandibular teeth 209, **2.36**
   maxillary teeth 209
   surgical endodontics 190

Angioneurotic oedema **14.144–14.145**
Ankylosis
   following thermocompaction **9.109**
   replacement resorption **13.25**
Anterior teeth restoration 244, 252–260, **15.21–15.26**, **15.77–15.154**
Anterior nasal spine 63
Antibiotics
   intracanal medication 146
   prophylactic 39, 85
Anticurvature filing 113–114, **7.102**, **7.122–7.124**
Apex locators, electronic 105–106, **7.61–7.68**
Apical abscess 48, 196, 199, **2.43–2.44**, **12.7–12.8**
Apical constriction 89
Apical control zone 129, **7.247**
Apical foramina
   irregular **9.21–9.25**
   microorganisms 24, **1.117**
   multiple 177, **9.26–9.28**, **10.1**
   transportation **7.100–7.101**
Apical root
   perforation **7.48–7.49**
   resorption 102–103, **7.46–7.47**
Apical seal 187, **11.20**
Apical surgery 186–187, **11.13–11.21**
Apit (Endex) apex locator 106, **7.66**
Atropine 84
Autoclaves 81, **5.18**
B lymphocytes 27
Bay cysts 31, **1.142–1.143**
Bead sterilizers 81, **5.17**
Beechwood creosote 276
Benzodiazepines 84
Bisecting angle projections 57, **3.27–3.31**
Bleaching 271–272, **15.238–15.246**
Bone removal 191
Briault probe 78
Bridges
   decemented **5.32–5.33**
   rubber dam placement **14.9–14.10**
Browne's tubes 81, **5.19**
Burs **7.13**
   Prepi **9.153–9.154**
   safe-ended **14.41**
   Trepan **14.173**, **14.175**, **14.190–14.191**
Calcific bridge formation **1.112**
Calcium hydroxide
   bony repair **13.30–13.31**
   cavity base 13–14, **1.70**

   direct pulp capping **1.96**, **1.103**
   indirect pulp capping 16–17, **1.89**
   internal resorption 202
   intracanal medication 146–147, **8.1–8.13**
   persistently weeping canal 221
   placement 148, **8.15–8.19**
   preparations 147–148, **8.14**
   pulpotomy 19, **1.109–1.110**
   removal/replacement 148–149, **8.20–8.25**
   reparative surgery 188
   root fractures **12.13**
Camphorated monochlorophenol (CMCP) 145
Canal Leader 142, **7.326**
Canal Master 119, **7.175–7.177**, **7.320–7.321**
Canal probe 78
Cancellous bone 62, **3.56**
Carbamide peroxide 124
Carbon dioxide probe 46, **2.34–2.35**
Caries **1.67**, **2.6**, **2.40**
   dressings 46, **4.3**
   primary dentition **16.1–16.2**
   pulp **1.49**
   radiography **2.15–2.16**
   removal 46, 85
   restoration **1.68–1.72**
   restoration failure **4.39**
   root canal **4.40**
   unrestorable tooth **4.1**
Cast cores 265–267, **15.191–15.207**
Cavit 150
Cavities
   access *see* Access cavities
   pulp damage 11, **1.51–1.52**
Cell-free zone 4, **1.2**
Cellulitis, acute periradicular 29, **1.118**, **1.120**, **1.129–1.139**
Cemental dysplasia (cementoma) 67, **3.83**
Cementocytes **1.29**
Cemento–enamel junction **1.4**
Cementoma 67, **3.83**
Cementum 7–8, **1.28–1.32**
Cermet 264–265, **15.188–15.190**
Cervical resorption 204–205, 208, **13.18–13.24**, **13.37–13.39**
Cervical tray 77, **5.1**
Chelating agents
   cavity cleaning 13
   root canal preparation 124
Chlorhexidine gel/mouthwash 39, 85
Chloroform dip technique **9.29**, **9.31–9.32**, **13.13–13.14**

errors 14.134–14.135
Chloropercha technique **9.187–9.188**
Chlororesin **9.186**
Cholesterol clefts **14.158**
Clamps 87, **5.37–5.38, 5.51**
Cleaning 80, **5.15**
Clinical area 77–82
Clinical examination 40–42
Clinical review **11.18**
Clinical tests 43–47
Cold lateral condensation 154–159, **9.11–9.59**
    causing root fractures 228–229, **14.139–14.143**
    technical problems **14.133–14.136**
Composite materials
    cores 264
    cusp restoration **15.43–15.44**
    MOD cavity restorations 250–251, **15.61–15.65**
    splint **12.20**
Condensing osteitis 30, **1.140**
    radiographic appearance 67, **3.81**
Congenital groove 178, **10.9–10.15**
Consent, informed 279
Consultation 39, **2.1**
Contamination zones 77
Copper band **5.40–5.44, 14.6–14.7**
Cores 260–264, **15.155–15.187**
    materials 264–267, **15.188–15.207**
Cortical trephination 186
Cross-infection control 82
Crown forms **14.6**
Crown fractures 49, 197, **12.9–12.10**
Crown-root fractures 198, **12.11**
Currettage, periradicular 187
Cysts, periradicular 30–33, **1.142–1.146**
Debridement 202, **13.8**
Decompression 192–193, **11.40–11.44**
Dental nurse 82–83, **5.22**
Dental pulp *see* Pulp
Dental state, general **2.8**
Dentinal tubules 2, **1.5–1.6**
    aspiration of odontoblasts **1.54**
    microorganisms 24, **1.58–1.60, 1.119**
    permeability 178
    sclerosis **1.57**
Dentine 2, **1.4–1.6**
    attrition **1.50**
    peritubular 3, **1.10**
    pins 261–262, **15.160–15.168**
    primary 3, **1.12–1.13**
    sclerosis **1.7–1.8, 1.11**
    secondary 3, **1.12–1.15, 1.56**
    sensitive 195
Dentures, fractured **15.15**
DG16 probe 214, **14.48–14.49**

Diagnosis 47–50
Diaket 153
Diamond bur **7.13**
Diffusion techniques 175, **9.186–9.188**
Discoloured teeth 271–272, **15.236–15.246**
Disinfection
    primary dentition 276, **16.19**
    root canals 219–220, **14.90–14.100**
Dowels 254, **15.93–15.94, 15.97–15.116**
    diameter 258, **15.137–15.140**
    diaphragm 260, **15.152–15.154**
    length 257–258, **15.126–15.136**
    shape 254–256, **15.117–15.124**
    surface configuration 259–260, **15.141–15.151**
    see also Posts
EDTA *see* Ethylenediaminetetra-acetic acid
Eggler post remover **14.184**
Electric pulp tester 44, **2.25–2.29**
Electronic apex locators 105–106, **7.61–7.68**
Electrosurgery **5.36, 5.39**
Emergencies 195–200
Endex apex locator 106, **7.66**
Endocarditis, infective 39, 85
Endodontic flora **1.117–1.118**
Endodontic locking tweezers 78, **5.5**
Endodontic treatment 1
    ease of access 41, **2.10**
    emergencies 199–200
    failed **11.1–11.11**
    informed consent 279
    medicolegal aspects 279
    planned review 74–75, 279, **4.32–4.42**
    planning 69–75
    record keeping 279
Endodontology 1
Endogrip 88
Endometric probe **7.58–7.60**
Endotec 160, **9.65, 9.67–9.68**
Endotoxins 24, 27
Epithelial rests of Malassez *see* Rests of Malassez
Equipment
    location 77
    sterilization *see* Sterilization
    see also Instruments
Ethylenediaminetetra-acetic acid (EDTA) **1.65**
    root canal preparation 124, 218, **14.87**
Excalibur 142, **7.328**
External resorption
    root 49, 72, **4.20**
    tooth 203–208, **13.12–13.39**
Extraradicular infection **14.156–14.158**
Facial pain, atypical 50, **2.46–2.47**
Facial swelling **2.2–2.3, 14.144–14.145**
Fibreoptic light 44, **2.22–2.24**
Fibrous tissue formation **1.163**

Files
    calcified canals **14.76–14.87**
    diagnostic 101–104, **7.39–7.43, 7.53–7.60**
        stops **7.69–7.70**
    dimensional formula 115, **7.137**
    flexible 113
    Golden medium **7.119, 7.150–7.152**
    intermediate 112–113, **7.117–7.119**
    too large 112, **7.115–7.116**
    modified use 114, **7.125**
    pathfinder 218, **14.77–14.83**
    precurving 111–112, **7.107–7.114**
    root canal preparation **7.105–7.106**
    see also Instruments
Flaps
    design/reflection 190–191, **11.32–11.34**
    full 190–191, **11.32**
    limited 191, **11.33–11.34**
    reflection **11.16**
Flex-R file 119, **7.169–7.171**
Flexofile 116, **7.147–7.152**
Flexogates 120, **7.178–7.180**
Foreign bodies
    peri-endo lesions 181, **10.26–10.28**
    reactions (giant cell lesions) **14.159–14.160**
Formaldehyde 38
    obturation 176, **9.199–9.200**
Formocresol pulpotomy 274–276, **16.6–16.13, 16.20**
Fractures
    dentures **15.15**
    instruments *see* Instruments: fractured
    posts **11.5, 14.180, 15.138**
    roots *see* Root fractures
    tooth
        crown fractures 49, 197, **12.9–12.10**
        crown-root fractures 198, **12.11**
        cusps **15.34–15.46**
        dentine pins **15.162–15.164**
        diagnosis 43, 49, **2.21, 2.37–2.38**
        fibreoptic light 44, **2.22–2.24**
        molar tooth **4.2**
        pulp exposure 18, **1.105**
        root-filled teeth 241–242, **15.1–15.9**
        treatment 197–198
        undiagnosed 195–196, **12.4–12.6**
        wood stick test **2.21**
Front surface mirror 78
Furcation bone loss **10.5**
Gag reflex 84
Gates Glidden **7.320–7.321**
Giant cell lesions **14.159–14.160**
Gingival fibres **1.34**
Gingival tissue, proliferative **5.35**
Giromatic 142, **6.324**
Glass ionomer cement

direct pulp capping **1.104**
temporary seal 150
Glutaraldehyde 81, 275
Golden medium files **7.119, 7.150–7.152**
Granulomas
periapical **14.155**
periradicular 30–33, **1.145**
Ground substance 4, **1.17**
Gumboil 28–29, **1.127–1.128**
Gutta percha
pellets 167
points
accessory **9.36, 9.40–9.42**
customizing 155, **9.33–9.35**
master points 154–155, **9.19–9.20**
non-standardized **9.12–9.12**
probing **10.21–10.22**
standardized **9.11**
transfer **5.25**
pulp testing 45, **2.30**
removal 235–236, **14.164–14.168**
root fillings 151–152, **9.1–9.4**
technical problems 227, **14.137–14.138**
thermoplasticized
carried on solid core 168–174, **9.137–9.185, 14.137–14.138**
injection 165–168, **9.113–9.136**
ultrasonic lateral compaction 160, **9.69–9.70**
Haemostasis
direct pulp capping 17, **1.101–1.102**
internal resorption 202, **13.8**
pulpotomy **1.108**
Halides 145–146
Healing
fibrous tissue formation **1.163**
periradicular lesions 33–34, **1.147–1.155**
Heart valves, prosthetic 39
Heat carriers **9.62–9.64**
Hedstrom file 117–118, **7.156–7.168**
Heliapical 119, **7.172–7.174**
Helisonic **7.181–7.183**
Hemisected tooth restoration 268–271, **15.220–15.235**
Hepatitis B infection 82, 85
HIV infection 82, 85
Hot air sterilizers 81, **5.16**
Howship's lacunae **1.47**
Hydrodynamic theory 6, **1.27**
Hydrogen peroxide
bleaching 271, **15.242**
cavity cleaning 13, **1.66**
root canal irrigation 124, **7.213–7.214**
Hypersensitivity reactions 27
paraformaldehyde 229–230, **14.147–14.148, 14.151**
Hypodermic needle **7.193–7.200**

Ice sticks 46, **2.31–2.33**
Impacted tooth resorption **13.15**
Incandescence **1.52**
Incision and drainage 186, **11.12**
Incisions
for flaps 190–191
surgical **11.14–11.15**
Incisive foramen 64, **3.60–3.61**
Infection
apical foramina 24, **1.117**
control of 82
dentinal tubules 24, **1.58–1.60, 1.119**
extraradicular **14.156–14.158**
periradicular lesions 20–24, **1.117–1.121**
primary dentition 273, **16.5**
root canals 97, **7.2–7.3**
see also Disinfection
Infective endocarditis 39, 85
Inferior dental canal (mandibular canal) 64, **3.62–3.63**
Inflammatory resorption 203, **13.12–13.14**
Instruments 78–79, **5.4–5.7**
fractured **11.4**
removal 237, **14.176–14.179**
root canal preparation 115–121, **7.137–7.192**
setting working lengths **5.26**
sodium hypochlorite **7.211**
sterilization see Sterilization
storage 79–80, **5.8–5.14**
surgical endodontics 189, **11.30**
transfer 83, **5.27–5.29**
see also Files
Intentional replantation see Replantation, intentional
Intermediate plexus **1.37**
Internal resorption
root see Root resorption: internal
tooth 201–203, **13.2–13.11**
Iodine–potassium iodide 146
Irrigants
canal preparation design 108, **7.76–7.77**
hydrodynamic method 108
simple canal systems 108
K-File 116, **7.138–7.140**
K-Flex file 116, **7.144–7.146**
K-Reamer 116, **7.141–7.143**
Lamina dura 62
Lateral canals
incidence 177, **10.2–10.4, 10.6**
lesions, radiographic appearance 66, **3.74–3.76**
morphology 89–90, **6.11–6.14**
Lateral condensation see Cold lateral condensation; Warm lateral condensation
Ledging **7.99**

Leubke–Ochsenbein flap 191, **11.33**
Light-proof box 53, **3.10–3.11**
Lignocaine 190
Lingual foramen 65, **3.66**
Long-shanked excavators 79
Ludwig's angina 29, **1.134–1.135**
McSpadden Engine file 120–121, **7.190–7.192**
McSpadden nickel–titanium thermocompactor **9.96–9.97, 9.100–9.101**
Magnetostrictive unit **7.332**
Maillefer Gutta condensor **9.96–9.99**
Mandible, sagittal splitting **14.148–14.152**
Mandibular canal (inferior dental canal) 64, **3.62–3.63**
Mandibular teeth
analgesia 209, **2.36**
canines
access cavities **7.30–7.31**
anatomical variations 94, **6.36–6.37**
first molars
access cavities 100, **7.35**
anatomical variations 94, **6.41–6.47**
root resection 182, **10.32–10.34**
first premolars
access cavities **7.32**
anatomical variations 94, **6.38**
incisors
access cavities **7.28–7.29**
anatomical variations 93, **6.34–6.35**
resection 188, **11.27**
second molars
access cavities 100, **7.36–7.37**
anatomical variations 95, **6.48–6.51**
second premolars
access cavities **7.33–7.34**
anatomical variations 94, **6.39–6.40**
third molars
access cavities 100
anatomical variations 95, **6.52–6.55**
Masel precision paralleling instrument **3.7**
Masserann kit 237, **14.172, 14.176–14.179**
Maxillary antrum 63, **3.57–3.58**
Maxillary teeth
analgesia 209
canines
access cavities **7.21–7.22**
anatomical variations 92, **6.19–6.20**
irregular wide root canal **7.81**
first molars
access cavities 99, **7.25–7.26**
anatomical variations 92–93, **6.26–6.30**
first premolars
access cavities **7.23–7.24**
anatomical variations 92, **6.21–6.23**
incisors
access cavities **7.20**

anatomical variations 91, **6.17–6.18**
molars
    root resection 188, **11.24–11.25**
    tooth resection 188, **11.26**
second molars
    access cavities 99, **7.27**
    anatomical variations 93, **6.31**
second premolars 92, **6.24–6.25**
third molars
    access cavities 99
    anatomical variations 93, **6.32–6.33**
Median suture **3.59**
Medical history 39–40
Medication
  intracanal 145–149, 202, **8.1–8.25**
  postoperative 84
Mental foramen 64, **3.64–3.65**
Mesiobuccal canals **6.26–6.28**
Messing Gun **8.15**
Metacresyl acetate 145
Microleakage 13–14, **1.61–1.62**
Microorganisms *see* Disinfection; Endodontic flora; Infection
Mobility 43, **2.20**
Mucoperiosteal flaps *see* Flaps
Nasal septum 63
Nayyar amalgam/dowel core 262, **15.169–15.180**
Necrosis
  local following root filling **14.146**
  pulp *see* Pulp necrosis
NiTiMatic 141, **7.322**
Non-endodontic lesions **14.161**
Nutrient canals 65, **3.67**
Oblique fibres **1.35–1.36**
Obtura system 167, **9.128–9.130**
Obturation *see* Root fillings
Occlusal loading 267
Occlusal space **15.10–15.14**
Odontoblastic processes 2, **1.9**
Odontoblasts
  aspiration into dentinal tubules **1.54**
  cell bodies 4, **1.16**
Oral hygiene **2.4**
Orthodontic band **5.40–5.44, 12.6, 14.6**
  cemented **15.36**
Orthodontic treatment **13.16**
Osteomyelitis, periradicular 29–30
Osteosclerosis, periradicular *see* Condensing osteitis
Overdenture
  elective endodontics **4.6–4.7**
  temporary 244, **15.25–15.26**
Paget's disease **13.17**
Pain
  atypical facial 50, **2.46–2.47**
  control *see* Anaesthesia; Analgesia

immediate relief 69, **4.1–4.2**
postoperative 84
Palpation 43, **2.18**
Parachute chain 88, **5.57**
Paraformaldehyde
  hypersensitivity 229–230, **14.147–14.148, 14.151**
  pulpotomy, primary dentition 275–276
Parallax techniques 58, **3.32–3.36**
Parallel periapical projections 55–56, **2.11, 3.20–3.26, 7.38–7.43**
Pathfinder files 218, **14.77–14.83**
Patients
  education/information 83, **5.30**
  protective clothing 82, **5.21, 5.45**
    for radiography 54–55, **3.16–3.18**
Peeso reamer **7.320–7.321**
Percussion 43, **2.19**
Perforations
  apical root **7.48–7.49**
  dentine pins **15.161**
  iatrogenic 179, **10.18–10.19**
  internal resorption 202, **10.16–10.17**
  postoperative **4.42**
  pulp chamber floor 212, **14.17–14.23**
  radiographic appearances 67, **3.79–3.80**
  reparative surgery 188, **11.22–11.23**
  root canal preparation **7.102–7.104**
  root canals 224–225, **14.118–14.125, 14.128**
Periapical granuloma **14.155**
Periapical inflammation, acute 48, **2.40–2.42**
Periapical radiolucent areas, non-resolution 230, **14.155–14.161**
Peri-endo lesions 177–184
  classification 179–180
  diagnosis/treatment 180–182
  endodontic 181, **10.24**
  necrotic pulp 182, **10.29–10.31**
  periodontal 181–182, **10.26–10.31**
  pulp vitality testing 181, **10.26–10.28**
  root canal treatment/root resection 182–184, **10.32–10.38**
  treatment flow chart **10.23**
Periodontal abscess 196, **12.7–12.8**
Periodontal condition **2.5**
Periodontal lesions
  pulp necrosis **15.29**
  radiographic appearance 67, **3.82**
Periodontal ligament 8–10, **1.33–1.44**
  acute inflammation 196
  disused **1.43**
  local analgesia 46, **2.36**
  overload **1.42, 1.44**
  radiographic appearance 62
Periodontal probe **5.7, 10.20**
Periodontal support 71, **4.12**

Periodontal tissue management 87
Periodontitis
  acute apical 196, 199
  chronic apical 48–49, **2.45**
Periodontium, thermocompaction effects **9.106–9.109**
Periradicular abscess/cellulitis 29, **1.118, 1.120, 1.129–1.139**
Periradicular currettage 187
Periradicular cysts 30–33, **1.142–1.146**
Periradicular granulomas 30–33, **1.145**
Periradicular inflammation
  acute 28, **1.124–1.125**
  chronic 28, **1.126**
  chronic suppurative 28–29, **1.127–1.128**
Periradicular lesions
  cells 27–28, **1.123**
  chemomechanical debridement 33, **1.147–1.152**
  decompression 192–193, **11.40–11.44**
  devitalized pulp 20, **1.75–1.76**
  endotoxins 24, 27
  healing 33–34, **1.147–1.155**
  host defence factors 27, **1.122**
  host tissue 20
  microorganisms 20–24, **1.117–1.121**
  mummification 38, **1.175**
  pathogenesis 20–28
  radiographic appearance 65–66, **3.68–3.73**
  retrograde seal 34–38, **1.165–1.172**
  surgery 34–38, **1.156–1.174**
  treatment 33–38
  types 28–32
Periradicular osteomyelitis 29–30
Periradicular osteosclerosis *see* Condensing osteitis
Periradicular surgery 34–38, **1.156–1.174**
Periradicular tissues 7–11
Phenol 145
Phosphoric acid **1.64**
Piezoelectric unit **7.333**
Pink spot 201, 204–205, **13.24**
Plexus of Raschow 6, **1.25**
Pluggers
  amalgam 79
  warm vertical condensation **9.71–9.78**
Pocket measuring probe **5.7**
Polymorphonuclear leucocyctes (PMNLs) 24, 27, **1.117**
Polyvinyl splint **12.18–12.19**
Porcelain veneers 253, 272, **15.85–15.86**
Post crown, temporary 244, **15.21–15.24**
Post systems, prefabricated **15.97–15.110**
Posterior teeth restoration 245–251, 260–267, **15.27–15.76, 15.155–15.207**
Posts
  deformation **15.137**

fractured **11.5, 14.180, 15.138**
reinforcement of intact root-filled teeth 252, **15.81–15.84**
removal 238, **14.180–14.193**
see also Dowels
Predentine 4, **1.16**
Prepi burs **9.153–9.154**
Primary dentition 273–277, **16.1–16.23**
Protective clothing
    operators 85
    patients *see* Patients: protective clothing
Pulp 1–4, **1.1**
    attrition **1.50**
    capping *see* Pulp capping
    caries **1.49**
    chamber *see* Pulp chamber
    concussed 47
    damage by restorative materials 11–14, **1.53–1.72**
    devitalized 20, **1.75–1.76**
    exposure by tooth fracture 18, **1.105**
    extirpated **2.42**
    fin **6.9**
    functions 4
    horn **14.25**
    hyperaemic **2.41**
    inflammation 14–15, **1.73–1.78, 1.86**
        localized **1.55**
    mineral deposits (calcification; stones) 15–16, **1.79–1.85, 14.42–14.51**
    necrosis *see* Pulp necrosis
    nerve supply 6–7, **1.25–1.27**
    normal 47
    pathology 11–20
        primary dentition 273, **16.1–16.2**
    polyp 18
    radiographic appearance 63
    removal *see* Pulpotomy
    space configurations 89, **6.1–6.10**
    stones 15–16, **1.79–1.85, 14.42–14.51**
    therapy 16–19
        assessment of success 19–20, **1.112–1.116**
    vascular supply 5–6, **1.18–1.24**
    wound irrigation **1.107**
Pulp capping
    crown fractures 197
    direct 17–18, **1.93–1.104**
    indirect 16–17, **1.87–1.91**
    primary dentition 274
Pulp chamber
    calcification 214, **14.24–14.25, 14.52**
    cross-sections **14.26–14.38**
    floor **14.39**
        avoiding damage **7.8–7.9**
        maintaining integrity **14.40–14.41**
        perforation 212, **14.17–14.23**
    primary dentition **16.3**
    roof 211, **14.12–14.16**
        removing **7.5–7.6**
    vital pulp tissue **1.75–1.76**
Pulp–dentine complex 1, **1.2–1.3**
Pulp necrosis **1.77–1.78, 1.86, 1.92**
    caused by orthognathic surgery **15.31, 15.78**
    caused by periodontal disease **15.29**
    caused by transplantation **15.79**
    diagnosis 47–48, **2.38**
    peri–endo lesions 182, **10.29–10.31**
    periodontal disease **15.29**
    root resection 184
    superficial, removal **1.106**
    traumatic **15.30, 15.77**
Pulp testing 44–46, **2.25–2.35**
    electric 44, **2.25–2.29**
    peri–endo lesions 181, **10.26–10.28**
    thermal 45–46, **2.30–2.35**
Pulpectomy, primary dentition 276, **16.14**
Pulpitis
    analgesia 209
    irreversible 47, 195–196, **2.37, 12.2–12.3**
    reversible 47, 195–196, **12.112.2–12.3**
Pulpotomy 18–19, 219, **1.105–1.111, 7.4, 14.88–14.89**
    calcific bridge formation **1.112**
    crown fractures 197
    elective devitalization 20, **1.115–1.116**
    primary dentition 274–276, **16.6–16.13, 16.20**
    root formation **1.113–1.114**
Quickfill 174, **9.179–9.185**
Quickfill compactor **9.96–9.97, 9.104–9.105**
Radiography 51–68
    bisecting angle projections 57, **3.27–3.31**
    caries **2.15–2.16**
    collimator 51, **3.3**
    equipment safety 55
    film holders 52, **3.5–3.8**
    film processing 58–60, **3.37–3.49**
    films 52
    grids **7.57**
    interpretation 61–68, **3.50–3.84**
    landmarks 62–65, **3.55–3.65**
    mounts 54, **3.14–3.15**
    operator safety 55, **3.19**
    parallax techniques 58, **3.32–3.36**
    parallel periapical projections 55–56, **2.11, 3.20–3.26, 7.38–7.43**
    patient assessment 41–42, **2.11–2.17**
    patient safety 54–55, **3.16–3.18**
    postoperative **11.19**
    preoperative **11.13**
    processing equipment 53–54, **3.9–3.12**
    safety regulations 54–55
    sinus tract 41–42, **2.12–2.14**
    spacer cone 51–52, **3.4**
    techniques 55–58
    treatment review **4.32–4.39, 4.41–4.42**
    tube head 51, **3.2–3.3**
    viewers 54, **3.13**
    X-ray machine 51, **3.1**
Radiovisiography 68, **3.85–3.87**
RAF tray 79, **5.8**
Recapitulation 122, **7.204**
Record keeping 279
Reparative surgery 188, **11.22–11.23**
Replacement resorption 205–206, **12.17, 13.25–13.31**
Replantation, intentional 189, **11.28–11.29**
    splints 199
Resistance form **7.11–7.12**
Resorption
    root *see* Root resorption
    tooth 201–208
        cervical 204–205, 208, **13.18–13.24, 13.37–13.39**
        external 203–208, **13.12–13.39**
        idiopathic 207–208, **13.32–13.39**
        impacted tooth **13.15**
        inflammatory 203, **13.12–13.14**
        internal 201–203, **13.2–13.11**
        primary dentition 273
        replacement 205–206, **12.17, 13.25–13.31**
        surface 204, **13.15–13.17**
Restorations
    access 70, **4.10**
    access cavities 246, **15.32–15.33, 15.80**
    anterior teeth 244, 252–260, **15.21–15.26, 15.77–15.154**
    with auxiliary aids 254–267, **15.93–15.207**
    capped cusp cast onlay **15.51–15.60, 15.66–15.76**
    cast onlay 246–247, **15.37–15.46**
    cast pins **15.41–15.42**
    ceramometal 251, **15.74–15.76, 15.90–15.92**
    cores *see* Cores
    dowels *see* Dowels
    gold 251
    hemisected tooth 268–271, **15.220–15.235**
    intact anterior teeth 252–253, **15.77–15.86**
    intact posterior teeth 245–247, **15.29–15.46**
    leaking 199, **14.90–14.92**
    materials, pulp damage 11–14, **1.53–1.72**
    mesio–occluso–distal cavities 250–251, **15.61–15.76**
    occlusal protection **12.4**
    overall plan 70, **4.5–4.9**
    plastic cores/cuspal coverage 248, **15.53–15.60**
    porcelain veneers 253, **15.85–15.86**

posterior teeth 245–251, 260–267, **15.27–15.76, 15.155–15.207**
proximal cavities 253, **15.87–15.92**
proximo-occlusal cavities 248, **15.47–15.60**
pulpal pathology 11, **1.51–1.52**
removal 85, **5.31–5.33**
restorability 71, **4.11**
root-filled tooth 241–272
timing after endodontic treatment 244–245, **15.21–15.28**
tooth with resected root 267–268, **15.211–15.219**
tooth tissue requirements 242, **15.16–15.20**
Rests of Malassez **1.38–1.39**
proliferation 30–32, **1.141**
Retreatment 235–238, **14.162–14.193**
Retrograde seal 34–38, **1.165–1.172**
Rheumatic fever 39
Rinn EndoRay 52, **3.8**
Rinn film holders **3.6**
Rispisonic **7.184–7.186**
Root canals
accessory 89–90, **6.11–6.14**
anatomy 71, **4.15–4.17**
anatomy and preparation/cleaning 107–110, **7.72–7.94**
apical widening **14.117, 14.126–14.127**
blockage 223, **14.111–14.112**
blunderbuss 102–103, **7.46–7.47, 7.82**
caries **4.40**
chemomechanical preparation 97
cleaning 219–220, **14.88–14.105**
complex systems 108–110, **7.72–7.73, 7.88–7.94**
configurations 89–91, **6.1–6.16**
curved, shaping 224
elimination of microorganisms 219–220, **14.90–14.100**
inaccurate instrumentation 222–224, **14.111–14.115**
infection 97, **7.2–7.3**
irrigation 97, **7.4**
lateral *see* Lateral canals
ledging 223, **14.113, 14.116**
length change during instrumentation 107, **7.71**
location 212–217, **14.24–14.72**
loss of working length 223, **14.114**
lubrication 218, **14.87**
mesiobuccal **6.26–6.28**
negotiating calcified 217–218, **14.73–14.87**
obturation *see* Root fillings
open apex 222, **14.106–14.109**
orifices **14.24**
perforations 224–225, **14.118–14.125, 14.128**

persistently weeping 221, **14.101–14.105**
preparation 97–144, 219–226, **14.88–14.128**
apical–coronal techniques 124, 125–130, **7.215, 7.217–7.247**
automated devices 141–144, **7.320–7.336**
Canal Master technique 138, **7.303–7.319**
coronal–apical techniques 124, 130–140, **7.216, 7.248–7.319**
crown-down pressureless technique 135, **7.277–7.302**
double-flared technique 132, **7.262–7.276**
errors 110–115, 224–226, **7.99–7.136, 14.116–14.128**
instruments 115–121, **7.137–7.192**
irrigation 121–124, **7.193–7.214**
mechanical (shaping) 110–121, **7.95–7.192**
modified instruments 114–115, **7.126–7.136**
preflaring 113, **7.120–7.121**
Roane technique 128, **7.236–7.246**
standardized 125, **7.217–7.222**
step-back 126, **7.223–7.235**
step-down technique 130–131, **7.248–7.261**
techniques 124–141
radicular access **7.76–7.77**
recontamination 230, **14.153–14.154**
relationships **14.56–14.63**
removal of dentine spur 214, **14.53–14.55**
sclerosed 73, 90, 215, **4.25–4.27, 6.15–6.16, 14.65–14.72**
sensitivity to instrumentation 222
shaping 222–226, **14.106–14.128**
simple systems 108, **7.78–7.87**
straight line access **7.7**
sudden apical curve **7.50–7.51**
widely flared **7.1**
width of taper 107, **7.74–7.75**
working length 101–104, **7.38–7.60**
Root fillings 151–176
causing root fractures 228–229, **12.22, 14.139–14.143**
failed **11.3**
to fracture lines **12.14**
hypersensitivity 229–230, **14.144–14.152**
internal resorption 202, **13.9**
local necrosis **14.146**
materials 151–152, **9.1–9.4**
removal 235–237, **14.162–14.175**
overextended **11.9–11.10, 12.21**
retreating 73–74, **4.28–4.31**

single visit approach 151
technical problems 226–227, **14.129–14.138**
Root fractures 72, **4.21–4.24**
caused by posts 15.139–15.140, 15.153–15.154
cold lateral compaction 9.55
during obturation 228–229, **12.22, 14.139–14.143**
horizontal **10.7**
postoperative **4.41**
radiographic appearance 66, **3.77–3.78**
surgical removal of apical portion **12.15–12.16**
treatment 198, **12.12–12.16**
undiagnosed **12.12**
vertical 187, **10.8, 11.21**
Root perforations *see* Perforations
Root resection 182–184, 188, 191, **10.32–10.38, 11.24–11.25**
Root resorption 72
apical root 102–103, **7.46–7.47**
external 49, 72, **4.20**
internal 49, 72, **4.18–4.19**
perforated 202, **10.16–10.17**
multinucleated cells **13.1**
thermocompaction **9.107–9.108**
Root sheath of Hertwig 9
Root ZX apex locator **7.67**
Roots, radiographically obscure 222, **14.110**
Rubber dam 83, 87–88, **2.26, 5.45**
applying 88, **5.52–5.56**
bridges **14.9–14.10**
forceps **5.49**
frames **5.50**
placement **5.23**
problems 209–210, **14.1–14.10**
punch **5.46**
sealing **14.4**
sodium hypochlorite **7.212**
stamp **5.47–5.48**
Russell bodies 27
Seals
apical 187, **11.20**
retrograde 34–38, **1.165–1.172**
temporary 149–150, **8.26–8.30**
Sealapex 152–153, **9.5–9.6**
Sealers 152–153, **9.5–9.6**
preparation/application 153, **9.7–9.10**
surgical endodontics 193
Sedation 84
Semilunar flap 191, **11.33–11.34**
Sensory innervation 6–7
Shaper **7.187–7.189**
Sharpey's fibres **1.30**
Silver point technique 175–176, **9.189–9.198**

removal 236, **14.169–14.175**
Sinus tract 28–29, **1.127–1.128**
    radiography 41–42, **2.12–2.14**
Smear layer 13, 122–123, **1.63–1.66**,
    7.205–7.206
Sodium hypochlorite
    intracanal medication 145–146
    root canal irrigation 123, **7.207–7.212**
Sodium perborate **15.243**
Sonic air **7.329**
Sonic oscillation 143, **7.329–7.331**
Spectacles, protective **5.21**, **5.45**
Splints 199, **12.18–12.20**
    mandibular **14.148–14.152**
Sponges 80, **5.14**
Spreaders **9.13–9.18**
Stabilization 69, **4.3–4.4**
Steiglitz forceps **14.169**
Sterilization 80–82, **5.16–5.20**
    instrument box 79, **5.10**
Steroids 146
Successfil 171–174
Suction **5.24**
Super X-30 film 53, **3.9**
Surface resorption 204, **13.15–13.17**
Surgery
    apical 186–187, **11.13–11.21**
    incisions **11.14–11.15**
    internal resorption 202–203, **13.10–13.11**
    orthognathic, causing pulp necrosis **15.31**,
        15.78
    periradicular lesions 34–38, **1.156–1.174**
    reparative 188, **11.22–11.23**
Surgical endodontics 185–193
Sutures 192, **11.17**
    anchor **11.38**
    interrupted **11.35**

removal 192
single sling **11.36**
vertical mattress 192, **11.37**
Symptom relief 69
T lymphocytes 27
Teeth
    anatomical variations 91–95, **6.17–6.55**
    average values 91
    avulsed 199
    broken down
        provisional restoration 86, **5.34–5.44**
        restoration 209–210, **14.1–14.10**
    discoloured 271–272, **15.236–15.246**
    fractured *see* Fractures: tooth
    missing/unapposed **2.7**, **4.13**
    mobility 43, **2.20**
    morphology, primary dentition 273,
        16.3–16.5
    non-restorable 183, **4.1**, **10.35–10.36**
    open drainage 221, **14.101–14.105**
    primary dentition 273–277, **16.1–16.23**
    resection 188, **11.26–11.27**
    resorption *see* Resorption
    restorability 71, 242, **4.11**, **15.10–15.20**
    strategic importance 71, **4.13–4.14**
    tooth substance conservation **7.10**
    wear **2.9**
Temporary seal 149–150, **8.26–8.30**
Term 150
Test cavity 47
Test tubes 80, **5.11–5.13**
Thermafil endodontic obturators 168–171,
    9.137–9.157
ThermaPrep oven **9.142**
Thermocompaction 163–165, **9.96–9.112**
Tooth *see* Teeth
Touch n'Heat 160, **9.66–9.67**

Transillumination 215, **14.64**
Transseptal fibres **1.34**
Trauma 196–199
    pulp necrosis **15.30**, **15.77**
    replacement resorption 205–206,
        13.26–13.29
Trepan bur **14.173**, **14.175**, **14.190–14.191**
Tubliseal 152
Tungsten-carbide bur **7.13**
Ultrafil system 167–168, **9.131–9.136**
Ultrasonic bath **5.15**
Ultrasonic oscillation 143–144, **7.332–7.336**
Ultrasonic units 77, **5.2–5.3**
Ultrasound post removal **14.181–14.183**
Velopex automatic processing machine 53–54,
    3.12
Veneers 253, 272, **15.85–15.86**
Warm lateral condensation 159–160, **9.60–9.70**
Warm vertical condensation 161–162,
    9.71–9.95
Work surfaces 77
Working length estimation 101–104, **7.38–7.60**
X-rays *see* Radiography
Xeroradiography 68
Zinc oxide/eugenol
    cavity base 13–14, **1.71**
    direct pulp capping **1.97**
    pulp capping 16–17, **1.90**
    pulpotomy 19, **1.111**
    sealers 152
    temporary seal 150, **8.28–8.30**
Zinc phosphate **15.240**
Zipperer Flexicut 117, **7.153–7.155**
Zipperer thermocompactor **9.96–9.97**,
    9.102–9.103
Zones of Fish 27, **1.123**